Breast Cancer
SOURCEBOOK

Third Edition

Health Reference Series

Third Edition

Breast Cancer
SOURCEBOOK

Basic Consumer Health Information about Breast Health and Breast Cancer, Including Facts about Environmental, Genetic, and Other Risk Factors, Prevention Efforts, Screening and Diagnostic Methods, Surgical Treatment Options and Other Care Choices, Complementary and Alternative Therapies, and Post-Treatment Concerns

Along with Statistical Data, News about Research Advances, a Glossary of Related Terms, and Directories of Resources for Additional Information and Support

Edited by
Karen Bellenir

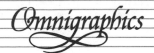

Omnigraphics

P.O. Box 31-1640, Detroit, MI 48231

Bibliographic Note

Because this page cannot legibly accommodate all the copyright notices, the Bibliographic Note portion of the Preface constitutes an extension of the copyright notice.

Edited by Karen Bellenir

Health Reference Series

Karen Bellenir, Managing Editor
David A. Cooke, M.D., Medical Consultant
Elizabeth Collins, Research and Permissions Coordinator
Cherry Edwards, Permissions Assistant
EdIndex, Services for Publishers, Indexers

* * *

Omnigraphics, Inc.

Matthew P. Barbour, Senior Vice President
Kevin M. Hayes, Operations Manager

* * *

Peter E. Ruffner, Publisher

Copyright © 2009 Omnigraphics, Inc.

ISBN 978-0-7808-1030-3

Library of Congress Cataloging-in-Publication Data

Breast cancer sourcebook : basic consumer health information about breast health and breast cancer ... / edited by Karen Bellenir.
     p. cm.
   Summary: "Provides basic consumer health information on risk factors, prevention, diagnosis, and treatment of breast cancer, along with facts about coping after treatment. Includes index, glossary of related terms and directory of resources"--Provided by publisher.
   Includes bibliographical references and index.
   ISBN 978-0-7808-1030-3 (hardcover : alk. paper) 1. Breast--Cancer--Popular works. I. Bellenir, Karen.
   RC280.B8B6887 2009
   616.99'449--dc22
                                                              2008048392

Table of Contents

Visit www.healthreferenceseries.com to view *A Contents Guide to the Health Reference Series*, a listing of more than 14,000 topics and the volumes in which they are covered.

Part III: Breast Cancer Screening and Diagnosis

Part V: Recurrent and Metastatic Cancer: Special Considerations

Part VI: Breast Cancer Research

Part VII: Moving Forward

Part VIII: Additional Help and Information

Preface

About This Book

Breast cancer, the second-most common type of cancer among women in the United States (after skin cancer), is diagnosed in more than 211,000 women and 1,700 men each year. According to the National Cancer Institute, 35 years ago approximately 75% of women diagnosed with breast cancer survived their disease at least five years. Today, that number is up to nearly 90%. In addition, recent advances in gene expression analysis have led to the identification of five subtypes of breast cancer that have distinct features. Medical researchers hope this knowledge will allow the development of treatment strategies based on an individual's tumor characteristics and that this will continue to improve treatment outcomes in the future.

Breast Cancer Sourcebook, Third Edition, provides updated information about breast health and breast cancer risk factors. It explains the different types of breast cancer, including breast cancer associated with different genes, inflammatory breast cancer, Paget disease of the nipple, and breast cancer in men. It discusses how screening for breast cancer with mammography, clinical breast exams, and self-exams may help doctors find and treat cancer early when treatments are more likely to be effective. Cancer treatment options, including surgery, radiation therapy, chemotherapy, and biological therapy are described, and the emotional concerns of women in and after treatment are addressed. A section on research advances offers information from recent clinical trials, and the book concludes with a glossary and directories of resources for additional help and support.

Readers interested in other topics related to cancer concerns among women may wish to consult these additional books within the *Health Reference Series*:

- *Cancer Sourcebook for Women, Third Edition* presents comprehensive information about other cancers that are of special concern to women, including cancer of the cervix, fallopian tubes, ovaries, uterus, vagina, vulva, lung, colon, and thyroid.

- *Cancer Sourcebook, Fifth Edition* provides information about the major forms and stages of cancers affecting specific body organs and systems and describes concerns related to metastatic, recurrent, and advanced cancers.

- *Cancer Survivorship Sourcebook* discusses the challenges of maintaining wellness during and after cancer treatment, including tips for researching specific types of cancer and treatment advances, suggestions for coping with the side effects and complications of cancer treatments, and facts about emotional, cognitive, and mental health issues in cancer care.

- *Cosmetic and Reconstructive Surgery Sourcebook, Second Edition* includes information about breast prostheses and post-mastectomy breast reconstruction.

- *Pregnancy and Birth Sourcebook, Second Edition* contains information for women concerned about high-risk pregnancies and pregnancy complications, including maternal cancers.

- *Smoking Concerns Sourcebook* provides facts about the health effects of tobacco use, including lung and other cancers, and offers information about smoking cessation.

- *Women's Health Concerns Sourcebook, Second Edition* includes facts about the medical and mental concerns of women.

How to Use This Book

This book is divided into parts and chapters. Parts focus on broad areas of interest. Chapters are devoted to single topics within a part.

Part I: Breast Health provides information to help women understand breast anatomy and to become familiar with the unique characteristics of their own breasts through the self-examination process. It describes the types of normal changes that may occur during aging, and it explains non-cancerous breast conditions, such as hyperplasia, cysts, and fibroadenomas.

Part II: Breast Cancer Fundamentals offers information about how breast cancer begins and spreads. It describes the various forms and stages of breast cancer, recounts how breast cancer affects different groups of people, and explains the factors that place people at increased risk for developing breast cancer. Efforts to help prevent breast cancer through lifestyle changes, the avoidance of things known to cause cancer, the use of medicines to treat precancerous conditions, and the practice of preventive mastectomy are also discussed.

Part III: Breast Cancer Screening and Diagnosis describes the risks and benefits associated with tests commonly used to screen for breast cancer, including mammography, clinical exam, and self-exam. It explains follow-up procedures and additional diagnostic tests that may be used if a screening exam leads to the discovery of a lump or other sign that may be indicative of breast cancer.

Part IV: Breast Cancer Treatment explains surgical options, including breast-conserving surgeries and mastectomies, radiation treatment, chemotherapy, and hormone therapies. Biological, complementary, and other nontraditional treatments that may be used to combat cancer or to lessen side effects associated with standard cancer treatments are also explained. The part concludes with information about the important role nutrition plays in helping patients feel better, stay stronger, and support the body's healing processes.

Part V: Recurrent and Metastatic Cancer: Special Considerations discusses issues that arise when cancer comes back. It explains the differences between local, regional, and distant recurrences, and it discusses the causes, symptoms, and treatments of metastatic cancer. Readers dealing with advanced cancer will find a discussion about identifying treatment goals and discussing such options as clinical trials, palliative therapies, hospice care, and home care with their families and health care team members.

Part VI: Breast Cancer Research provides facts about efforts currently underway to help reduce mortality from breast cancer by identifying risk factors, studying the effects of prevention efforts, and improving treatments based on new information in the fields of genetics, molecular biology, and immunology. For readers interested in taking part in breast cancer research, the part concludes with facts about searching for and participating in clinical trials.

Part VII: Moving Forward discusses the emotional responses and body changes that may arise during and after treatment for breast cancer, including coping with feelings, finding support, and discussing cancer with family members and friends. It offers guidelines for follow-up medical care, and addresses such other issues as intimacy, sexuality, and pregnancy in breast cancer survivors.

Part VIII: Additional Help and Information provides a glossary of breast cancer terms, a directory of resources for information and support, and a list of state contacts for breast and cervical cancer early detection programs.

Bibliographic Note

This volume contains documents and excerpts from publications issued by the following U.S. government agencies: Centers for Disease Control and Prevention; National Cancer Institute; National Institute of Arthritis and Musculoskeletal and Skin Diseases; National Institute of Environmental Health Sciences; National Institutes of Health; National Library of Medicine; Office of Minority Health; U.S. Department of Labor; and the U.S. Food and Drug Administration.

In addition, this volume contains copyrighted documents from the following organizations: A.D.A.M., Inc.; American Association for Clinical Chemistry; Breast Cancer Fund; Breast Cancer Network of Strength; CancerConsultants.com; Imaginis Corporation; Johns Hopkins Avon Foundation Breast Center; Susan G. Komen for the Cure; Lawrence Berkeley National Laboratory; Living Beyond Breast Cancer; and the Missouri Department of Health and Senior Services.

Full citation information is provided on the first page of each chapter or section. Every effort has been made to secure all necessary rights to reprint the copyrighted material. If any omissions have been made, please contact Omnigraphics to make corrections for future editions.

Acknowledgements

In addition to the organizations who have contributed to this *Sourcebook*, special thanks are due to research and permissions coordinator, Liz Collins; permissions assistant, Cherry Stockdale; editorial assistants, Elizabeth Bellenir and Nicole Salerno; and prepress technician, Stephen G. Wesley.

About the Health Reference Series

The *Health Reference Series* is designed to provide basic medical information for patients, families, caregivers, and the general public. Each volume takes a particular topic and provides comprehensive coverage. This is especially important for people who may be dealing with a newly diagnosed disease or a chronic disorder in themselves or in a family member. People looking for preventive guidance, information about disease warning signs, medical statistics, and risk factors for health problems will also find answers to their questions in the *Health Reference Series*. The *Series*, however, is not intended to serve as a tool for diagnosing illness, in prescribing treatments, or as a substitute for the physician/patient relationship. All people concerned about medical symptoms or the possibility of disease are encouraged to seek professional care from an appropriate health care provider.

A Note about Spelling and Style

Health Reference Series editors use *Stedman's Medical Dictionary* as an authority for questions related to the spelling of medical terms and the *Chicago Manual of Style* for questions related to grammatical structures, punctuation, and other editorial concerns. Consistent adherence is not always possible, however, because the individual volumes within the *Series* include many documents from a wide variety of different producers and copyright holders, and the editor's primary goal is to present material from each source as accurately as is possible following the terms specified by each document's producer. This sometimes means that information in different chapters or sections may follow other guidelines and alternate spelling authorities. For example, occasionally a copyright holder may require that eponymous terms be shown in possessive forms (Crohn's disease *vs.* Crohn disease) or that British spelling norms be retained (leukaemia *vs.* leukemia).

Locating Information within the Health Reference Series

The *Health Reference Series* contains a wealth of information about a wide variety of medical topics. Ensuring easy access to all the fact sheets, research reports, in-depth discussions, and other material contained within the individual books of the *Series* remains one of our

Chapter 1

Anatomy of the Breast

It is important for women to become familiar with the normal anatomy and physiology (function) of their breasts so that they can recognize early signs of possible abnormalities. This chapter outlines basic information on breast composition, development, and typical changes from puberty to pregnancy to menopause.

Breast Composition

The breast is a mass of glandular, fatty, and fibrous tissues positioned over the pectoral muscles of the chest wall and attached to the chest wall by fibrous strands called Cooper's ligaments. A layer of fatty tissue surrounds the breast glands and extends throughout the breast. The fatty tissue gives the breast a soft consistency.

The glandular tissues of the breast house the lobules (milk producing glands at the ends of the lobes) and the ducts (milk passages). Toward the nipple, each duct widens to form a sac (ampulla). During lactation, the bulbs on the ends of the lobules produce milk. Once milk is produced, it is transferred through the ducts to the nipple.

The breast is composed of:

- milk glands (lobules) that produce milk;
- ducts that transport milk from the milk glands (lobules) to the nipple;

After birth, estrogen and progesterone levels decrease and the production of prolactin declines. The breasts will usually begin to produce milk three to five days after a woman has given birth. During these few days before milk is produced, the body produces colostrum, a liquid substance that contains antibodies to help protect the infant against infections. Some physicians believe that colostrum also decreases an infant's chances of developing asthma and other allergies. Within a few days, the infant's own immune system will develop and he or she will not need colostrum.

The other hormone responsible for milk production, oxytocin, delivers the milk that prolactin has produced. When an infant suckles at the mother's breast, it brings milk out of the nipples. This suction signals the body to make more milk (using prolactin) and deliver more milk (using oxytocin). The body also produces a variety of other hormones (insulin, thyroid, cortisol) that provide the infant with nutrition when he or she takes the mother's milk. A woman's body will continue to produce milk until she stops breast-feeding, and even then, it may take several months for milk production to completely stop. The breasts will usually return to their previous size (or slightly smaller) after breast-feeding is completed.

Breast Changes after Menopause

When a woman reaches menopause (typically in her late 40s or early 50s), her body stops producing estrogen and progesterone. The loss of these hormones causes a variety of symptoms in many women including hot flashes, night sweats, mood changes, vaginal dryness, and difficulty sleeping. During this time, the breasts also undergo change. For some women, the breasts become more tender and lumpy, sometimes forming cysts (accumulated packets of fluid).

The breasts' glandular tissue, which has been kept firm so that the glands could produce milk, shrinks after menopause and is replaced with fatty tissue. The breasts also tend to increase in size and sag because the fibrous (connective) tissue loses its strength. Because the breasts become less dense after menopause, it is often easier for radiologists to detect breast cancer on an older woman's mammogram films, since abnormalities are not hidden by breast density. Since a woman's risk of breast cancer increases with age, all women should begin receiving annual screening mammograms at age 40, and continue monthly breast self-exams and physician-performed clinical breast exams every year.

Chapter 2

Breast Self-Examination

Important Questions

Why do a breast self-examination?

There are many good reasons for doing a breast self-examination each month. It is easy to do. When you get to know how your breasts normally feel, you may be able to feel a change. With practice, it should take about 15 minutes each month. Early detection is the key to successful treatment and cure.

When to do a breast self-examination?

The best time to do breast self-examination is right after your period, when breasts are least tender or swollen. If you do not have regular

From "How to Examine Your Breast—Monthly Breast Self Exam (BSE)," created by Missouri's Show Me Healthy Women, a breast and cervical cancer screening program. Reprinted with permission. Missouri Department of Health and Senior Services, 920 Wildwood Drive, P.O. Box 570, Jefferson City, MO 65102-0570. Web address: www.dhss.mo.gov/BreastCervCancer. The Show Me Healthy Women program is a joint program of the Missouri Department of Health and Senior Services and the Centers for Disease Control and Prevention, Grant Agreement #5U58DO000820-02. Alternative forms of this publication for persons with disabilities may be obtained by contacting Missouri Department of Health and Senior Services' Show Me Healthy Women program at 573-522-2845. Hearing impaired citizens telephone 1-800-735-2966. VOICE 1-800-735-2466. An Equal Opportunity/ Affirmative Action employer. Services provided on a nondiscriminatory basis.

periods or sometimes skip a month, choose a day and do it the same time every month.

Remember the ABCs of Breast Health

- **A** screening mammogram
- **B**reast self-examination
- **C**linical breast examination

A breast self-examination can save your life. Most breast lumps are found by women themselves or their partners. Most lumps in the breast are not cancer. Any lump or change should be checked by a doctor. Early detection is your best protection.

How to Examine Your Breast

Look for changes in front of a mirror.

View front and each side in each of the 3 positions:

1. Relax arms at your sides. Look for changes in shape and color. View for puckering, dimpling, skin changes, nipple discharge.

2. Raise hands above your head. Check again for puckering, dimpling and skin changes.

3. Place hands on hips, press down, bend forward. Check nipple direction and general appearance.

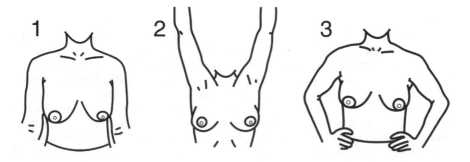

Figure 2.1. View front and each side in each of the three positions.

Feel for changes lying down.

Remember the seven "Ps":

1. Palpation: A) Use the pads of the middle three fingers of each hand to examine the breast on the opposite side. Do not use fingertips. Keep fingers together. B) Move fingers in dime-size circles using the three levels of pressure (see below) in each spot. Keep fingers, knuckles, and wrists straight. C) "Walk and slide" finger pads along so no breast tissue is missed.

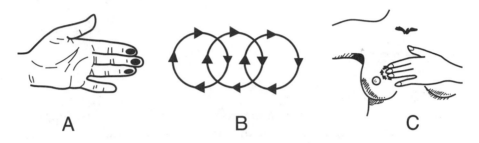

Figure 2.2. *Palpation.*

2. Pressure: Lumps can occur at any depth. Use three levels of pressure to examine each spot thoroughly.

- *Light:* Use very light pressure on the first dime-size circle. Pressure should be just enough to move the skin without disturbing the tissue underneath. Pressing too hard at first could cause a lump to move out of the way.

- *Medium:* On the second circle, use medium pressure to feel for changes below the surface to mid-level of the breast tissue.

- *Deep:* On the third circle, check for lumps deep in the breast tissue.

Press as firmly as you can without discomfort. The goal is to feel the ribs with the deep pressure.

3. Pattern: Start the exam under the arm (A).Use a vertical strip pattern to check the entire breast area. Imagine mowing a lawn with straight, vertical, overlapping rows. When you reach the end of each row, move over about one finger width and start the next row.

Once you start, do not lift fingers from the breast area. Be sure to examine the nipple with the same palpation technique you use to examine the rest of the breast tissue (B).

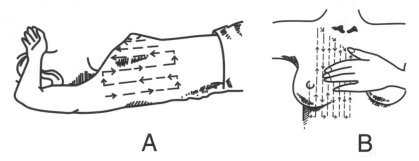

A   **B**

Figure 2.3. Pattern.

4. Perimeter: The area to be examined includes sides, top, and bottom of breast. Sides include the line from the middle of arm pit (axilla), that includes the area beyond breast fullness, down to the bottom bra line, and over to the middle of the breast bone. The top starts two finger-widths above the collarbone. Two finger-widths below the bra line indicates the bottom of the breast.

Figure 2.4. Perimeter.

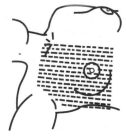

5. Position

- *Position 1*: Spread the breast tissue evenly over rib cage. Turn on your side with knees bent. Lean shoulder back toward the outside (away from your hip) and put your hand on your forehead. Place a pillow under your lower back to make it more comfortable. You are in the right position when your nipple seems to "float" at the top of the mound of your breast tissue.

- *Position 2*: When search pattern reaches the nipple, hold fingers in place on the nipple and roll back into a position flat on your back. The arm on the side being examined should now be extended directly away from the body (at a right angle).

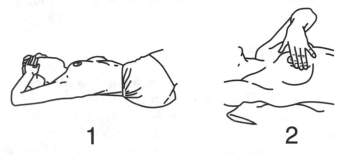

Figure 2.5. *Position.*

6. Pace: Go slowly. Take your time. Cover every square inch of the breast tissue. Performing breast self-exam every month could potentially save your life.

7. Practice: With monthly practice, you can become skilled at looking and feeling for changes in your breasts. Perform breast self-exam every month.

Check the lymph nodes.

Lymph nodes drain breast tissue. The lymph nodes that drain the breast tissue are located in three areas:

Figure 2.6. *Location of the lymph nodes.*

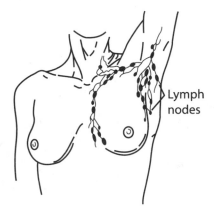

Lymph nodes

- Above your collar bone
- Below your collar bone
- In the armpit

You will want to know if any nodes are enlarged, movable, or unmovable.

Free Cancer Screenings

Are you eligible for free cancer screenings? In Missouri, you may qualify for Show Me Healthy Women if you are age 35–64 and you meet income guidelines. Call Show Me Healthy Women at 573-522-2845 or visit http://www.dhss.mo.us/BreastCervCancer.

Women in other states can find information about local programs by consulting the list of state contacts for breast and cervical cancer early detection programs provided at the end of this book or by calling the National Cancer Institute's Cancer Information Service at 800-4-CANCER (800-422-6237).

Chapter 3

Understanding
Breast Changes

About Your Breasts

The breast is a gland that produces milk in late pregnancy and after childbirth. Breasts consist of the following:

- Each breast is made of lobes.

- Lobes are groups of milk glands called lobules.

- Lobules are arranged around thin tubes called ducts.

- Ducts carry the milk to the nipple.

- These lobules and ducts make up the glandular tissue.

The breasts also contain lymph vessels, which carry a clear fluid called lymph.

- The lymph vessels lead to small, round organs called lymph nodes. Groups of lymph nodes are found near the breast in the underarm, above the collarbone, in the chest behind the breastbone, and in many other parts of the body.

- The lymph nodes trap bacteria, cancer cells, or other harmful substances that may be in the lymphatic system. Their job is to make sure harmful substances are safely removed from the body.

Excerpted from "Understanding Breast Changes: A Health Guide for Women," National Cancer Institute (www.cancer.gov); 2004.

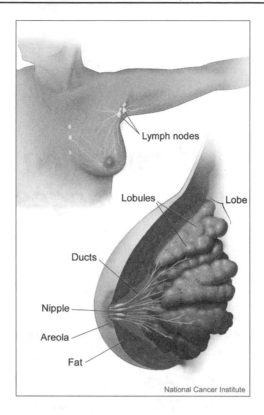

National Cancer Institute

Figure 3.1. *The Breast and Adjacent Lymph Nodes (Source: Don Bliss, National Cancer Institute).*

See your health care provider about a breast change when you have any of the following:

- A lump in or near your breast or under your arm
- Thick or firm tissue in or near your breast or under your arm
- Nipple discharge or tenderness
- A nipple pulled back (inverted) into the breast
- Itching or skin changes such as redness, scales, dimples, or puckers
- A change in breast size or shape

If you notice a lump in one breast, check the other breast. If both breasts feel the same, it may be normal. You should still see your health care provider for a clinical breast exam to see if more tests are needed.

Types of Breast Changes

Breast changes occur in almost all women. Most of these changes are not cancer. However, some breast changes may be signs of cancer. Breast changes that are not cancer are called benign.

Lumpiness: Most women have some type of lumpiness in their breasts. Some areas may be more dense than others and can feel lumpy in an exam. What you are feeling may be glandular breast tissue.

Breast changes due to your period: Many women have swelling, tenderness, and pain in their breasts before and sometimes during their periods. You may also feel one or more lumps during this time because of extra fluid in your breasts.

Because some lumps are caused by normal hormone changes, your health care provider may suggest watching the lump for a month or two to see if it changes or goes away.

Single lumps: Single lumps can appear at any time and come in various types and sizes. Most lumps are not cancer, but your health care provider should always check the lump carefully. He or she may do more tests to make sure the lump is not cancer.

Check with your health care provider if you notice any kind of lump. Even if you had a lump in the past that turned out to be benign, you can't be sure that a new lump is also benign.

Nipple discharge: Nipple discharge is common for some women. It is fluid that comes from the nipple in different colors or textures. Usually, it is not a sign of cancer. For example, birth control pills and other medicines, such as sedatives, can cause a little discharge. Certain infections also cause nipple discharge. However, for women who are going through or have passed menopause, nipple discharge can be a sign of cancer.

See your doctor if you have nipple discharge for the first time, or a change in your discharge's color or texture. He or she may send a sample of the discharge to be checked at a lab.

Finding Breast Changes

There are two ways to find breast changes:

- **Clinical breast exams:** A breast exam done by your health care provider.

- **Mammograms:** An x-ray of your breasts.

One way to find breast changes is with a clinical breast exam done by your health care provider. He or she will check your breasts and underarms for any lumps, nipple discharge, or other possible changes. This breast exam should be part of a routine medical check-up.

The best tool for finding breast cancer is a mammogram. A mammogram is a picture of the breast that is made by using low-dose x-rays. It is currently recommended that women over age 40 receive a mammogram every one to two years.

Some women check their own breasts for changes. If you find a change, it's important to call your health care provider for an appointment. Make sure to watch the change you found until you see your provider. But a breast self-exam and a clinical breast exam are not substitutes for mammograms.

Here are some questions to ask your health care provider about breast changes:

- How can I tell the difference between my usual lumps and lumps I need to do something about?
- How will you be able to tell what kind of breast change I have?
- What should we do to watch this change over time?

Mammograms

Mammograms are used for both screening and diagnosis.

A screening mammogram is used to find breast changes in women who have no signs of breast cancer. Most women get two x-rays of each breast. (Tip: Take your original mammogram and copy of the medical report with you if you change doctors or centers or need a second opinion.)

If your recent screening mammogram revealed a breast change since your last one, or if you or your health care provider noticed a change, he or she will probably recommend a diagnostic mammogram. More x-rays are taken during a diagnostic mammogram than a screening mammogram to get clearer, more detailed pictures of the breast. It is also used to rule out other breast problems.

A digital mammogram is another way to take a picture of your breasts. The procedure for having a digital mammogram is the same as a screening mammogram, except that it records the x-ray images in computer code instead of on x-ray film.

Figure 3.2 shows mammograms of two different women. Doctors look at these x-rays for any breast changes that don't look normal.

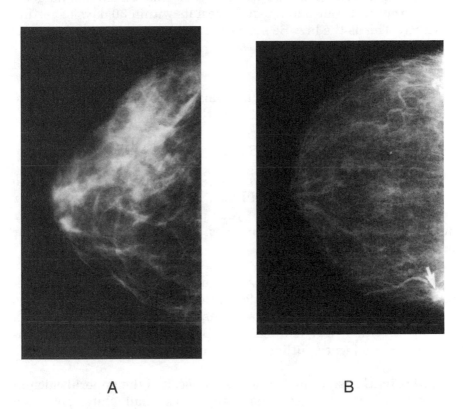

A   B

Figure 3.2. Two Mammograms: A. Mammogram of a normal breast (Source: American College of Radiology, AV-9004-3717, National Cancer Institute); B. Mammogram of a fatty breast with an obvious cancer, indicated by an arrow (Source: Dr. Dwight Kaufman, National Cancer Institute).

Mammograms and breast implants: When you go for your mammogram, tell staff if you have a breast implant. A technologist who is trained in x-raying patients with implants will do your mammogram. Breast implants can hide some breast tissue and make it harder to read your mammograms.

If you got implants for cosmetic reasons you still need to get screening mammograms, with extra pictures to help get an accurate reading.

If you got an implant after having a mastectomy for breast cancer you should continue to get mammograms of your other breast. Ask your doctor if you still need mammograms of the breast with the implant.

Getting Your Mammogram Results

Ask your doctor when you will get your results. You should get a written report of your mammogram results within 30 days of getting the x-ray. This is the law. Be sure the mammogram facility has your current address.

If your results were normal, it means the radiologist did not find anything that needs follow-up.

If your results were abnormal, it means the radiologist found a change from a past mammogram, or a change that needs more follow-up.

What a Mammogram Can Show

The radiologist will look at your x-rays for breast changes that do not look normal. The doctor will look for differences between your breasts. He or she will compare your past mammograms with your most recent one to check for changes. The doctor will also look for lumps and calcifications.

Lumps (or "mass"): The size, shape, and edges of a lump sometimes can give doctors more information about whether or not it is cancer. On a mammogram, a growth that is benign often looks smooth and round with a clear, defined edge. On the other hand, breast cancer often has a jagged outline and an irregular shape.

Calcifications: A calcification is a deposit of the mineral calcium in the breast tissue. Calcifications appear as small white spots on a mammogram. There are two types:

- Macrocalcifications are large calcium deposits often caused by aging. These are usually not cancer.

- Microcalcifications are tiny specks of calcium that may be found in an area of rapidly dividing cells. If they are found grouped together in a certain way, it may be a sign of cancer.

Depending on how many calcium specks you have, how big they are, and what they look like, your doctor may suggest that you have a different type of mammogram that allows the radiologist to have a closer look at the area; have another screening mammogram, usually within six months; or have a test called a biopsy.

Calcium in the diet does not create calcium deposits (calcifications) in the breast.

Are Mammogram Results Always Right?

No. Although they are not perfect, mammograms are the best method to find breast changes. If your mammogram shows a breast change, sometimes other tests are needed to better understand it. Even if the doctor sees something on the mammogram, it does not mean it is cancer.

Changes That Need More Follow-Up

Sometimes your doctor needs more information about a change on your mammogram. Your doctor may do follow-up tests such as an ultrasound or more mammograms. The only way to find out if an abnormal result is cancer is to do a biopsy. It is important to know that most abnormal findings are not cancer.

Breast Changes during Your Lifetime That Are Not Cancer

You might notice different kinds of breast changes at different times in your life. Many of these are caused by changes in your hormone levels and are a normal part of getting older.

Younger women may have more glandular (more dense, less fatty) breast tissue than older women who have stopped having their period (menopause). This kind of tissue is where breast changes usually occur.

Before or during your period, you might have lumpiness, tenderness, and pain in your breasts. The lumpiness and pain usually go away by the end of your period.

During pregnancy, your breasts may feel lumpy, as the glands that produce milk increase in number and get larger. Still, breast cancer has been found in pregnant women, so talk with your doctor if you have questions about any breast lumps.

While breastfeeding, you may get an infection called mastitis that happens when a milk duct becomes blocked. Mastitis causes the breast to look red and feel lumpy, warm, and tender. Mastitis is often treated with antibiotics. Sometimes the duct may need to be drained. If the redness or mastitis does not go away with treatment, call your doctor, as you may need further care.

As you approach menopause, your periods may become less frequent. Changing hormone levels also can make your breasts feel tender, even when you are not having your period; feel more dense; or feel more "lumpy" than they did before.

As you age, other breast changes are more common:

- **Intraductal papilloma:** This is a growth inside the nipple that looks like a wart. It can be removed by surgery without changing the way the breast looks.

- **Mammary duct ectasia:** As you near menopause, ducts beneath the nipple can become swollen and clogged. This can be painful and cause nipple discharge. The problem is treated with warm packs, antibiotics, and sometimes surgery to remove the duct.

If you are taking hormones, such as hormone replacement therapy (HRT), birth control pills, or injections, when getting your mammogram be sure to let your doctor know. Hormones may cause your breasts to be more dense. This can limit your doctor's ability to read a mammogram.

When you stop having periods (menopause), your hormone levels drop, and your breast tissue becomes less dense and more fatty. You may stop having the lumps, pain, or nipple discharge you used to have. And because your breast tissue is less dense, mammograms can be easier to read. This means doctors are more likely to find breast changes or early breast cancer.

Chapter 4

What Are Benign Breast Conditions?

The term benign breast conditions, also known as benign breast disease, is used to describe a number of benign (non-cancerous) disorders that can affect the breast. Some cause discomfort or pain and require treatment, while others are of little concern and need no medical attention. Unfortunately, many breast conditions mimic the symptoms of cancer and so require tests and sometimes surgical biopsy to diagnose. Though the prospect of cancer is certainly scary, most biopsies find a benign breast condition instead of cancer.

Some of the more common benign breast conditions are hyperplasia, cysts, and fibroadenomas. The term "fibrocystic changes" is used by some health care providers to describe a broad range of benign breast conditions. There are many types of benign breast conditions that differ from each other in their cellular appearance under a microscope. If "fibrocystic changes" is used to describe someone's condition, it's important to ask about the specific type of fibrocystic change that was identified (for example, whether it is a cyst or hyperplasia). While benign breast conditions are not cancer, certain types do actually increase the risk of breast cancer.

Hormonal factors, such as the use of postmenopausal hormones, can increase the risk of benign breast conditions. Similar to the risk of breast cancer, risk of benign breast conditions is increased among women with inherited genetic susceptibilities including BRCA1 or BRCA2 mutations.

"What Are Benign Breast Conditions (Benign Breast Disease)?" © 2008. Material reprinted from www.komen.org, with permission from Susan G. Komen for the Cure®.

Hyperplasia: Hyperplasia is a term describing the excessive accumulation or build up (sometimes called proliferation) of cells. It is usually found on the inside of the lobules or ducts in the breast tissue. Hyperplasia usually occurs among women in their 20s and often is associated with breast pain. There are two main types of hyperplasia—usual and atypical. Both raise the risk of breast cancer, though atypical hyperplasia does so to a greater degree.

Cysts: Cysts are fluid-filled sacs that are almost always benign. Often they can be left alone, or if painful, they can be drained of the fluid (aspirated). They may also be drained if they are palpable (can be felt) and could potentially interfere with clinical exams. Up to a third of women between the ages of 35 and 50 have cysts in their breasts, though most cysts are too small to feel and can be detected only by examination with ultrasound.

If cysts are large enough, they may feel like lumps in the breast. Breast pain and nipple discharge may also be present. In a small proportion of patients, the cysts will recur after being aspirated. If this happens repeatedly, patients may want to have them removed. Cysts are more common in women as they approach menopause, but they are not associated with an increased risk of cancer. After menopause, cysts occur much less frequently.

It is unknown exactly what causes cysts to develop. Although certain dietary factors, such as caffeine intake, have been discussed as possible risk factors for developing breast cysts, there are currently very little data backing up any link between cyst development and either dietary or lifestyle factors.

Fibroadenomas: Fibroadenomas, another type of benign lump, are most common in younger women. They are usually not removed because they pose no risk. Sometimes they are uncomfortable and produce a lump that can be felt in the breast. If a fibroadenoma is large, a woman will probably want it removed. In older women, fibroadenomas are generally removed to be certain they are not cancerous. Fibroadenomas are not generally associated with an increased risk of cancer.

Sclerosing adenosis: Sclerosing adenosis most commonly occurs in women in their 30s. It is characterized by small breast nodules that are composed of distorted, elongated glandular cells. Sclerosing adenosis may increase the risk of atypical hyperplasia, lobular carcinoma in situ and ductal carcinoma in situ.

Radial scars: Radial scars are discovered most often during a biopsy on a breast tumor removed for other reasons. They can look like breast cancer on a mammogram, but they are not actual cancer. Although some studies have found that radial scars increase the risk of breast cancer, this may be because they are typically identified alongside existing disease.

Intraductal papillomas: Intraductal papillomas occur in the lactation ducts of the breasts. These small masses may appear with or without nipple discharge. There are two types of intraductal papillomas—solitary and multiple (or peripheral). Solitary intraductal papillomas usually occur among women in their 30s and 40s and do not increase the risk of breast cancer unless atypical cells are present. Multiple intraductal papillomas occur among even younger women and are associated with a small increase in breast cancer risk.

Benign phyllodes tumor: Phyllodes tumors are very rare, comprising less than one percent of all breast tumors in women. There are several sub-types. Benign phyllodes tumor is most common, accounting for more than 50 percent of all phyllodes tumors, and the least aggressive of these sub-types. These benign tumors are similar to fibroadenomas and typically occur among women younger than 50. Because phyllodes tumors are so rare, it is unclear whether or not they increase the risk of breast cancer.

Sclerosing lymphocytic lobulitis/ductitis (diabetic mastopathy, lymphocytic mastitis): Sclerosing lymphocytic lobulitis (also called diabetic mastopathy and lymphocytic mastitis) are benign breast masses that most often appear in women with insulin-dependent (type 1) diabetes. These tumors are typically small, hard masses and can appear in the ducts (lymphocytic ductitis) or in the lobules (lymphocytic lobulitis). This type of benign breast condition does not appear to increase the risk of breast cancer.

Chapter 5

Breast Lumps: What You Should Know

Definition: A breast lump is a swelling, protuberance, or lump in the breast.

Alternative Names: Breast mass

Considerations

Normal breast tissue is present in both males and females of all ages. This tissue responds to hormonal changes and, therefore, certain lumps can come and go.

Breast lumps may appear at all ages:

- Infants may have breast lumps related to estrogen from the mother. The lump generally goes away on its own as the estrogen clears from the baby's body. It can happen to boys and girls.

- Young girls often develop "breast buds" that appear just before the beginning of puberty. These bumps may be tender. They are common around age nine but may happen as early as age six.

- Teenage boys may develop breast enlargement and lumps because of hormonal changes in mid-puberty. Although this may distress the teen, the lumps or enlargement generally go away on their own over a period of months.

- Breast lumps in an adult woman raise concern for breast cancer, even though most lumps turn out to be not cancerous.

Causes

Lumps in a woman are often caused by fibrocystic changes, fibroadenomas, and cysts.

Fibrocystic changes can occur in either or both breasts. These changes are common in women (especially during the reproductive years), and are considered a normal variation of breast tissue. Having fibrocystic breasts does not increase your risk for breast cancer. It does, however, make it more difficult to interpret lumps that you or your doctor find on exam. Many women feel tenderness in addition to the lumps and bumps associated with fibrocystic breasts.

Fibroadenomas are non-cancerous lumps that feel rubbery and are easily moveable within the breast tissue. Like fibrocystic changes, they occur most often during the reproductive years. Usually, they are not tender and, except in rare cases, do not become cancerous later. A doctor may feel fairly certain from an exam that a particular lump is a fibroadenoma. The only way to be sure, however, is to remove or biopsy it.

Cysts are fluid-filled sacs that often feel like soft grapes. These can sometimes be tender, especially just before your menstrual period. Cysts may be drained in the doctor's office. If the fluid removed is clear or greenish, and the lump disappears completely after it is drained, no further treatment is needed. If the fluid is bloody, it is sent to the lab to look for cancer cells. If the lump doesn't disappear, or recurs, it is usually removed surgically.

Other causes of breast lumps include:

- Milk cysts (sacs filled with milk) and infections (mastitis), which may turn into an abscess. These typically occur if you are breastfeeding or have recently given birth.

- Breast cancer, found on mammogram or ultrasound, then a biopsy. Men also can get breast cancer.

- Injury—sometimes if your breast is badly bruised, there will be a collection of blood that feels like a lump. These lumps tend to get better on their own in a matter of days or weeks. If not, your doctor may have to drain the blood.

- Lipoma—a collection of fatty tissue.

- Intraductal papilloma—a small growth inside a milk duct of the breast. This often occurs near the areola, the colored part of the breast surrounding the nipple, in women ages 35–55. It is harmless and often cannot be felt. In some cases the only symptom is a watery, pink discharge from the nipple. Since a watery or bloody discharge can also be a sign of breast cancer, your doctor should check this.

Home Care

For fibrocystic changes, birth control pills are often helpful. Other women are helped by:

- avoiding caffeine and chocolate;
- limiting fat and increasing fiber in the diet;
- taking vitamin E, vitamin B complex, or evening primrose oil supplements.

When to Contact a Medical Professional

Call your doctor if:

- the skin on your breast appears dimpled or wrinkled (like the peel of an orange);
- you find a new breast lump during your monthly self-exam;
- you have bruising on your breast, but did not experience any injury;
- you have nipple discharge, especially if it is bloody or pinkish (blood-tinged);
- your nipple is inverted (turned inward) but normally is not inverted.

Also call if:

- you are a woman, age 20 or older, and want guidance on how to perform a breast self-examination;
- you are a woman over age 40 and have not had a mammogram in the past year.

What to Expect at Your Office Visit

Your doctor will get a complete history from you, with special attention to factors that may increase your risk of breast cancer. The health care provider will perform a thorough breast examination. If you don't know how to perform breast self-examination, ask your health care provider to teach you the proper method.

Medical history questions regarding breast lumps include:

- When and how did you first notice the lump?

- Do you have other symptoms such as pain, nipple discharge, or fever?

- Where is the lump located?

- Do you do self-breast exams and is this lump a recent change?

- Have you had any type of injury to your breast?

- Are you taking any hormones, medications, or supplements?

Tests that may be performed include:

- Biopsy of the lump
- Mammogram
- Needle aspiration of a cyst and examination of the fluid under a microscope
- Study of nipple discharge under a microscope
- Ultrasound to see if the lump is solid or a cyst

Treatment of a breast lump depends on the cause. Solid breast lumps are often removed surgically. Cysts can be drained. Breast infections require antibiotics. If breast cancer is diagnosed, most women receive surgery, radiation, chemotherapy, or hormonal therapy. Discuss these options carefully and thoroughly with your doctor.

If you have a family history of breast cancer, your doctor may also suggest testing for genes that make you more likely to get breast cancer.

Prevention

Breast cancer screening is an important way to find breast cancer early, when it is most easily treated and cured.

- Get regular mammograms.
- If you are over age 20, consider doing a monthly breast self-exam.

- If you are over age 20, have a complete breast exam by your provider at least every three years—every year if you are over 40.

Having fibrocystic breast tissue, mastitis, or breast tenderness related to PMS does not put you at greater risk for breast cancer. Having fibrocystic breasts does, however, make your self-exam more confusing, because there are many normal lumps and bumps.

To prevent breast cancer:

- Exercise regularly
- Reduce fat intake
- Eat lots of fruits, vegetables, and other high fiber foods
- Do not drink more than one or one and a half glasses of alcohol a day

References

Saslow D, Boetes C, Burke W, et al. American cancer society guidelines for breast screening with MRI as an adjunct to mammography. *CA Cancer J Clin*. 2007 Mar-Apr; 57(2): 75–89.

Marchant DJ. Benign breast disease. *Obstet Gynecol Clin North Am*. 2002; 29(1): 1–20.

Klein S. Evaluation of palpable breast masses. *Am Fam Physician*. 2005; 71(9): 1731–1738.

Part Two

Breast Cancer Fundamentals

Chapter 6

What You Need to Know about Breast Cancer

Breast cancer is the most common type of cancer among women in this country (other than skin cancer). Each year, more than 211,000 American women learn they have this disease. Each year, about 1,700 men in this country learn they have breast cancer.

Scientists are studying breast cancer to find out more about its causes. And they are looking for better ways to prevent, find, and treat it.

The Breasts

The breasts sit on the chest muscles that cover the ribs. Each breast is made of 15 to 20 lobes. Lobes contain many smaller lobules. Lobules contain groups of tiny glands that can produce milk. Milk flows from the lobules through thin tubes called ducts to the nipple. The nipple is in the center of a dark area of skin called the areola. Fat fills the spaces between the lobules and ducts.

The breasts also contain lymph vessels. These vessels lead to small, round organs called lymph nodes. Groups of lymph nodes are near the breast in the axilla (underarm), above the collarbone, in the chest behind the breastbone, and in many other parts of the body. The lymph nodes trap bacteria, cancer cells, or other harmful substances.

Excerpted from "What You Need to Know about Breast Cancer," National Cancer Institute (www.cancer.gov), November 2007.

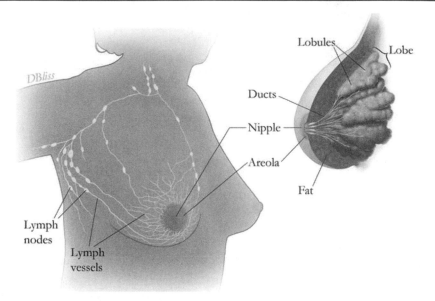

Figure 6.1. This picture shows the parts of the breast and the lymph nodes and lymph vessels near the breast. (Source: Don Bliss, CDR415520, National Cancer Institute).

Understanding Cancer

Cancer begins in cells, the building blocks that make up tissues. Tissues make up the organs of the body.

Normally, cells grow and divide to form new cells as the body needs them. When cells grow old, they die, and new cells take their place.

Sometimes, this orderly process goes wrong. New cells form when the body does not need them, and old cells do not die when they should. These extra cells can form a mass of tissue called a growth or tumor.

Tumors can be benign or malignant:

- Benign tumors are not cancer:

  - Benign tumors are rarely life-threatening.

  - Generally, benign tumors can be removed. They usually do not grow back.

  - Cells from benign tumors do not invade the tissues around them.

  - Cells from benign tumors do not spread to other parts of the body.

- Malignant tumors are cancer:

  - Malignant tumors are generally more serious than benign tumors. They may be life-threatening.

  - Malignant tumors often can be removed. But sometimes they grow back.

  - Cells from malignant tumors can invade and damage nearby tissues and organs.

  - Cells from malignant tumors can spread (metastasize) to other parts of the body. Cancer cells spread by breaking away from the original (primary) tumor and entering the bloodstream or lymphatic system. The cells invade other organs and form new tumors that damage these organs. The spread of cancer is called metastasis.

When breast cancer cells spread, the cancer cells are often found in lymph nodes near the breast. Also, breast cancer can spread to almost any other part of the body. The most common are the bones, liver, lungs, and brain. The new tumor has the same kind of abnormal cells and the same name as the primary tumor. For example, if breast cancer spreads to the bones, the cancer cells in the bones are actually breast cancer cells. The disease is metastatic breast cancer, not bone cancer. For that reason, it is treated as breast cancer, not bone cancer. Doctors call the new tumor "distant" or metastatic disease.

Risk Factors

No one knows the exact causes of breast cancer. Doctors often cannot explain why one woman develops breast cancer and another does not. They do know that bumping, bruising, or touching the breast does not cause cancer. And breast cancer is not contagious. You cannot "catch" it from another person.

Research has shown that women with certain risk factors are more likely than others to develop breast cancer. A risk factor is something that may increase the chance of developing a disease.

Studies have found the following risk factors for breast cancer:

- Age
- Personal history of breast cancer
- Family history
- Certain breast changes

- Gene changes
- Reproductive and menstrual history
- Race
- Radiation therapy to the chest
- Breast density
- Taking DES (diethylstilbestrol)
- Being overweight or obese after menopause
- Lack of physical activity
- Drinking alcohol

Other possible risk factors are under study. Researchers are studying the effect of diet, physical activity, and genetics on breast cancer risk. They are also studying whether certain substances in the environment can increase the risk of breast cancer.

If you think you may be at risk, you should discuss this concern with your doctor. Your doctor may be able to suggest ways to reduce your risk and can plan a schedule for checkups.

Screening

Screening for breast cancer before there are symptoms can be important. Screening can help doctors find and treat cancer early. Treatment is more likely to work well when cancer is found early.

You should ask your doctor about when to start and how often to check for breast cancer.

Screening Mammogram

To find breast cancer early, the National Cancer Institute offers the following guidelines:

- Women in their 40s and older should have mammograms every one to two years. A mammogram is a picture of the breast made with x-rays.
- Women who are younger than 40 and have risk factors for breast cancer should ask their health care provider whether to have mammograms and how often to have them.

Mammograms can often show a breast lump before it can be felt. They also can show a cluster of tiny specks of calcium. These specks are called microcalcifications. Lumps or specks can be from cancer, precancerous cells, or other conditions. Further tests are needed to find out if abnormal cells are present.

If an abnormal area shows up on your mammogram, you may need to have more x-rays. You also may need a biopsy. A biopsy is the only way to tell for sure if cancer is present.

Clinical Breast Exam

During a clinical breast exam, your health care provider checks your breasts. You may be asked to raise your arms over your head, let them hang by your sides, or press your hands against your hips.

Your health care provider looks for differences in size or shape between your breasts. The skin of your breasts is checked for a rash, dimpling, or other abnormal signs. Your nipples may be squeezed to check for fluid.

Using the pads of the fingers to feel for lumps, your health care provider checks your entire breast, underarm, and collarbone area. A lump is generally the size of a pea before anyone can feel it. The exam is done on one side, then the other. Your health care provider checks the lymph nodes near the breast to see if they are enlarged.

Breast Self-Exam

You may perform monthly breast self-exams to check for any changes in your breasts. It is important to remember that changes can occur because of aging, your menstrual cycle, pregnancy, menopause, or taking birth control pills or other hormones. It is normal for breasts to feel a little lumpy and uneven. Also, it is common for your breasts to be swollen and tender right before or during your menstrual period.

You should contact your health care provider if you notice any unusual changes in your breasts.

Symptoms

Common symptoms of breast cancer include the following:

- A change in how the breast or nipple feels:
    - A lump or thickening in or near the breast or in the underarm area
    - Nipple tenderness

- A change in how the breast or nipple looks:
  - A change in the size or shape of the breast
  - A nipple turned inward into the breast
  - The skin of the breast, areola, or nipple may be scaly, red, or swollen. It may have ridges or pitting so that it looks like the skin of an orange.
- Nipple discharge (fluid)

Early breast cancer usually does not cause pain. Still, a woman should see her health care provider about breast pain or any other symptom that does not go away. Most often, these symptoms are not due to cancer. Other health problems may also cause them. Any woman with these symptoms should tell her doctor so that problems can be diagnosed and treated as early as possible.

Diagnosis

If you have a symptom or screening test result that suggests cancer, your doctor must find out whether it is due to cancer or to some other cause. Your doctor may ask about your personal and family medical history. You may have a physical exam. Your doctor also may order a mammogram or other imaging procedure. These tests make pictures of tissues inside the breast. After the tests, your doctor may decide no other exams are needed. Your doctor may suggest that you have a follow-up exam later on. Or you may need to have a biopsy to look for cancer cells.

Clinical Breast Exam

Your health care provider feels each breast for lumps and looks for other problems. If you have a lump, your doctor will feel its size, shape, and texture. Your doctor will also check to see if it moves easily. Benign lumps often feel different from cancerous ones. Lumps that are soft, smooth, round, and movable are likely to be benign. A hard, oddly shaped lump that feels firmly attached within the breast is more likely to be cancer.

Diagnostic Mammogram

Diagnostic mammograms are x-ray pictures of the breast. They take clearer, more detailed images of areas that look abnormal on a screening mammogram. Doctors use them to learn more about unusual breast changes, such as a lump, pain, thickening, nipple discharge, or change in breast size or shape. Diagnostic mammograms may focus on a specific area of the breast. They may involve special techniques and more views than screening mammograms.

Ultrasound

An ultrasound device sends out sound waves that people cannot hear. The waves bounce off tissues. A computer uses the echoes to create a picture. Your doctor can view these pictures on a monitor. The pictures may show whether a lump is solid or filled with fluid. A cyst is a fluid-filled sac. Cysts are not cancer. But a solid mass may be cancer. After the test, your doctor can store the pictures on video or print them out. This exam may be used along with a mammogram.

Magnetic Resonance Imaging

Magnetic resonance imaging (MRI) uses a powerful magnet linked to a computer. MRI makes detailed pictures of breast tissue. Your doctor can view these pictures on a monitor or print them on film. MRI may be used along with a mammogram.

Biopsy

Your doctor may refer you to a surgeon or breast disease specialist for a biopsy. Fluid or tissue is removed from your breast to help find out if there is cancer.

Some suspicious areas can be seen on a mammogram but cannot be felt during a clinical breast exam. Doctors can use imaging procedures to help see the area and remove tissue. Such procedures include ultrasound-guided, needle-localized, or stereotactic biopsy.

Staging

To plan your treatment, your doctor needs to know the extent (stage) of the disease. The stage is based on the size of the tumor and whether the cancer has spread. Staging may involve x-rays and lab tests. These tests can show whether the cancer has spread and, if so, to what parts of your body. When breast cancer spreads, cancer cells are often found in lymph nodes under the arm (axillary lymph nodes). The stage often is not known until after surgery to remove the tumor in your breast and the lymph nodes under your arm.

41

These are the stages of breast cancer:

Stage 0 is carcinoma in situ.

- **Lobular carcinoma in situ (LCIS):** Abnormal cells are in the lining of a lobule. LCIS seldom becomes invasive cancer. However, having LCIS in one breast increases the risk of cancer for both breasts.

- **Ductal carcinoma in situ (DCIS):** Abnormal cells are in the lining of a duct. DCIS is also called intraductal carcinoma. The abnormal cells have not spread outside the duct. They have not invaded the nearby breast tissue. DCIS sometimes becomes invasive cancer if not treated.

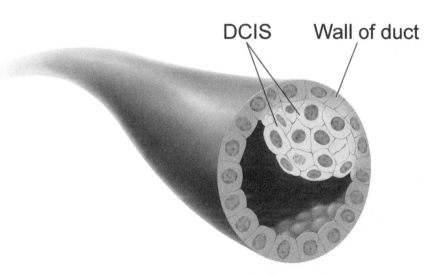

DCIS   Wall of duct

Figure 6.2. This picture shows ductal carcinoma in situ. (Source: Don Bliss, National Cancer Institute).

Stage I is an early stage of invasive breast cancer. The tumor is no more than two centimeters (three-quarters of an inch) across. Cancer cells have not spread beyond the breast.

Stage II is one of the following:

- The tumor is no more than two centimeters (three-quarters of an inch) across. The cancer has spread to the lymph nodes under the arm.

- The tumor is between two and five centimeters (three-quarters of an inch to two inches). The cancer has not spread to the lymph nodes under the arm.

- The tumor is between two and five centimeters (three-quarters of an inch to two inches). The cancer has spread to the lymph nodes under the arm.

- The tumor is larger than five centimeters (two inches). The cancer has not spread to the lymph nodes under the arm.

Stage III is locally advanced cancer. It is divided into Stage IIIA, IIIB, and IIIC. Stage IIIA is one of the following:

- The tumor is no more than five centimeters (two inches) across. The cancer has spread to underarm lymph nodes that are attached to each other or to other structures. Or the cancer may have spread to lymph nodes behind the breastbone.

- The tumor is more than five centimeters across. The cancer has spread to underarm lymph nodes that are either alone or attached to each other or to other structures. Or the cancer may have spread to lymph nodes behind the breastbone.

Stage IIIB is a tumor of any size that has grown into the chest wall or the skin of the breast. It may be associated with swelling of the breast or with nodules (lumps) in the breast skin.

- The cancer may have spread to lymph nodes under the arm.

- The cancer may have spread to underarm lymph nodes that are attached to each other or other structures. Or the cancer may have spread to lymph nodes behind the breastbone.

- Inflammatory breast cancer is a rare type of breast cancer. The breast looks red and swollen because cancer cells block the lymph vessels in the skin of the breast. When a doctor diagnoses inflammatory breast cancer, it is at least Stage IIIB, but it could be more advanced.

Stage IIIC is a tumor of any size. It has spread in one of the following ways:

- The cancer has spread to the lymph nodes behind the breastbone and under the arm.

- The cancer has spread to the lymph nodes above or below the collarbone.

Stage IV is distant metastatic cancer. The cancer has spread to other parts of the body.

Recurrent cancer is cancer that has come back (recurred) after a period of time when it could not be detected. It may recur locally in the breast or chest wall. Or it may recur in any other part of the body, such as the bone, liver, or lungs.

Treatment

Many women with breast cancer want to take an active part in making decisions about their medical care. It is natural to want to learn all you can about your disease and treatment choices. Knowing more about breast cancer helps many women cope.

Getting a Second Opinion

Before starting treatment, you might want a second opinion about your diagnosis and treatment plan. Many insurance companies cover a second opinion if you or your doctor requests it. It may take some time and effort to gather medical records and arrange to see another doctor. You may have to gather your mammogram films, biopsy slides, pathology report, and proposed treatment plan. Usually it is not a problem to take several weeks to get a second opinion. In most cases, the delay in starting treatment will not make treatment less effective. To make sure, you should discuss this delay with your doctor. Some women with breast cancer need treatment right away.

Treatment Methods

Women with breast cancer have many treatment options. These include surgery, radiation therapy, chemotherapy, hormone therapy, and biological therapy. Many women receive more than one type of treatment.

The choice of treatment depends mainly on the stage of the disease. Your doctor can describe your treatment choices and the expected results. You and your doctor can work together to develop a treatment plan that reflects your medical needs and personal values.

Cancer treatment is either local therapy or systemic therapy:

- **Local therapy:** Surgery and radiation therapy are local treatments. They remove or destroy cancer in the breast. When breast cancer has spread to other parts of the body, local therapy may be used to control the disease in those specific areas.

- **Systemic therapy:** Chemotherapy, hormone therapy, and biological therapy are systemic treatments. They enter the bloodstream and destroy or control cancer throughout the body. Some women with breast cancer have systemic therapy to shrink the tumor before surgery or radiation. Others have systemic therapy after surgery and/or radiation to prevent the cancer from coming back. Systemic treatments also are used for cancer that has spread.

Because cancer treatments often damage healthy cells and tissues, side effects are common. Side effects depend mainly on the type and extent of the treatment. Side effects may not be the same for each woman, and they may change from one treatment session to the next.

Breast Reconstruction

Some women who plan to have a mastectomy decide to have breast reconstruction. Other women prefer to wear a breast form (prosthesis). Others decide to do nothing. All of these options have pros and cons. What is right for one woman may not be right for another. What is important is that nearly every woman treated for breast cancer has choices.

Breast reconstruction may be done at the same time as the mastectomy, or later on. If you are thinking about breast reconstruction, you should talk to a plastic surgeon before the mastectomy, even if you plan to have your reconstruction later on.

Which type of reconstruction is best depends on your age, body type, and the type of surgery you had. The plastic surgeon can explain the risks and benefits of each type of reconstruction.

Complementary and Alternative Medicine

Some women with breast cancer use complementary and alternative medicine (CAM):

- An approach is generally called complementary medicine when it is used along with standard treatment.

- An approach is called alternative medicine when it is used instead of standard treatment.

Acupuncture, massage therapy, herbal products, vitamins or special diets, visualization, meditation, and spiritual healing are types of CAM.

Many women say that CAM helps them feel better. However, some types of CAM may change the way standard treatment works. These changes could be harmful. And some types of CAM could be harmful even if used alone.

Some types of CAM are expensive. Health insurance may not cover the cost.

Nutrition and Physical Activity

It is important for women with breast cancer to take care of themselves. Taking care of yourself includes eating well and staying as active as you can.

You need the right amount of calories to maintain a good weight. You also need enough protein to keep up your strength. Eating well may help you feel better and have more energy.

Sometimes, especially during or soon after treatment, you may not feel like eating. You may be uncomfortable or tired. You may find that foods do not taste as good as they used to. In addition, the side effects of treatment (such as poor appetite, nausea, vomiting, or mouth sores) can make it hard to eat well. Your doctor, dietitian, or other health care provider can suggest ways to deal with these problems.

Many women find they feel better when they stay active. Walking, yoga, swimming, and other activities can keep you strong and increase your energy. Exercise may reduce nausea and pain and make treatment easier to handle. It also can help relieve stress. Whatever physical activity you choose, be sure to talk to your doctor before you start. Also, if your activity causes you pain or other problems, be sure to let your doctor or nurse know about it.

Follow-Up Care

Follow-up care after treatment for breast cancer is important. Recovery is different for each woman. Your recovery depends on your treatment, whether the disease has spread, and other factors.

Even when the cancer seems to have been completely removed or destroyed, the disease sometimes returns because undetected cancer cells remained somewhere in the body after treatment. Your doctor will monitor your recovery and check for recurrence of the cancer.

You should report any changes in the treated area or in your other breast to the doctor right away. Tell your doctor about any health problems, such as pain, loss of appetite or weight, changes in menstrual cycles, unusual vaginal bleeding, or blurred vision. Also talk to your doctor about headaches, dizziness, shortness of breath, coughing or hoarseness, backaches, or digestive problems that seem unusual or that don't go away. Such problems may arise months or years after treatment. They may suggest that the cancer has returned, but they can also be symptoms of other health problems. It is important to share your concerns with your doctor so problems can be diagnosed and treated as soon as possible.

Follow-up exams usually include the breasts, chest, neck, and underarm areas. Since you are at risk of getting cancer again, you should have mammograms of your preserved breast and your other breast. You probably will not need a mammogram of a reconstructed breast or if you had a mastectomy without reconstruction. Your doctor may order other imaging procedures or lab tests.

Sources of Support

Learning you have breast cancer can change your life and the lives of those close to you. These changes can be hard to handle. It is normal for you, your family, and your friends to have many different and sometimes confusing feelings.

You may worry about caring for your family, keeping your job, or continuing daily activities. Concerns about treatments and managing side effects, hospital stays, and medical bills are also common. Doctors, nurses, and other members of the health care team can answer questions about treatment, working, or other activities. Meeting with a social worker, counselor, or member of the clergy can be helpful if you want to talk about your feelings or concerns. Often, a social worker can suggest resources for financial aid, transportation, home care, or emotional support.

Friends and relatives can be very supportive. Also, you may find it helps to discuss your concerns with others who have cancer. Women with breast cancer often get together in support groups to share what they have learned about coping with their disease and the effects of their treatment. It is important to keep in mind, however, that each woman is different. Ways that one woman deals with cancer may not be right for another. You may want to ask your health care provider about advice you receive from other women with breast cancer.

Several organizations offer special programs for women with breast cancer. Women who have had the disease serve as trained volunteers. They may talk with or visit women with breast cancer, provide information, and lend emotional support. They often share their experiences with breast cancer treatment, breast reconstruction, and recovery.

Chapter 7

Inflammatory Breast Cancer

What is inflammatory breast cancer (IBC)?

Inflammatory breast cancer is a rare but very aggressive type of breast cancer in which the cancer cells block the lymph vessels in the skin of the breast. This type of breast cancer is called "inflammatory" because the breast often looks swollen and red, or "inflamed." IBC accounts for one to five percent of all breast cancer cases in the United States.[1] It tends to be diagnosed in younger women compared to non-IBC breast cancer. It occurs more frequently and at a younger age in African Americans than in Whites. Like other types of breast cancer, IBC can occur in men, but usually at an older age than in women. Some studies have shown an association between family history of breast cancer and IBC, but more studies are needed to draw firm conclusions.[2]

What are the symptoms of IBC?

Symptoms of IBC may include redness, swelling, and warmth in the breast, often without a distinct lump in the breast. The redness and warmth are caused by cancer cells blocking the lymph vessels in the skin. The skin of the breast may also appear pink, reddish purple, or bruised. The skin may also have ridges or appear pitted, like the skin of an orange (called peau d'orange), which is caused by a buildup of fluid and edema (swelling) in the breast. Other symptoms include

"Inflammatory Breast Cancer: Questions and Answers," National Cancer Institute (www.cancer.gov), August 29, 2006.

heaviness, burning, aching, increase in breast size, tenderness, or a nipple that is inverted (facing inward).[3] These symptoms usually develop quickly—over a period of weeks or months. Swollen lymph nodes may also be present under the arm, above the collarbone, or in both places. However, it is important to note that these symptoms may also be signs of other conditions such as infection, injury, or other types of cancer.[1]

How is IBC diagnosed?

Diagnosis of IBC is based primarily on the results of a doctor's clinical examination.[1] Biopsy, mammogram, and breast ultrasound are used to confirm the diagnosis. IBC is classified as either stage IIIB or stage IV breast cancer.[2] Stage IIIB breast cancers are locally advanced; stage IV breast cancer is cancer that has spread to other organs. IBC tends to grow rapidly, and the physical appearance of the breast of patients with IBC is different from that of patients with other stage III breast cancers. IBC is an especially aggressive, locally advanced breast cancer.

Cancer staging describes the extent or severity of an individual's cancer. (More information on staging is available in the National Cancer Institute's fact sheet "Staging: Questions and Answers" at http://www.cancer.gov/cancertopics/factsheet/Detection/staging on the internet.) Knowing a cancer's stage helps the doctor develop a treatment plan and estimate prognosis (the likely outcome or course of the disease; the chance of recovery or recurrence).

How is IBC treated?

Treatment consisting of chemotherapy, targeted therapy, surgery, radiation therapy, and hormonal therapy is used to treat IBC. Patients may also receive supportive care to help manage the side effects of the cancer and its treatment. Chemotherapy (anticancer drugs) is generally the first treatment for patients with IBC, and is called neoadjuvant therapy. Chemotherapy is systemic treatment, which means that it affects cells throughout the body. The purpose of chemotherapy is to control or kill cancer cells, including those that may have spread to other parts of the body.

After chemotherapy, patients with IBC may undergo surgery and radiation therapy to the chest wall. Both radiation and surgery are local treatments that affect only cells in the tumor and the immediately surrounding area. The purpose of surgery is to remove the tumor from the body, while the purpose of radiation therapy is to destroy remaining cancer cells. Surgery to remove the breast (or as much of the breast tissue as possible) is called a mastectomy. Lymph node dissection (removal of the lymph nodes in the underarm area for examination under a microscope) is also done during this surgery.

After initial systemic and local treatment, patients with IBC may receive additional systemic treatments to reduce the risk of recurrence (cancer coming back). Such treatments may include additional chemotherapy, hormonal therapy (treatment that interferes with the effects of the female hormone estrogen, which can promote the growth of breast cancer cells), targeted therapy (such as trastuzumab, also known as Herceptin®), or all three. Trastuzumab is administered to patients whose tumors over express the HER–2 tumor protein.

Supportive care is treatment given to improve the quality of life of patients who have a serious or life-threatening disease, such as cancer. It prevents or treats as early as possible the symptoms of the disease, side effects caused by treatment of the disease, and psychological, social, and spiritual problems related to the disease or its treatment. For example, compression garments may be used to treat lymphedema (swelling caused by excess fluid buildup) resulting from radiation therapy or the removal of lymph nodes. Additionally, meeting with a social worker, counselor, or member of the clergy can be helpful to those who want to talk about their feelings or discuss their concerns. A social worker can often suggest resources for help with recovery, emotional support, financial aid, transportation, or home care.

Are clinical trials (research studies with people) available? Where can people get more information about clinical trials?

Yes. The NCI is sponsoring clinical trials that are designed to find new treatments and better ways to use current treatments. Before any new treatment can be recommended for general use, doctors conduct clinical trials to find out whether the treatment is safe for patients and effective against the disease. Participation in clinical trials is a treatment option for many patients with IBC, and all patients with IBC are encouraged to consider treatment in a clinical trial.

People interested in taking part in a clinical trial should talk with their doctor. Information about clinical trials is available from the NCI's Cancer Information Service (CIS) at 800-4-CANCER and in the NCI booklet "Taking Part in Clinical Trials: What Cancer Patients Need To Know," which is available at http://www.cancer.gov/publications on the internet. This booklet describes how research studies are carried out and explains their possible benefits and risks. Further information about clinical trials is available at http://www.cancer.gov/clinicaltrials on the NCI's website. The website offers detailed information about specific ongoing studies by linking to PDQ®, the NCI's comprehensive cancer information database. The CIS also provides information from PDQ.

What is the prognosis for patients with IBC?

Prognosis describes the likely course and outcome of a disease—that is, the chance that a patient will recover or have a recurrence. IBC is more likely to have metastasized (spread to other areas of the body) at the time of diagnosis than non-IBC cases.[3] As a result, the 5-year survival rate for patients with IBC is between 25 and 50 percent, which is significantly lower than the survival rate for patients with non-IBC breast cancer. It is important to keep in mind, however, that these statistics are averages based on large numbers of patients. Statistics cannot be used to predict what will happen to a particular patient because each person's situation is unique. Patients are encouraged to talk to their doctors about their prognosis given their particular situation.

Where can a person find more information about breast cancer and its treatment?

To learn more about IBC, other types of breast cancer, and breast health in general, please refer to the following resources:

- NCI's Breast Cancer Home Page (http://www.cancer.gov/breast)

- Breast Cancer (PDQ®): Treatment (http://www.cancer.gov/cancertopics/pdq/treatment/breast/patient)

- Understanding Breast Changes: A Health Guide for All Women (http://www.cancer.gov/cancertopics/understanding-breast-changes)

- What You Need To Know About™ Breast Cancer (http://www.cancer.gov/cancertopics/wyntk/breast)

Selected References

1. Merajver SD, Sabel MS. Inflammatory breast cancer. In: Harris JR, Lippman ME, Morrow M, Osborne CK, editors. *Diseases of the Breast. 3rd ed.* Philadelphia: Lippincott Williams and Wilkins, 2004.

2. Anderson W, Schairer C, Chen B, Hance K, Levine P. Epidemiology of inflammatory breast cancer (IBC). *Breast Disease 2005*; 22:9–23.

3. Chittoor SR, Swain SM. Locally advanced breast cancer: Role of medical oncology. In: Bland KI, Copeland EM, editors. *The Breast: Comprehensive Management of Benign and Malignant Diseases.* Vol. 2. 2nd ed. Philadelphia: W.B. Saunders Company, 1998.

Chapter 8

Paget Disease of the Nipple

What is Paget disease of the nipple?

Paget disease of the nipple, also called Paget disease of the breast, is an uncommon type of cancer that forms in or around the nipple.[1, 2, 3] More than 95 percent of people with Paget disease of the nipple also have underlying breast cancer; however, Paget disease of the nipple accounts for less than five percent of all breast cancers.[1] For instance, of the 211,240 new cases of breast cancer projected to be diagnosed in 2005, fewer than 11,000 will also involve Paget disease of the nipple.[4]

Most patients diagnosed with Paget disease of the nipple are over age 50, but rare cases have been diagnosed in patients in their 20s.[1] The average age at diagnosis is 62 for women and 69 for men. The disease is rare among both women and men.

Paget disease of the nipple was named after Sir James Paget, a scientist who noted an association between changes in the appearance of the nipple and underlying breast cancer.[1, 5] There are several other unrelated diseases named after Paget, including Paget disease of the bone and Paget disease of the vulva; this fact sheet discusses only Paget disease of the nipple.

What are the possible causes of Paget disease of the nipple?

Scientists do not know exactly what causes Paget disease of the nipple, but two major theories have been suggested for how it develops.[1, 2] One

---

"Paget's Disease of the Nipple: Questions and Answers," National Cancer Institute (www.cancer.gov), June 27, 2005.

theory proposes that cancer cells, called Paget cells, break off from a tumor inside the breast and move through the milk ducts to the surface of the nipple, resulting in Paget disease of the nipple. This theory is supported by the fact that more than 97 percent of patients with Paget disease also have underlying invasive breast cancer or ductal carcinoma in situ (DCIS).[1] DCIS, also called intraductal carcinoma, is a condition in which abnormal cells are present only in the lining of the milk ducts in the breast, and have not invaded surrounding tissue or spread to the lymph nodes. DCIS sometimes becomes invasive breast cancer. Invasive breast cancer is cancer that has spread outside the duct into the breast tissue, and possibly into the lymph nodes under the arm or into other parts of the body.

The other theory suggests that skin cells of the nipple spontaneously become Paget cells. This theory is supported by the rare cases of Paget disease in which there is no underlying breast cancer, and the cases in which the underlying breast cancer is found to be a separate tumor from the Paget disease.[1]

What are the symptoms of Paget disease of the nipple?

Symptoms of early Paget disease of the nipple include redness and mild scaling and flaking of the nipple skin.[1] Early symptoms may cause only mild irritation and may not be enough to prompt a visit to the doctor.[3] Improvement in the skin can occur spontaneously, but this should not be taken as a sign that the disease has disappeared. More advanced disease may show more serious destruction of the skin.[1] At this stage, the symptoms may include tingling, itching, increased sensitivity, burning, and pain. There may also be discharge from the nipple, and the nipple can appear flattened against the breast.[1, 2]

In approximately half of patients with Paget disease of the nipple, a lump or mass in the breast can be felt during physical examination.[1] In most cases, Paget disease of the nipple is initially confined to the nipple, later spreading to the areola or other regions of the breast.[1, 2] The areola is the circular area of darker skin that surrounds the nipple. Paget disease of the nipple can also be found only on the areola, where it may resemble eczema, a noncancerous itchy red rash.[1] Although rare, Paget disease of the nipple can occur in both breasts.[2]

How is Paget disease of the nipple diagnosed?

If a health care provider suspects Paget disease of the nipple, a biopsy of the nipple skin is performed.[1, 2, 3] In a biopsy, the doctor removes a small sample of tissue. A pathologist examines the tissue under a microscope to see if Paget cells are present. The pathologist may use a technique called immunohistochemistry (staining tissues to identify specific cells) to differentiate Paget cells from other cell types.[1] A sample of nipple discharge may also be examined under a microscope for the presence of Paget cells.[3]

Because most people with Paget disease of the nipple also have underlying breast cancer, physical examination and mammography (x-ray of the breast) are used to make a complete diagnosis.

How is Paget disease of the nipple treated?

Surgery is the most common treatment for Paget disease of the nipple.[1, 2, 5] The specific treatment often depends on the characteristics of the underlying breast cancer.

A modified radical mastectomy may be recommended when invasive cancer or extensive DCIS has been diagnosed.[5] In this operation, the surgeon removes the breast, the lining over the chest muscles, and some of the lymph nodes under the arm. In cases where underlying breast cancer is not invasive, the surgeon may perform a simple mastectomy to remove only the breast and the lining over the chest muscles.[2, 5]

Alternatively, patients whose disease is confined to the nipple and the surrounding area may undergo breast-conserving surgery or lumpectomy followed by radiation therapy.[1, 2, 5] During breast-conserving surgery, the surgeon removes the nipple, areola, and the entire portion of the breast believed to contain the cancer. In most cases, radiation therapy is also used to help prevent recurrence (return of the cancer).

During surgery, particularly modified radical mastectomy, the doctor may perform an axillary node dissection to remove the lymph nodes under the arm.[1, 5] The lymph nodes are then examined to see if the cancer has spread to them. In some cases, a sentinel lymph node biopsy may be performed to remove only one or a few lymph nodes.

Adjuvant treatment (treatment that is given in addition to surgery to prevent the cancer from coming back) may be part of the treatment plan, depending on the type of cancer and whether cancer cells have spread to the lymph nodes. Radiation treatment is a common adjuvant therapy for Paget disease of the nipple following breast-conserving surgery. Adjuvant treatment with anticancer drugs or hormone therapies may also be recommended, depending on the extent of the disease and prognostic factors (estimated chance of recovery from the disease or chance that the disease will recur).

Are clinical trials (research studies) available? Where can people get more information about clinical trials?

Yes. The National Cancer Institute (NCI) is currently sponsoring many clinical trials for all types of breast cancer. These studies are designed to find new treatments and better ways to use current treatments. As new and improved treatments are found for breast cancer, the treatment options for Paget disease of the nipple will also improve.[2, 5]

People interested in taking part in a clinical trial should talk with their doctor. Information about clinical trials is available from the NCI's Cancer Information Service (CIS) at 800-4-CANCER and in the NCI booklet "Taking Part in Clinical Trials: What Cancer Patients Need To Know," which can be found at http://www.cancer.gov/publications on the internet. This booklet describes how research studies are carried out and explains their possible benefits and risks. Further information about clinical trials is available at http://www.cancer.gov/clinicaltrials on the NCI's website. The website offers detailed information about specific ongoing studies by linking to PDQ®, the NCI's cancer information database. The CIS also provides information from PDQ.

Selected References

1. Kaelin CM. Paget's Disease. In: Harris JR, Lippman ME, Morrow M, Osborne CK, editors. *Diseases of the Breast*. 3rd ed. Philadelphia: Lippincott Williams and Wilkins, 2004.

2. DeVita, VT Jr., Hellman S, Rosenberg SA, editors. Cancer: *Principles and Practice of Oncology*. 7th ed. Philadelphia: Lippincott Williams and Wilkins, 2004.

3. Beers MH, Berkow R, editors. *The Merck Manual of Diagnosis and Therapy*. 17th ed. Whitehouse Station, NJ: Merck & Company, Inc., 1999.

4. American Cancer Society (2005). *Cancer Facts and Figures 2005*. Atlanta, GA: American Cancer Society. Retrieved April 20, 2005, from http://www.cancer.org/downloads/STT/CAFF2005f4PWSecured.pdf.

5. Marcus E. *The management of Paget's disease of the breast*. Current Treatment Options in Oncology 2004; 5:153–160.

Chapter 9

Male Breast Cancer

General Information about Breast Cancer in Men

Breast cancer may occur in men. Men at any age may develop breast cancer, but it is usually detected (found) in men between 60 and 70 years of age. Male breast cancer makes up less than 1% of all cases of breast cancer.

The following types of breast cancer are found in men:

- **Infiltrating ductal carcinoma:** Cancer that has spread beyond the cells lining ducts in the breast. Most men with breast cancer have this type of cancer.

- **Ductal carcinoma in situ:** Abnormal cells that are found in the lining of a duct; also called intraductal carcinoma.

- **Inflammatory breast cancer:** A type of cancer in which the breast looks red and swollen and feels warm.

- **Paget disease of the nipple:** A tumor that has grown from ducts beneath the nipple onto the surface of the nipple.

Lobular carcinoma in situ (abnormal cells found in one of the lobes or sections of the breast), which sometimes occurs in women, has not been seen in men.

From PDQ® Cancer Information Summary. National Cancer Institute; Bethesda, MD. Male Breast Cancer (PDQ®): Treatment - Patient. Updated 07/2008. Available at: http://cancer.gov. Accessed September 15, 2008.

Risk Factors

Anything that increases your risk of getting a disease is called a risk factor. Having a risk factor does not mean that you will get cancer; not having risk factors doesn't mean that you will not get cancer. People who think they may be at risk should discuss this with their doctor. Risk factors for breast cancer in men may include the following:

- Being exposed to radiation.

- Having a disease related to high levels of estrogen in the body, such as cirrhosis (liver disease) or Klinefelter syndrome (a genetic disorder).

- Having several female relatives who have had breast cancer, especially relatives who have an alteration of the BRCA2 gene.

Male breast cancer is sometimes caused by inherited gene mutations (changes). The genes in cells carry the hereditary information that is received from a person's parents. Hereditary breast cancer makes up approximately 5% to 10% of all breast cancer. Some altered genes related to breast cancer are more common in certain ethnic groups. Men who have an altered gene related to breast cancer have an increased risk of developing this disease.

Tests have been developed that can detect altered genes. These genetic tests are sometimes done for members of families with a high risk of cancer.

Symptoms and Diagnosis

Men with breast cancer usually have lumps that can be felt. Lumps and other symptoms may be caused by male breast cancer. Other conditions may cause the same symptoms. A doctor should be seen if changes in the breasts are noticed.

Tests that examine the breasts are used to detect (find) and diagnose breast cancer in men. The following tests and procedures may be used:

- **Biopsy:** The removal of cells or tissues so they can be viewed under a microscope by a pathologist to check for signs of cancer. The following are different types of biopsies:

  - Fine-needle aspiration (FNA) biopsy: The removal of tissue or fluid using a thin needle.

  - Core biopsy: The removal of tissue using a wide needle.

- Excisional biopsy: The removal of an entire lump of tissue.

- **Estrogen and progesterone receptor test:** A test to measure the amount of estrogen and progesterone (hormones) receptors in cancer tissue. If cancer is found in the breast, tissue from the tumor is checked in the laboratory to find out whether estrogen and progesterone could affect the way cancer grows. The test results show whether hormone therapy may stop the cancer from growing.

- **HER2 test:** A test to measure the amount of HER2 in cancer tissue. HER2 is a growth factor protein that sends growth signals to cells. When cancer forms, the cells may make too much of the protein, causing more cancer cells to grow. If cancer is found in the breast, tissue from the tumor is checked in the laboratory to find out if there is too much HER2 in the cells. The test results show whether monoclonal antibody therapy may stop the cancer from growing.

Prognosis

Survival for men with breast cancer is similar to that for women with breast cancer when their stage at diagnosis is the same. Breast cancer in men, however, is often diagnosed at a later stage. Cancer found at a later stage may be less likely to be cured.

The prognosis (chance of recovery) and treatment options depend on the following:

- The stage of the cancer (whether it is in the breast only or has spread to other places in the body)

- The type of breast cancer

- Estrogen-receptor and progesterone-receptor levels in the tumor tissue

- Whether the cancer is also found in the other breast

- The patient's age and general health

Stages of Male Breast Cancer

After breast cancer has been diagnosed, tests are done to find out if cancer cells have spread within the breast or to other parts of the body. This process is called staging. The information gathered from the staging process determines the stage of the disease. It is important to know the stage in order to plan treatment. Breast cancer in men is staged the same as it is in women. The spread of cancer from the breast to lymph nodes and other parts of the body appears to be similar in men and women. (See Chapter 6 for more information.)

Recurrent male breast cancer: Recurrent breast cancer is cancer that has recurred (come back) after it has been treated. The cancer may come back in the breast, in the chest wall, or in other parts of the body.

Treatment Options

Different types of treatment are available for men with breast cancer. Some treatments are standard (the currently used treatment), and some are being tested in clinical trials. A treatment clinical trial is a research study meant to help improve current treatments or obtain information on new treatments for patients with cancer. When clinical trials show that a new treatment is better than the standard treatment, the new treatment may become the standard treatment.

Standard Treatment

Four types of standard treatment are used to treat men with breast cancer:

- **Surgery:** Surgery for men with breast cancer is usually a modified radical mastectomy (removal of the breast, many of the lymph nodes under the arm, the lining over the chest muscles, and sometimes part of the chest wall muscles). Breast-conserving surgery, an operation to remove the cancer but not the breast itself, is also used for some men with breast cancer. A lumpectomy is done to remove the tumor (lump) and a small amount of normal tissue around it. Radiation therapy is given after surgery to kill any cancer cells that are left.

- **Chemotherapy:** Chemotherapy is a cancer treatment that uses drugs to stop the growth of cancer cells, either by killing the cells or by stopping them from dividing. When chemotherapy is taken by mouth or injected into a vein or muscle, the drugs enter the bloodstream and can reach cancer cells throughout the body (systemic chemotherapy). When chemotherapy is placed directly into the spinal column, an organ, or a body cavity such as the abdomen, the drugs mainly affect cancer cells in those areas (regional chemotherapy). The way the chemotherapy is given depends on the type and stage of the cancer being treated.

- **Hormone therapy:** Hormone therapy is a cancer treatment that removes hormones or blocks their action and stops cancer cells from growing. Hormones are substances made by glands in the body and circulated in the bloodstream. Some hormones can cause certain cancers to grow. If tests show that the cancer cells have places where hormones can attach (receptors), drugs, surgery, or radiation therapy are used to reduce the production of hormones or block them from working.

- **Radiation therapy:** Radiation therapy is a cancer treatment that uses high-energy x-rays or other types of radiation to kill cancer cells or keep them from growing. There are two types of radiation therapy. External radiation therapy uses a machine outside the body to send radiation toward the cancer. Internal radiation therapy uses a radioactive substance sealed in needles, seeds, wires, or catheters that are placed directly into or near the cancer. The way the radiation therapy is given depends on the type and stage of the cancer being treated.

Breast cancer in men is treated the same as breast cancer in women.

Initial surgery: Treatment for men diagnosed with breast cancer is usually modified radical mastectomy. Breast-conserving surgery with lumpectomy may be used for some men.

Adjuvant therapy: Therapy given after an operation when cancer cells can no longer be seen is called adjuvant therapy. Even if the doctor removes all the cancer that can be seen at the time of the operation, the patient may be given radiation therapy, chemotherapy, hormone therapy, and/or monoclonal antibody therapy after surgery to try to kill any cancer cells that may be left.

- **Node-negative:** For men whose cancer is node-negative (cancer has not spread to the lymph nodes), adjuvant therapy should be considered on the same basis as for a woman with breast cancer because there is no evidence that response to therapy is different for men and women.

- **Node-positive:** For men whose cancer is node-positive (cancer has spread to the lymph nodes), adjuvant therapy may include chemotherapy plus tamoxifen (to block the effect of estrogen), other hormone therapy, or a clinical trial of trastuzumab (Herceptin).

These treatments appear to increase survival in men as they do in women. The patient's response to hormone therapy depends on whether there are hormone receptors (proteins) in the tumor. Most breast cancers in men have these receptors. Hormone therapy is usually recommended for male breast cancer patients, but it can have many side effects, including hot flashes and impotence (the inability to have an erection adequate for sexual intercourse).

Distant metastases: Treatment for men with distant metastases (cancer that has spread to other parts of the body) may be hormone therapy, chemotherapy, or both. Hormone therapy may include the following:

- Orchiectomy (the removal of the testicles to decrease hormone production)

- Luteinizing hormone-releasing hormone agonist with or without total androgen blockade (to decrease the production of sex hormones)

- Tamoxifen for cancer that is estrogen-receptor positive

- Progesterone (a female hormone)

- Aromatase inhibitors (to lessen the amount of estrogen produced)

Hormone therapies may be used in sequence (one after the other). Standard chemotherapy regimens may be used if hormone therapy does not work. Men usually respond to therapy in the same way as women who have breast cancer.

Treatment Options for Locally Recurrent Male Breast Cancer

For men with locally recurrent disease (cancer that has come back in a limited area after treatment), treatment is usually either surgery combined with chemotherapy or radiation therapy combined with chemotherapy.

Clinical Trials

For some patients, taking part in a clinical trial may be the best treatment choice. Many of today's standard treatments for cancer are based on earlier clinical trials. Patients who take part in a clinical trial may receive the standard treatment or be among the first to receive a new treatment.

Patients who take part in clinical trials also help improve the way cancer will be treated in the future. Even when clinical trials do not lead to effective new treatments, they often answer important questions and help move research forward.

Some clinical trials only include patients who have not yet received treatment. Other trials test treatments for patients whose cancer has not gotten better. There are also clinical trials that test new ways to stop cancer from recurring (coming back) or reduce the side effects of cancer treatment.

Clinical trials are taking place in many parts of the country. Information about clinical trials is available from the National Cancer Institute (NCI) website at http://www.cancer.gov/clinicaltrials. Choosing the most appropriate cancer treatment is a decision that ideally involves the patient, family, and health care team.

New Types of Treatment

This summary section describes a treatment that is being studied in clinical trials. It may not mention every new treatment being studied. Information about clinical trials is available from the NCI website.

Monoclonal antibodies as adjuvant therapy: Monoclonal antibody therapy is a cancer treatment that uses antibodies made in the laboratory, from a single type of immune system cell. These antibodies can identify substances on cancer cells or normal substances that may help cancer cells grow. The antibodies attach to the substances and kill the cancer cells, block their growth, or keep them from spreading. Monoclonal antibodies are given by infusion. They may be used alone or to carry drugs, toxins, or radioactive material directly to cancer cells. Monoclonal antibodies are also used in combination with chemotherapy as adjuvant therapy (treatment given after surgery to increase the chances of a cure).

Trastuzumab (Herceptin) is a monoclonal antibody that blocks the effects of the growth factor protein HER2.

Chapter 10

Breast Cancer Statistics

Trends

Incidence Trends

In the United States, incidence of breast cancer has:

- decreased significantly by 3.5% per year from 2001 to 2004 among women.

- remained level from 1992 to 2004 among African-American women.

- remained level from 1995 to 2004 among Asian/Pacific Islander women.

- remained level from 1995 to 2004 among American Indian/ Alaska Native women.

- remained level from 1995 to 2004 among Hispanic women.

This chapter includes excerpts from the following documents produced by the Centers for Disease Control and Prevention (CDC): "Trends," August 8, 2007; "Risk of Breast Cancer by Age," October 4, 2007; and "Comparing Breast Cancer in Different U.S. States," December 10, 2007. Also included is text excerpted from "Decline in Breast Cancer Incidence—United States, 1999–2003," *MMWR*, June 8, 2007.

Mortality Trends

In the United States, deaths from breast cancer have:

- decreased significantly by 2.2% per year from 1990 to 2004 among women.

- decreased significantly by 1.3% per year from 1992 to 2004 among African-American women.

- remained level from 1995 to 2004 among Asian/Pacific Islander women.

- remained level from 1995 to 2004 among American Indian/ Alaska Native women.

- decreased significantly by 2.4% per year from 1995 to 2004 among Hispanic women.

Source for trend data: Ries LAG, Melbert D, Krapcho M, Mariotto A, Miller BA, Feuer EJ, Clegg L, Horner MJ, Howlader N, Eisner MP, Reichman M, Edwards BK (eds*). SEER Cancer Statistics Review, 1975–2004*, National Cancer Institute. Bethesda, MD, based on November 2006 SEER data submission, posted to the SEER website, 2007.

Risk of Breast Cancer by Age

The risk of getting breast cancer increases with age. Table 10.1 shows the percentage of women (how many out of 100) who will get breast cancer over different time periods. The time periods are based on the person's current age.

For example, go to current age 60. The table shows 3.5% of women who are now 60 years old will get breast cancer sometime during the next 10 years. That is, three to four out of every 100 women who are 60 years old today will get breast cancer by the age of 70.

Deaths from Breast Cancer by Age

The risk of dying from breast cancer increases with age. Table 10.2 shows the percentage of women (how many out of 100) who will die from breast cancer over different time periods. The time periods are based on the person's current age.

Table 10.1. Percent of U.S. Women Who Develop Breast Cancer Over 10-, 20-, and 30-Year Intervals According to Their Current Age, 2002–2004

Current Age	10 Years	20 Years	30 Years
30	0.4	1.8	4.2
40	1.4	3.9	7.0
50	2.5	5.8	8.9
60	3.5	6.9	8.8
70	3.9	6.1	N/A

Source: Data are from 17 Surveillance, Epidemiology, and End Results (SEER) registries covering 25% of the U.S. population. Age-specific data are not available for women over 95 years old. SEER Fast Stats, National Cancer Institute.

Table 10.2. Percent of U.S. Women Who Die from Breast Cancer Over 10-, 20-, and 30-Year Intervals According to Their Current Age, 2002–2004

Current Age	10 Years	20 Years	30 Years
30	0.1	0.3	0.7
40	0.2	0.6	1.2
50	0.4	1.1	1.8
60	0.7	1.4	2.2
70	0.9	1.7	N/A

Source: Data are from National Center for Health Statistics (NCHS). Age-specific data are not available for women over 95 years old. SEER Fast Stats, National Cancer Institute.

Comparing Breast Cancer in Different U.S. States

Rates of Getting Breast Cancer by State

The number of people who get breast cancer is called the breast cancer incidence. In the United States, the risk of getting breast cancer varies from state to state.

The states with the breast cancer incidence rates in the first interval (102.9 to 110.7 per 100,000) include Alabama, Arizona, Arkansas, Florida, Idaho, Indiana, Mississippi, Nevada, New Mexico, South Dakota, Tennessee, and Texas. The states with incidence rates in the second interval (110.8 to 118.5 per 100,000) include Alaska, California, Colorado, Delaware, Illinois, Kentucky, Missouri, Montana, North Carolina, South Carolina, Utah, West Virginia, Wisconsin, and Wyoming. The states with incidence rates in the third interval (118.6 to 126.2 per 100,000) include Georgia, Hawaii, Iowa, Kansas, Louisiana,

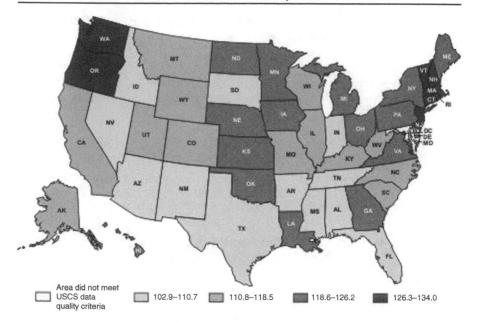

Figure 10.1. Female Breast Cancer Incidence Rates by State, 2004. Rates are per 100,000 and are age-adjusted to the 2000 U.S. standard population. (Source: U.S. Cancer Statistics Working Group. United States Cancer Statistics: 2004 Incidence and Mortality. Atlanta (GA): Department of Health and Human Services, Centers for Disease Control and Prevention, and National Cancer Institute; 2007.)

Maine, Michigan, Minnesota, Nebraska, New York, North Dakota, Ohio, Oklahoma, Pennsylvania, and Virginia. The states with incidence rates in the fourth interval (126.3 to 134.0 per 100,000) include Connecticut, Massachusetts, New Hampshire, New Jersey, Oregon, Rhode Island, Vermont, and Washington; the District of Columbia is in the fourth interval. Maryland did not meet U.S. Cancer Statistics Working Group (USCS) publication criteria. (See Figure 10.1.)

Deaths from Breast Cancer by State

The state with the breast cancer death rate in the first interval (15.6 to 18.6 per 100,000) is Hawaii. The states with death rates in the second interval (18.7 to 21.6 per 100,000) include Alaska, Maine, and Rhode Island. The states with death rates in the third interval (21.7 to 24.6 per 100,000) include Alabama, Arizona, California, Colorado, Florida, Idaho, Indiana, Iowa, Kansas, Kentucky, Massachusetts, Michigan, Minnesota, Montana, Nebraska, New Hampshire, New Mexico, New

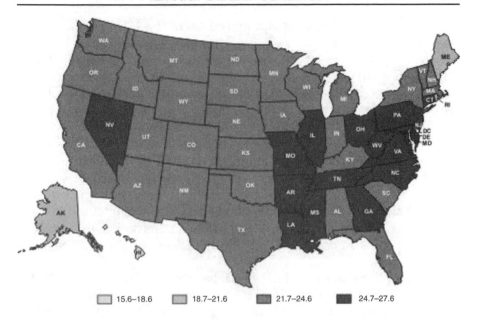

| 15.6–18.6 | 18.7–21.6 | 21.7–24.6 | 24.7–27.6 |

Figure 10.2. *Female Breast Cancer Death Rates, by State, 2004. Rates are per 100,000 and are age-adjusted to the 2000 U.S. standard population. (Source: U.S. Cancer Statistics Working Group. United States Cancer Statistics: 2004 Incidence and Mortality. Atlanta (GA): Department of Health and Human Services, Centers for Disease Control and Prevention, and National Cancer Institute; 2007.)*

York, North Dakota, Oklahoma, Oregon, South Carolina, South Dakota, Texas, Utah, Vermont, Washington, Wisconsin, and Wyoming. The states with the death rates in the fourth interval (24.7 to 27.6 per 100,000) include Arkansas, Connecticut, Delaware, Georgia, Illinois, Louisiana, Maryland, Mississippi, Missouri, Nevada, New Jersey, North Carolina, Ohio, Pennsylvania, Tennessee, Virginia, and West Virginia; the District of Columbia is in the fourth interval. (See Figure 10.2.)

Decline in Breast Cancer Incidence—United States, 1999–2003

The 2006 *Annual Report to the Nation on the Status of Cancer*[2] described a stabilization in female breast cancer incidence rates during 2001–2003, ending increases that began in the 1980s, and a decline in the number of breast cancer cases diagnosed in 2003. In addition, researchers who used 1990–2003 data from the National Cancer Institute (NCI)'s Surveillance, Epidemiology, and End Results (SEER) program, representing approximately 14% of the U.S. population, reported a 7% decrease in invasive breast cancer rates from 2002 to 2003.[3] To further assess breast cancer annual incidence rates during 1999–2003, CDC analyzed data collected by CDC's National Program of Cancer Registries (NPCR) and the NCI SEER program. These combined data account for approximately 86% of the U.S. population.[1] The results of this analysis indicated that age-adjusted incidence rates for invasive breast cancer decreased each year during 1999–2003, with the greatest decrease (6.1%) occurring from 2002 to 2003; women aged 50 years or older experienced a significant decrease during this period. Rates of in situ (that is, noninvasive) breast cancer increased each year during 1999–2002 and then decreased from 2002 to 2003; women aged 50–79 years experienced a significant decrease during this period. Future studies should focus on determining potential causes for these decreases.

Reported by: SL Stewart, PhD, SA Sabatino, MD, SL Foster, MPH, LC Richardson, MD, Division of Cancer Prevention and Control, National Center for Chronic Disease Prevention and Health Promotion, CDC.

Discussion

The findings in this report suggest that invasive female breast cancer rates have been decreasing in recent years, with a sharper decline occurring from 2002 to 2003. Furthermore, both in situ and invasive female breast cancer rates decreased from 2002 to 2003 across several age and stage groups and across most racial/ethnic populations. Decreases in 2003 occurred primarily among women aged 50 years and older, a finding consistent with those of other studies.[3] The overall decrease from 2002 to 2003 occurred in 24 states.

Decreases in rates of invasive female breast cancer from 2002 to 2003 were detected for all racial/ethnic populations analyzed except American Indian/Alaska Natives (AI/ANs), although this population had the lowest overall incidence rate throughout the five years examined. In addition, the decrease in rates for black females was smaller than the decreases for other populations. Additional study is needed to determine possible reasons for these differences.

From 2002 to 2003, significant decreases occurred in incidence rates for localized, regional, and unstaged breast cancer but not distant breast cancer; the reason for the absence of a decrease in distant breast cancer is unknown. The 9.5% decrease in unstaged breast cancer cases might have resulted, in part, from more complete data collection about stage of disease at diagnosis, resulting in fewer unstaged cases. This finding is consistent with a SEER data analysis that attributed improvements in tumor staging to the substantial decrease (13.5 per 100,000 in 1975 to 4.9 per 100,000 in 2003) in unknown staged cases observed over the duration of the SEER program.[4]

Several factors might affect breast cancer incidence and contribute to differences in rates over time and among populations. One such factor is hormone replacement therapy (HRT). Evidence collected, in part, through the National Institute of Health's Women's Health Initiative suggested an increased risk for invasive breast cancer among women who used HRT.[5] The same year, the United States Preventive Services Task Force began recommending against the routine use of HRT (primarily combined estrogen and progestin regimens) for the prevention of chronic conditions, such as cardiovascular disease, in postmenopausal women.§ The mechanism by which HRT use might result in an increase in breast cancer incidence is unknown. One study suggested that hormones play a role in the promotion of breast carcinogenesis, increasing the rate at which certain preexisting but undetectable cancers grow.[6] A population-based study in California of women aged 50–74 years who were members of a health-care plan determined that age-adjusted rates of hormone therapy decreased 68% from 2001 to 2003; during the same period, breast cancer incidence rates decreased 10% among the health-plan members and 11% among all women in California.[7]

Because the breast cancer incidence rate began decreasing before 2002 (that is, before the decrease in HRT use), other factors (for example, differences in risk-factor prevalence, diet, and lifestyle) might be used to explain changes in breast cancer incidence rates. Mammography screening rates also might influence breast cancer incidence. A study in Connecticut that analyzed breast cancer incidence rates during 1943–2002 indicated that although incidence rates increased over time, they increased more quickly after initiation of mammography screening recommendations in the early 1980s, suggesting that more cases were being detected through screening.[8] Data from another recent report indicate that the number of women aged 40 years and older who reported having received a mammogram within the preceding two years decreased significantly, by 2.4%, from 2000 to 2005.[9] Similar decreases were indicated by National Health Interview Survey data; in 2003, 69.5% of women aged 40 years and older had a mammogram within the preceding two years, compared with 70.4% in 2000.** Moreover, similar decreases in mammography screening rates were reported among persons enrolled in several types of health plans (that is, commercial, Medicare, and Medicaid).†† The extent to which the decreases in mammography screening rates might affect breast cancer incidence is unknown.

The findings in this report are subject to at least four limitations. First, although the data are the most geographically comprehensive data available, data are not included from all U.S. states; therefore, some populations might not be well represented. Second, data for Asian/Pacific Islanders (A/PIs), AI/ANs, and Hispanic populations might be underestimated because of misclassification in medical records. Third, no additional information about tumor characteristics (for example, estrogen receptor status), screening, and risk factors was available in the data set used in this analysis; therefore, the role of such factors in the observed changes cannot be assessed. Finally, reporting delays for cancers, such as breast cancer, that are commonly diagnosed in outpatient settings might result in numerous additional cases being added to totals from previous years. NPCR and SEER registries require two to three years to compile and report complete information about cancer cases in their respective CDC and NCI databases. Revised and updated information about cancer cases for previous years are submitted to CDC and NCI each year along with current statistics. However, a recent study demonstrated no statistically significant difference between breast cancer incidence in the delay-adjusted trend compared with the non-delay-adjusted trend.[2] Therefore, the non-delay-adjusted rates and trends described in this report are not expected to vary significantly because of reporting delays.

Analyses of future breast cancer incidence rates are needed to confirm the findings in this report.

References

1. US Cancer Statistics Working Group. *United States cancer statistics: 2002 incidence and mortality*. Atlanta, GA: US Department of Health and Human Services, CDC, and National Cancer Institute; 2005. Available at http://apps.nccd.cdc.gov/uscs.

2. Howe HL, Wu X, Ries LAG, et al. Annual report to the nation on the status of cancer, 1975–2003, featuring cancer among U.S. Hispanic/Latino populations. *Cancer* 2006; 107:1711–42.

3. Ravdin PM, Cronin KA, Howlander N, Chlebowski RT, Berry DA, MD Anderson Cancer Center, National Cancer Institute, UCLA Medical Center. A decrease in breast cancer incidence in the United States in 2003. 29th Annual San Antonio Breast Cancer Symposium. December 2006. San Antonio, TX. Available

at http://www.abstracts2view.com/sabcs06/
view.php?nu=SABCS06L_766.

4. Jemal A, Ward E, Thun MJ. Recent trends in breast cancer incidence rates by age and tumor characteristics among U.S. women. *Breast Cancer Res* 2007; 9:R28.

5. Writing Group for the Women's Health Initiative Investigators. Risks and benefits of estrogen plus progestin in healthy postmenopausal women. Principal results from the Women's Health Initiative randomized controlled trial. *JAMA* 2002; 288:321–33.

6. Dietel M, Lewis MA, Shapiro S. Hormone replacement therapy: pathobiological aspects of hormone-sensitive cancers in women relevant to epidemiological studies on HRT: a mini-review. *Human Repro* 2005; 20:2052–60.

7. Clarke CA, Glaser SL, Uratsu CS, Selby JV, Kushi LH, Herrinton LJ. Recent declines in hormone therapy utilization and breast cancer incidence: clinical and population-based evidence [Letter to the editor]. *J Clin Oncol* 2006; 24:e49–50.

8. Anderson WF, Jatoi I, Devesa SS. Assessing the impact of screening mammography: breast cancer incidence and mortality rates in Connecticut (1943–2002). *Breast Cancer Res Treat* 2006; 99:333–40.

9. CDC. Use of mammograms among women aged >40 years–United States, 2000–2005. *MMWR* 2007; 56:49–51.

Notes

• Medical records are the primary source of cancer incidence data. Staff members at health-care facilities abstract cancer incidence data from patients' medical records, enter the data into the facility's own cancer registry, if it has one, and then send the data to the regional or state registry. Both NPCR and SEER registries collect data using uniform data items and codes as documented by the North American Association of Central Cancer Registries. Additional information on NPCR and SEER methodology is available at http://www.cdc.gov/cancer/npcr/npcrpdfs/uscs_2003_technical_notes.pdf.

§ United States Preventive Services Task Force. Recommendations and rationale: hormone replacement therapy for primary

prevention of chronic conditions. Available at http://www.ahrq
.gov/clinic/uspstf/uspspmho.htm.

** National Center for Health Statistics. Health, United States,
2005. Available at http://www.cdc.gov/nchs/data/hus/hus05.pdf
#086.

†† National Committee for Quality Assurance. The state of health
care quality: industry trends and analysis. 2006. Available at
http://www.ncqa.org/communications/sohc2006/sohc_2006.pdf.

Chapter 11

Breast Cancer in Minority Populations

Chapter Contents

Section 11.1

Breast Cancer Incidence and Mortality by Race and Ethnicity

Breast cancer incidence and mortality rates vary widely among racial/ethnic groups, among various age groups and among the populations of counties, states, and countries. Globally, incidence is highest among white women of European descent who live in industrialized countries.

Although diversity is increasing in the U.S., medical and scientific research on diverse populations has not kept pace. Much of current breast cancer diagnosis and treatment is based on research in white women. Breast cancer among women of color is only beginning to be addressed. Even so, evidence shows genetic variations affect susceptibility to environmental exposures as well as the characteristics of the tumors themselves. It is also clear that breast cancer is more aggressive in some racial/ethnic groups than in others.

Incidence

White (non-Hispanic) women of all ages have the highest incidence of breast cancer of any racial/ethnic group in the United States. American Indian/Alaska Natives have the lowest incidence of the disease. Latinas have a much lower incidence of breast cancer than either black or white women, but the figure is rising.

Black women younger than age 35 have a higher incidence of breast cancer than their white counterparts, and a less favorable prognosis. They have more aggressive tumors: typically estrogen-receptor negative, progesterone receptor negative, HER2-negative, and basal-type tumors, sometimes referred to as "triple-negative" tumors. Triple-negative tumors do not respond to hormonal therapies such as tamoxifen. In addition, young black women present with more advanced breast cancer at diagnosis, including larger tumors and more lymph node involvement.

Throughout the 1990s, the incidence of inflammatory breast cancer (IBC), a rare type that primarily affects premenopausal women, increased in both black women and white women. However, the incidence of IBC is higher among black women. Because IBC does not cause a lump in the breast, it may be misdiagnosed as an infection, leading to delays in treatment.

And research suggests that breast cancer risk factors are different for black women and white women. Early age at first birth and having four or more children before age 45 appears to increase the risk of breast cancer in black women, while in white women early childbearing reduces breast cancer risk. Use of oral contraceptives may increase the risk of breast cancer in black women, apparently by raising levels of insulin-like growth factor-1 (IGF-1), which is associated with increased risk of breast cancer. On the other hand, oral contraceptive use suppresses levels of IGF-1 in white women.

Mortality

Black women have the highest breast cancer mortality rate of any racial/ethnic group. Asian Americans, particularly Japanese Americans and Chinese Americans, have the best survival rates. The reasons for these disparities are not clearly understood. However, socioeconomic factors undoubtedly play a role in both environmental exposures and access to care. According to Centers for Disease Control (CDC) scientists, blacks have higher body burden levels than whites or Mexican Americans of some chemicals, such as PCBs [polychlorinated biphenyls], mercury, lead, PAHs [polycyclic aromatic hydrocarbons], dioxin, and phthalates. Mexican Americans have higher levels of the pesticides DDT/DDE dichlorodiphenyltrichloroethane/dichlorodiphenyldichloroethylene], lindane, and 2,4,5,TCP [trichlorophenol]. Biomonitoring can provide important information about differences in exposures that must be considered in investigating the causes of breast cancer.

Breast cancer is the leading cause of cancer death in Latinas in the U.S. Like young black women, Latinas are also disproportionately affected by aggressive triple-negative tumors. Environmental exposures may be contributing to the rising rates, particularly among farm workers. Research also shows that hormone therapy may pose a greater risk of breast cancer in postmenopausal Latinas than in their white counterparts.

American Indian/Alaska Native (AI/AN) women have the lowest incidence of breast cancer and one of the lowest mortality rates. However, the American Cancer Society urges caution in interpreting these statistics, stating: "Cancer incidence rates among the American Indian population have been monitored more systematically in the Southwest than in other geographic regions and may not reflect the cancer experience of American Indians or Alaska Natives residing elsewhere." The National Cancer Institute's SEER (Surveillance, Epidemiology, and End Results) data for AI/AN populations predominantly reflect the cancer rates for those living on reservations covered by the New Mexico registry and in urban areas in California. Therefore, it is possible that many cases of breast cancer may go unreported, particularly among women living in rural reservations with limited access to health care.

Research Implications

Research on breast cancer in racial/ethnic populations needs to recognize that genetic, cultural, and historical diversity exists within those populations. For example, African Americans comprise a heterogeneous group, based on the region of Africa from which their ancestors came. Hispanic/Latino Americans include people from Cuba, Mexico, Puerto Rico, Central and South America, Dominican Republic, and other countries. Asian/Pacific Islander Americans include many nationalities—Chinese, Filipinos, Koreans, Hawaiians, Indians, Japanese, Samoans, Vietnamese, and others. The American Indian/Alaska Native population represents more than 500 diverse tribes with different cultures, sociodemographic factors, and languages.

Reporting cancer statistics according to broad racial and ethnic groupings may mask wide variations for specific groups within those broad categories. For example, a study of Asian American women in Los Angeles found that breast cancer risk among women of Japanese and Filipino ancestry is twice that of Chinese and Korean women. Asian women, who have relatively low breast cancer rates in their native countries, experience increasing breast cancer incidence after immigrating to the U.S.

A more detailed understanding of breast cancer among women of color is urgently needed. Research needs to move beyond examining patterns of mammography screening among various ethnic groups. Future research should include occupational studies and biomonitoring to determine exposures, as well as analyses to determine tumor characteristics within various racial/ethnic groups.

Section 11.2

Breast Cancer Health Disparities: Questions and Answers

Excerpted from "Cancer Health Disparities: Questions and Answers,"
National Cancer Institute (www.cancer.gov), March 11, 2008.

How does the National Cancer Institute (NCI) define "cancer health disparities"?

The National Cancer Institute (NCI) defines "cancer health disparities" as adverse differences in cancer incidence (new cases), cancer prevalence (all existing cases), cancer death (mortality), cancer survivorship, and burden of cancer or related health conditions that exist among specific population groups in the United States. These population groups may be characterized by age, disability, education, ethnicity, gender, geographic location, income, or race. People who are poor, lack health insurance, and are medically underserved (have limited or no access to effective health care)—regardless of ethnic and racial background—often bear a greater burden of disease than the general population.

A close look at cancer incidence and death statistics reveals that certain groups in this country suffer disproportionately from cancer and its associated effects, including premature death. For example, African Americans/Blacks, Asian Americans, Hispanic/Latinos, American Indians, Alaska Natives, and underserved Whites are more likely than the general population to have higher incidence and death statistics for certain types of cancer.

What factors contribute to cancer health disparities?

Complex and interrelated factors contribute to the observed disparities in cancer incidence and death among racial, ethnic, and underserved groups. The most obvious factors are associated with a lack of health care coverage and low socioeconomic status (SES).

SES is most often based on a person's income, education level, occupation, and other factors, such as social status in the community and where he or she lives. Studies have found that SES, more than race or ethnicity, predicts the likelihood of an individual's or a group's access to education, certain occupations, health insurance, and living conditions—including conditions where exposure to environmental toxins is most common—all of which are associated with the risk of developing and surviving cancer. SES, in particular, appears to play a major role in influencing the prevalence of behavioral risk factors for cancer (for example, tobacco smoking, physical inactivity, obesity, and excessive alcohol intake, and health status), as well as in following cancer screening recommendations.

Research also shows that individuals from medically underserved populations are more likely to be diagnosed with late-stage diseases that might have been treated more effectively or cured if diagnosed earlier. Financial, physical, and cultural beliefs are also barriers that prevent individuals or groups from obtaining effective health care.

How does NCI gather data on cancer incidence and death for various population groups in the United States?

The Surveillance, Epidemiology, and End Results (SEER) Program is NCI's authoritative source for information about cancer incidence and survival. SEER collects cancer incidence and survival data from cancer registries that cover approximately 26 percent of the U.S. population. Over several decades, SEER has worked diligently to better represent racial, ethnic, and socioeconomic diversity and currently covers 23 percent of African Americans/Blacks, 40 percent of Hispanic/Latinos, 42 percent of American Indians and Alaska Natives, 53 percent of Asian Americans, and 70 percent of Hawaiian/Pacific Islanders living in the United States. In addition, SEER statistics reflect the U.S. population in regard to poverty and education, with both urban and rural groups represented. The Methods for Measuring Cancer Disparities report describes how data are collected to measure cancer health disparities.

The incidence and death statistics presented in this section are from the *SEER Cancer Statistics Review, 1975–2004*. These statistics are most often reported as the numbers of new cases of invasive cancer and cancer deaths per year per 100,000 persons in the U.S. population. When the statistics focus on cancer incidence and death in a single gender—for example, on female breast cancer or male prostate cancer—the numbers are per 100,000 persons of that gender. In addition, the SEER statistics are age-adjusted to the 2000 U.S. standard population. Age-adjustment is done because different population groups may not be comparable with respect to age. Age-adjustment allows cancer incidence and death statistics (expressed below as cancer incidence and death "rates") for these population groups to be compared.

What are the overall cancer incidence and death rates for different populations living in the United States?

Although cancer deaths have declined for both Whites and African Americans/Blacks living in the United States, African Americans/Blacks continue to suffer the greatest burden for each of the most common types of cancer. For all cancers combined, the death rate is 25 percent higher for African Americans/Blacks than for Whites. Incidence and death rates for all cancers among U.S. racial/ethnic groups are shown in Table 11.1.

Table 11.1. Overall Cancer Incidence and Death Rates

Racial/Ethnic Group	Incidence	Death
All	470.1	192.7
African American/Black	504.1	238.8
Asian/Pacific Islander	314.9	115.5
Hispanic/Latino	356.0	129.1
American Indian/Alaska Native	297.6	160.4
White	477.5	190.7

Statistics are for 2000–2004, age-adjusted to the 2000 U.S. standard million population, and represent the number of new cases of invasive cancer and deaths per year per 100,000 men and women.

How do breast cancer incidence and death rates differ for women from different racial or ethnic groups?

In the United States, White women have the highest incidence rate for breast cancer, although African American/Black women are most likely to die from the disease. Breast cancer incidence and death rates are lower for women from other racial and ethnic groups than for White and African American/Black women. Incidence and death rates for female breast cancer are shown in Table 11.2.

Table 11.2. Female Breast Cancer Incidence and Death Rates

Racial/Ethnic Group	Incidence	Death
All	127.8	25.5
African American/Black	118.3	33.8
Asian/Pacific Islander	89.0	12.6
Hispanic/Latino	89.3	16.1
American Indian/Alaska Native	69.8	16.1
White	132.5	25.0

Statistics are for 2000–2004, age-adjusted to the 2000 U.S. standard million population, and represent the number of new cases of invasive cancer and deaths per year per 100,000 women.

What factors might contribute to the higher breast cancer death rate observed in African American/Black women?

Lack of medical coverage, barriers to early detection and screening, and unequal access to improvements in cancer treatment may contribute to observed differences in survival between African American/ Black and White women. In addition, recent NCI-supported research indicates that aggressive breast tumors are more common in younger African American/Black and Hispanic/Latino women living in low SES areas. This more aggressive form of breast cancer is less responsive to standard cancer treatments and is associated with poorer survival.

Section 11.3

Estimating Breast Cancer Risk in African Americans

"Model More Accurately Estimates Breast-Cancer Risk in African Americans," by Sharon Reynolds, *NCI Cancer Bulletin*, Vol. 4, No. 31, National Cancer Institute, December 4, 2007.

A new model published online November 27, 2007, in the *Journal of the National Cancer Institute (JNCI)* more accurately estimates the risk of invasive breast cancer for African American women than the current NCI Breast Cancer Risk Assessment Tool.

The NCI tool is widely used for determining both risk for individual women and enrollment eligibility for clinical trials of breast cancer prevention agents, but was developed using data collected primarily from white women.

Researchers have long been concerned that the NCI tool may not be as precise in predicting risk for African American and other non-white women, and the online version of the tool currently conveys this concern in a disclaimer.

"A lot of the original work was done using white women and validated using white women, and there is a need for studies of this type to either validate or develop specific models for other groups," says Dr. Mitchell Gail, from NCI's Division of Cancer Epidemiology and

Genetics, lead author of the *JNCI* paper and developer of the original model behind the NCI risk-assessment tool, known as the Gail model.

Researchers based the new model on data collected for the Women's Contraceptive and Reproductive Experiences (CARE) study, from 1,607 African American women diagnosed with breast cancer and 1,647 African American women without breast cancer. Information was available for all participating women on the risk factors used to compute the Gail model: age at the start of menstruation; age at first live birth; number of previous benign breast biopsies; and number of first-degree relatives (mother or sisters) with breast cancer.

This information was combined with nationwide breast cancer incidence data from NCI's SEER program and with national mortality data. The researchers then validated the new CARE model using information from 14,059 African American women enrolled in the Women's Health Initiative. The CARE model predicted that 323 women in the group would develop invasive breast cancer. The actual number who developed cancer—350—was not statistically different, though the CARE model did underestimate risk among women with a previous benign breast biopsy.

Overall, the CARE model "tended to produce larger estimates of absolute invasive breast cancer risk than the NCI Breast Cancer Risk Assessment Tool in African American women aged 45 years or older," state the authors.

To see how this increased estimation of risk would affect enrollment into breast cancer prevention clinical trials, the investigators compared how many African American women would have been eligible to enroll in the STAR trial using the CARE model versus the number actually enrolled using the NCI Breast Cancer Risk Assessment Tool. Enrollment in the STAR trial required a five-year projected risk of at least 1.66 percent.

They found that while 14.5 percent of African American women screened using the NCI tool were eligible, this number rose to 30.3 percent using the CARE model. "While the average increase in five-year risk found with the CARE model compared to the NCI tool is less than one-half percent, the proportion eligible increased by more than twofold," said Dr. Joseph Costantino, director of the National Surgical Adjuvant Breast and Bowel Project Biostatistical Center and co-author of the CARE model.

Like the NCI tool, the CARE model would not be accurate in certain subpopulations, such as women with a prior history of breast cancer or with mutations in genes such as BRCA1 or BRCA2, which greatly increase the risk of breast cancer.

But while the CARE model would still benefit from further validation, especially in women under the age of 50, the authors recommend that clinicians adopt the CARE model "for counseling African American women and for determining their eligibility for breast cancer prevention trials." The CARE model will be included in a revision of the online NCI tool.

Section 11.4

Younger Black Women Develop a More Lethal Type of Breast Cancer

Reprinted from the *NCI Cancer Bulletin*, Vol. 3, No. 24, National Cancer Institute, June 13, 2006.

The incidence of breast cancer in premenopausal African American women is lower than in their white counterparts, but they are more likely to die from the disease. New findings reported in the June 7, 2006, issue of the *Journal of the American Medical Association* determined for the first time the population prevalence of a basal-like subtype of cancer in this group, say researchers, which may help to explain their higher mortality.

The risk of the less treatable, more deadly basal-type breast cancer was 2.1 times greater in African Americans than others: 39 percent in premenopausal African Americans, falling to 14 percent after they reached menopause. Risk for non-African American women was 16 percent, both before and after menopause.

Dr. Lisa A. Carey of the University of North Carolina at Chapel Hill and colleagues found the pattern by analyzing a subgroup of 469 women participating in the Carolina Breast Cancer Study, a population-based case-control study designed to look at molecular and environmental determinants of breast cancer risk. Study participants were sorted into two groups: those identifying themselves as African Americans and all others.

Immunohistochemical analysis of tumors was used to identify four main subtypes of breast cancer, which were then adjusted by age, race, and stage of cancer. Compared with the least threatening type, all women in the study had an 80-percent increase in mortality with the basal-like cancer. When these cases were removed from the analysis, however, younger African American women still had the highest mortality, "which may reflect the impact on prognosis of access to care, treatment, or other differences," wrote the authors.

Section 11.5

Hispanic Breast Cancer Differences Persist with Equal Access to Care

Adapted from the *NCI Cancer Bulletin*, Vol. 4, No. 15, National Cancer Institute, April 27, 2007.

Despite equal access to health care services, differences persist in the size, stage, and grade of breast cancer for Hispanic women compared with non-Hispanic white (NHW) women, according to results from a study published April 9, 2007 in *Cancer*.

The study compared 139 Hispanic women and 2,118 NHW women with breast cancer who were all established members of the Kaiser Permanente Colorado health plan. The Hispanic women were diagnosed at a younger age; at a later stage of disease; with larger, higher grade tumors; and with less treatable estrogen- and progesterone-negative tumors, reported the investigators led by Dr. A. Tyler Watlington at the University of Colorado Health Sciences Center.

"The results of this study confirm those of many previous studies that breast cancer presents differently in Hispanic women," the researchers noted. Previous research has suggested that the differences may be due to socioeconomic factors, especially lack of or inadequate health insurance and less access to care among low-income Hispanic women. However, the current study shows that "these differences were apparent even among a group of Hispanic women with equal access to care and similar health care utilization," they added.

"The results of this study, in our opinion, lend further support to the evidence for a biologic/genetic basis for these differences," the researchers stated. Future research should more carefully explore differences in clinical presentation as well as biologic differences in tumor genotypes and phenotypes, "as different strategies for breast cancer prevention may then be warranted for Hispanic women," they concluded.

Section 11.6

Triple-Negative Breast Cancer Disproportionately Affects African American and Hispanic Women

By Sharon Reynolds in *NCI Cancer Bulletin*, Vol. 4, No. 22,
National Cancer Institute, July 24, 2007.

A form of breast cancer shown to disproportionately affect young African American women has also recently been found to have an increased incidence in Hispanic women. Called "triple-negative" breast cancer because its cells lack the receptors for estrogen, progesterone, and human epidermal growth factor receptor 2 (HER2), it cannot be controlled with drugs such as tamoxifen or trastuzumab that target these receptors, limiting the effective treatment options for patients.

Triple-negative breast cancer primarily consists of a molecular subtype called the basal-like subtype. Different molecular subtypes of breast cancer can now be identified in patients by gene-expression profiling.

The first hints that molecular subtypes of breast cancer may not be distributed equally among populations in the United States emerged several years ago, and in 2006, results from the Carolina Breast Cancer Study (CBCS) showed that 39 percent of premenopausal African American women diagnosed with breast cancer had basal-like disease, compared with 14 percent of postmenopausal African American women and 16 percent of non-African American women of any age. In early 2007, a study from the California Cancer Registry confirmed the higher incidence of triple-negative breast cancer in young African American women and also identified a smaller but significant increased prevalence in Hispanic women.

Researchers are now attempting to answer the complex question of why this unequal distribution among various racial and ethnic groups exists. "The obvious question, if you recognize that there are subtypes of breast cancer," said Dr. Lisa Carey, medical director of the University of North Carolina Breast Center and lead author of the CBCS paper, "is to stop saying 'what causes breast cancer?' and say 'what causes different subtypes?'"

Intriguing data from the Nurses Health Study, the Women's Health Initiative, and smaller studies suggest that risk factors might be different for different subtypes of breast cancer. Follow-up results from the CBCS and from a large, population-based breast cancer case-control study conducted in Poland identified elevated waist-to-height ratio, excess weight gain since childhood, lack of breast-feeding after pregnancy and use of lactation suppressants, and several other variables as potential risk factors for basal-like breast cancer.

Now researchers led by Dr. Sarah Gehlert, director of the Center for Interdisciplinary Health Disparities Research (CIHDR) at the University of Chicago, have begun a unique, multidisciplinary study looking at the social environment (including crime) and other community factors that contribute to social isolation, reported perceptions of stress, and levels of salivary cortisol—a hormone involved in the response to stress—in a group of African American women in Chicago to determine if stress and social isolation contribute to breast carcinogenesis. "It's a completely integrated model," explained Dr. Gehlert.

"We realized from our animal work that social isolation was a very significant feature" in tumor development, said Dr. Gehlert. Their study hypothesis, she explained, is that "women who live in areas with...a lot of violent crime, and who live in unsafe housing, without a lot of community support to make it easier to deal with that stress, will be more likely to have sporadic mutations and will have [worse outcomes] with breast cancer."

An important part of this integrated model is the collection of tumor tissue from participants. Interim results from the study have already found glucocorticoid receptors in tumors of women who reported high stress levels, indicating that an altered stress response may contribute to failure of apoptosis and lead to tumor growth.

The tissue collected will be analyzed by Dr. Olufunmilayo Olopade, professor of medicine and human genetics at the University of Chicago and one of four project leaders in CIHDR. Dr. Olopade's previous work with African women in Nigeria and Senegal has shown an even higher incidence of estrogen-negative breast cancer than that found in African American women. Her laboratory is now deeply involved in determining if genetic mutations similar to BRCA1 and BRCA2 may contribute to the disparity in triple-negative disease under study by CIHDR.

Work is also now beginning across the U.S. to better understand the impact of triple-negative breast cancer in the Hispanic population. "We're concerned about this triple-negative phenomenon and whether Mexican Americans are also facing a similar [disparity]," explained Dr. Melissa Bondy, professor of epidemiology at the University of Texas M.D. Anderson Cancer Center. Dr. Bondy and her colleagues are starting a study to examine risk factors for triple-negative breast cancer in Mexican American women living in Texas and Arizona, and Mexican women from Northern Mexico and from the city of Guadalajara.

The next steps for researchers will be to figure out ways to help these populations reduce their risk and to develop new treatment options for triple-negative breast cancer, which are limited to traditional surgery, radiation therapy, and chemotherapy.

"The whole point [of the Carolina Breast Cancer Study] was…to figure out what the population frequencies were of these different subtypes and what some of the clinical associations were so that we could design trials for them," said Dr. Carey.

Dr. Carey's group and others around the country are now involved in large, multi-institution clinical trials testing therapies for triple-negative breast cancer. Drug regimens being examined in these trials include the antiangiogenesis agent bevacizumab given before surgery; new, targeted drugs that interfere with cell-signaling pathways other than those triggered by the estrogen, progesterone, and HER2 receptors; and platinum-based chemotherapy drugs, which may be effective in triple-negative disease.

Chapter 12

Pregnancy and Breastfeeding May Influence Breast Cancer Risk

Every woman's hormone levels change throughout her life for a variety of reasons, and hormone changes can lead to changes in the breasts. Hormone changes that occur during pregnancy may influence a woman's chances of developing breast cancer later in life. Research continues to help us understand reproductive events and breast cancer risk. The National Cancer Institute (NCI) is currently funding research that may lead to discoveries that identify ways to mimic pregnancy's protective effects and translate them into effective prevention strategies.

Pregnancy-Related Factors that Protect against Breast Cancer

Some factors associated with pregnancy are known to reduce a woman's chance of developing breast cancer later in life:

- The younger a woman has her first child, the lower her risk of developing breast cancer during her lifetime.

- A woman who has her first child after the age of 35 has approximately twice the risk of developing breast cancer as a woman who has a child before age 20.

"Pregnancy and Breast Cancer Risk," National Cancer Institute (www.cancer.gov), December 20, 2003. Supplemental information under the heading "Breastfeeding and Breast Cancer Risk" added by David A. Cooke, M.D., June 2008.

91

- A woman who has her first child around age 30 has approximately the same lifetime risk of developing breast cancer as a woman who has never given birth.

- Having more than one child decreases a woman's chances of developing breast cancer. In particular, having more than one child at a younger age decreases a woman's chances of developing breast cancer during her lifetime.

- Although not fully understood, research suggests that preeclampsia, a pathologic condition that sometimes develops during pregnancy, is associated with a decrease in breast cancer risk in the offspring, and there is some evidence of a protective effect for the mother.

Pregnancy-Related Factors that Increase Breast Cancer Risk

Some factors associated with pregnancy are known to increase a woman's chances of developing breast cancer:

- After a woman gives birth, her risk of breast cancer is temporarily increased. This temporary increase lasts only for a few years.

- A woman who during pregnancy took DES (diethylstilbestrol), a synthetic form of estrogen that was used between the early 1940s and 1971, has a slightly higher risk of developing breast cancer. (So far, research does not show an increased breast cancer risk for their female offspring who were exposed to DES before birth. Those women are sometimes referred to as "DES daughters.")

Breastfeeding and Breast Cancer Risk

Breastfeeding reduces a woman's risk of developing breast cancer. The reasons for this benefit to the mother are not completely clear, but multiple studies of large populations have found lower rates in women who have breastfed their infants than among those who did not. It is suspected that hormonal changes that occur during breastfeeding reduce the likelihood of cancer developing.

The duration of breastfeeding appears to be the major factor on degree of benefit. The largest study to date concluded that for every 12 months of breastfeeding over a woman's lifetime, breast cancer risk drops by about 4%. It has been speculated that breast cancer rates are higher in modern times than the past because women tend to have fewer children, and spend less of their lifetime breastfeeding.

It remains uncertain what effect pregnancy has upon women who have previously survived breast cancer. Some studies have suggested a higher risk of tumor recurrence, while others have suggested subsequent pregnancy may decrease risk. Until further studies have been done, it is difficult to make a general recommendation for or against pregnancy after breast cancer.

For women who do give birth after prior breast cancer, breast feeding is still usually an option. Breastfeeding from the untreated side is unaffected, although many experts recommend against feeding from the treated breast. This is based on concerns of reduced milk production and greater difficulty in treating mastitis, rather than any risk to the infant. Breastfeeding is considered safe after breast cancer unless the woman is undergoing chemotherapy at the time.

Other Breast Cancer Risk Factors Not Related to Pregnancy

At present, other factors known to increase a woman's chance of developing breast cancer include age (a woman's chances of getting breast cancer increase as she gets older), a family history of breast cancer in a first degree relative (mother, sister, or daughter), an early age at first menstrual period (before age 12), a late age at menopause (after age 55), use of menopausal hormone replacement drugs, and certain breast conditions.

Obesity is also a risk factor for breast cancer in postmenopausal women.

Misunderstandings about Breast Cancer Risk Factors

There are a number of misconceptions about what can cause breast cancer. These include, but are not limited to, using deodorants or antiperspirants, wearing an underwire bra, having a miscarriage or induced abortion, or bumping or bruising breast tissue. Even though doctors can seldom explain why one person gets cancer and another does not, it is clear that none of these factors increase a woman's risk of breast cancer. In addition, cancer is not contagious; no one can "catch" cancer from another person.

Preventing Breast Cancer

There are some things women can do to reduce their breast cancer risk.

Because some studies suggest that the more alcoholic beverages a woman drinks the greater her risk of breast cancer, it is important to limit alcohol intake. Maintaining a healthy body weight is important because being overweight increases risk of postmenopausal breast cancer. New evidence suggests that being physically active may also reduce risk. Physical activity that is sustained throughout lifetime or, at a minimum, performed after menopause, may be particularly beneficial in reducing breast cancer risk. Eating a diet high in fruits and vegetables, and energy and fat intake balanced to energy expended in exercise are useful approaches to avoiding weight gain in adult life.

Detecting Breast Cancer

A woman can be an active participant in improving her chances for early detection of breast cancer. NCI recommends that, beginning in their 40s, women have a mammogram every year or two. Women who have a higher than average risk of breast cancer (for example, women with a family history of breast cancer) should seek expert medical advice about whether they should be screened before age 40, and how frequently they should be screened.

Chapter 13

Medications and Breast Cancer Risk

Chapter Contents

Section 13.1

Antibiotics and Breast Cancer Risk

"Study Shows Link between Antibiotic Use and Increased Risk of
Breast Cancer," *NIH News*, National Institutes of Health news release
dated February 17, 2004.

A study published recently in the *Journal of the American Medical Association (JAMA)* provides evidence that use of antibiotics is associated with an increased risk of breast cancer. The authors—from Group Health Cooperative (GHC) in Seattle; the National Cancer Institute (NCI), a part of the National Institutes of Health in Bethesda, Maryland; the University of Washington, Seattle; and the Fred Hutchinson Cancer Center, also in Seattle—concluded that the more antibiotics the women in the study used, the higher their risk of breast cancer.

The results of this study do not mean that antibiotics cause breast cancer. "These results only show that there is an association between the two," explained co-author Stephen H. Taplin, M.D., of NCI's Division of Cancer Control and Population Sciences and formerly of the GHC. "More studies must be conducted to determine whether there is indeed a direct cause-and-effect relationship."

"This trial suggests another piece in the puzzle of factors that may potentially be involved in the development of breast cancer," said NCI Director Andrew C. von Eschenbach, M.D. "The NCI will continue to support research into underlying mechanisms of cancer risk."

The authors of this *JAMA* study found that women who took antibiotics for more than 500 days—or had more than 25 prescriptions—over an average period of 17 years had more than twice the risk of breast cancer as women who had not taken any antibiotics. The risk was smaller for women who took antibiotics for fewer days. However, even women who had between one and 25 prescriptions over an average period of 17 years had an increased risk; they were about 1.5 times more likely to be diagnosed with breast cancer than women who didn't take any antibiotics. The authors found an increased risk in all classes of antibiotics that they studied.

"Breast cancer is the second leading cause of cancer deaths among women in the United States—with an estimated 40,000 deaths this

96

year—and is the most common cancer in women worldwide," said first author Christine Velicer, Ph.D., of GHC's Center for Health Studies. "Antibiotics are used extensively in this country and in many parts of the world. The possible association between breast cancer and antibiotic use was important to examine."

To gather the necessary data, the researchers used computerized pharmacy and breast cancer screening databases at GHC, a large, nonprofit health plan in Washington state. They compared the antibiotic use of 2,266 women with breast cancer to similar information from 7,953 women without breast cancer. All the women in the study were age 20 and older, and the researchers examined a wide variety of the most frequently prescribed antibiotic medications.

The authors offer a few possible explanations for the observed association between antibiotic use and increased breast cancer risk. Antibiotics can affect bacteria in the intestine, which may impact how certain foods that might prevent cancer are broken down in the body. Another hypothesis focuses on antibiotics' effects on the body's immune response and response to inflammation, which could also be related to the development of cancer. It is also possible that the underlying conditions that led to the antibiotics prescriptions caused the increased risk, or that a weakened immune system—either alone, or in combination with the use of antibiotics—is the cause of this association.

The results of the study are consistent with an earlier Finnish study of almost 10,000 women. "Further studies must be conducted, though, for us to know why we see this increased risk and the full implications of these findings," said Velicer. Studies are also necessary to clarify whether specific indications for antibiotic use, such as respiratory infection or urinary tract infection, or times of use, such as adolescence, pregnancy or menopause, are associated with increased breast cancer risk. Additionally, breast cancer risks could differ between women who take low-dose antibiotics for a long period of time and women who take high-dose antibiotics only once in a while.

Antibiotics are regularly prescribed for conditions such as respiratory infections, acne, and urinary tract infections, in addition to a wide range of other conditions or illnesses. In this *JAMA* study, for example, more than 70 percent of women had used between one and 25 prescriptions for antibiotics to treat various conditions over an average 17-year period, and only 18 percent of women in the study had not filled any antibiotic prescriptions during their enrollment in the health plan.

Over the past decade, overuse of antibiotics has become a serious problem. According to the Centers for Disease Control and Prevention (CDC), tens of millions of antibiotics are prescribed for viral infections that are not treatable with antibiotics, contributing to the troubling growth of antibiotic resistance. Efforts are underway such as the "Get Smart: Know When Antibiotics Work" campaign—unveiled last year by the Department of Health and Human Services' CDC and the Food and Drug Administration (FDA) and other partners—to lower the rate of antibiotic overuse.

"These study results do not mean that women should stop using antibiotics to treat bacterial infections," stressed Taplin. "Until we understand more about the association between antibiotics and cancer, people should take into account the substantial benefits that antibiotics can have, but should continue to use these medicines wisely."

Section 13.2

Oral Contraceptives and Breast Cancer Risk

"Oral Contraceptives and Cancer Risk: Questions and Answers,"
National Cancer Institute (www.cancer.gov), May 4, 2006.

Oral contraceptives (OCs) first became available to American women in the early 1960s. The convenience, effectiveness, and reversibility of action of birth control pills (popularly known as "the pill") have made them the most popular form of birth control in the United States. However, concerns have been raised about the role that the hormones in OCs might play in a number of cancers, and how hormone-based OCs contribute to their development. Sufficient time has elapsed since the introduction of OCs to allow investigators to study large numbers of women who took birth control pills for many years.

This section addresses only what is known about OC use and the risk of developing cancer. It does not deal with other serious side effects of OC use, such as the increased risk of cardiovascular disease for certain groups of women. Recently, alternative methods of delivering hormones for contraception have been developed, including a topical patch, vaginal ring, and intrauterine delivery system, but these products are too new to have been tested in clinical trials (research studies) for long-term safety and other effects.

What types of oral contraceptives are available in the United States? Why do researchers believe that oral contraceptives may influence cancer risk?

Currently, two types of OCs are available in the United States. The most commonly prescribed OC contains two man-made versions of natural female hormones (estrogen and progesterone) that are similar to the hormones the ovaries normally produce. This type of pill is often called a "combined oral contraceptive." The second type of OC available in the United States is called the minipill. It contains only a type of progesterone.

Estrogen stimulates the growth and development of the uterus at puberty, causes the endometrium (the inner lining of the uterus) to thicken during the first half of the menstrual cycle, and influences breast tissue throughout life, but particularly from puberty to menopause.

Progesterone, which is produced during the last half of the menstrual cycle, prepares the endometrium to receive the egg. If the egg is fertilized, progesterone secretion continues, preventing release of additional eggs from the ovaries. For this reason, progesterone is called the "pregnancy-supporting" hormone, and scientists believe that it has valuable contraceptive effects. The man-made progesterone used in OCs is called progestogen or progestin.

Because medical research suggests that some cancers depend on naturally occurring sex hormones for their development and growth, scientists have been investigating a possible link between OC use and cancer risk. Researchers have focused a great deal of attention on OC users over the past 40 years. This scrutiny has produced a wealth of data on OC use and the development of certain cancers, although results of these studies have not always been consistent. The risk of endometrial and ovarian cancers is reduced with the use of OCs, while the risk of breast and cervical cancers is increased.

How do oral contraceptives affect breast cancer risk?

A woman's risk of developing breast cancer depends on several factors, some of which are related to her natural hormones. Hormonal factors that increase the risk of breast cancer include conditions that may allow high levels of hormones to persist for long periods of time, such as beginning menstruation at an early age (before age 12), experiencing menopause at a late age (after age 55), having a first child after age 30, and not having children at all.

A 1996 analysis of worldwide epidemiologic data conducted by the Collaborative Group on Hormonal Factors in Breast Cancer found that women who were current or recent users of birth control pills had a slightly elevated risk of developing breast cancer. The risk was highest for women who started using OCs as teenagers. However, 10 or more years after women stopped using OCs, their risk of developing breast cancer returned to the same level as if they had never used birth control pills, regardless of family history of breast cancer, reproductive history, geographic area of residence, ethnic background, differences in study design, dose and type of hormone, or duration of use. In addition, breast cancers diagnosed in women after 10 or more years of not using OCs were less advanced than breast cancers diagnosed in women who had never used OCs. To conduct this analysis, the researchers examined the results of 54 studies. The analysis involved 53,297 women with breast cancer and 100,239 women without breast cancer. More than 200 researchers participated in this combined analysis of their original studies, which represented about 90 percent of the epidemiological studies throughout the world that had investigated the possible relationship between OCs and breast cancer.

The findings of the Women's Contraceptive and Reproductive Experiences (Women's CARE) study were in contrast to those described above. The Women's CARE study examined the use of OCs as a risk factor for breast cancer in women ages 35 to 64. Researchers interviewed 4,575 women who were diagnosed with breast cancer between 1994 and 1998, and 4,682 women who did not have breast cancer. Investigators collected detailed information about the participants' use of OCs, reproductive history, health, and family history. The results, which were published in 2002, indicated that current or former use of OCs did not significantly increase the risk of breast cancer. The findings were similar for white and black women. Factors such as longer periods of use, higher doses of estrogen, initiation of OC use before age 20, and OC use by women with a family history of breast cancer were not associated with an increased risk of the disease.

In a National Cancer Institute (NCI)-sponsored study published in 2003, researchers examined risk factors for breast cancer among women ages 20 to 34 compared with women ages 35 to 54. Women diagnosed with breast cancer were asked whether they had used OCs for more than six months before diagnosis and, if so, whether the most recent use had been within five years, five to 10 years, or more than 10 years. The results indicated that the risk was highest for women who used OCs within five years prior to diagnosis, particularly in the younger group.

What screening tests are available for the breast cancer?

Studies have found that regular breast cancer screening with mammograms reduces the number of deaths from breast cancer for women ages 40 to 69. Women who are at increased risk for breast cancer should seek medical advice about when to begin having mammograms and how often to be screened. A high-quality mammogram, with a clinical breast exam (an exam done by a professional health care provider), is the most effective way to detect breast cancer early.

Section 13.3

Decrease in Breast Cancer Rates Related to Reduction in Use of Hormone Replacement Therapy

National Cancer Institute (www.cancer.gov), April 18, 2007.

The sharp decline in the rate of new breast cancer cases in 2003 may be related to a national decline in the use of hormone replacement therapy (HRT), according to a new report in the April 19, 2007, issue of the *New England Journal of Medicine*. The report used data from the Surveillance, Epidemiology and End Results (SEER) program of the National Cancer Institute (NCI), part of the National Institutes of Health.

Age-adjusted breast cancer incidence rates in women in the United States fell 6.7 percent in 2003. During this same period, prescriptions for HRT declined rapidly, following highly publicized reports from the Women's Health Initiative (WHI) study that showed an increased risk of breast cancer, heart disease, stroke, blood clots, and urinary incontinence among postmenopausal women who were using hormone replacement therapy that included both estrogen and progestin. The two most commonly prescribed forms of HRT in the United States, Premarin® and Prempro™, had their steepest declines starting in 2002–2003— from 61 million prescriptions written in 2001 to 21 million in 2004.

Led by senior investigator Donald Berry, PhD., of the University of Texas M.D. Anderson Cancer Center, Houston, Texas, the research team showed that the decrease in breast cancer incidence began in mid-2002 and leveled off after 2003. Comparing rates from 2001 and 2004 showed a decrease in annual age-adjusted incidence of 8.6 percent. The decrease occurred only in women over the age of 50 and was more evident in women with cancers that were estrogen receptor (ER) positive—tumors that need estrogen in order to grow and multiply. The speed at which breast cancer rates declined after the WHI announcements may indicate that extremely small ER-positive breast cancers may have stopped progressing, or even regressed, after HRT was stopped.

"Breast cancer is the most frequently diagnosed cancer among women in the United States, and we have made great strides in its treatment," said NCI Director John E. Niederhuber, M.D. "Still, we don't know all the causes of breast cancer, and breast cancer rates had been increasing for two decades up to 2002. Finding the simple ways, such as limiting HRT use to decrease breast cancer risk, is a step forward."

Preliminary findings of this report were presented at the 29th annual San Antonio Breast Cancer Symposium in 2006. Data from 2004, which was of great interest to those present for the meeting, were not available at that time. This report now includes the data from 2004, which show a leveling-off of breast cancer incidence from 2003 to 2004. This observation, combined with a stabilization of HRT use in 2004, further strengthens the association between breast cancer incidence and use of HRT.

Understanding the effect of cessation of HRT may be complex. Effects may vary depending on the type of HRT used and other factors specific to how the hormones affect the body. From the data in this report, it seems that the decline in breast cancer incidence that is related to a nationwide decline in use of HRT may have has run its course, and breast cancer incidence rates may stabilize or even begin to rise again. Researchers do not yet know if this reduction in HRT use will have a long-term effect on rates, or whether reduction in hormone levels simply slowed the growth of clinically detectable tumors, in which case as HRT use stabilizes, breast cancer incidence will begin to rise again.

Several other possibilities were considered to explain the sudden decrease in new breast cancer cases, including changes in reproductive factors, rates of mammography screening, environmental exposures, and changes in diet. HRT was the only risk factor that changed substantially from 2002 to 2003 and provides a possible explanation for this trend. "Recent reports have suggested a small decline in mammography use after 2000," said Kathy Cronin, Ph.D., of the Surveillance Research Program at NCI. "Screening may play a role as well, and the contribution of mammography to the observed decline in incidence is currently being investigated."

Because this analysis is based on population statistics, the study does not prove a link between HRT and breast cancer incidence. Only a randomized clinical trial could prove causation. When the link between breast cancer and HRT was first confirmed in the WHI, which was a randomized clinical trial, women in the study were asked to discontinue their study medications (either placebo or hormones), and were encouraged to continue undergoing annual mammography. These women are still being followed, and the WHI researchers are expected to release a follow-up report later this year about the group who received HRT (estrogen and progestin). This report will provide a much higher level of evidence about the influence of HRT (and cessation of HRT) on the incidence of breast cancer.

"The decision about use of HRT is complex," says study researcher Christine Berg, M.D., from the National Cancer Institute. "While HRT provides relief from the symptoms of menopause, it may also increase one's risk of breast cancer. It is important that women meet with their doctor to discuss what decision is right for them, particularly if they are at high risk for breast cancer."

Section 13.4

Hormone Replacement Therapy and Breast Cancer Relapse

Clinical Trial Results, National Cancer Institute (www.cancer.gov), May 10, 2006.

Breast cancer survivors who took hormone replacement therapy (HRT) to relieve menopausal symptoms had more than three times as many breast cancer recurrences as survivors who did not take HRT, a new study from Sweden has found. The study—which was stopped ahead of schedule because of these findings—was the first randomized clinical trial to examine the effect of HRT in women with breast cancer.

Improved survival among women with breast cancer has meant that more breast cancer survivors are going through menopause, which for some women causes severe symptoms such as hot flashes, night sweats, and loss of sexual desire. For many years, HRT (usually a combination of the hormones estrogen and progestin) was widely prescribed to women to relieve these menopausal symptoms. It was also thought that HRT might reduce the risk of breast cancer, heart disease, and other conditions.

However, in July 2002, a large randomized clinical trial of estrogen and progestin in healthy postmenopausal women (part of the Women's Health Initiative) was stopped early when researchers found that women who took the hormones had an increased risk of developing breast cancer and heart disease.

The U.S. Food and Drug Administration has since recommended that women discuss with their doctors whether the benefits of taking estrogen and progestin outweigh the risks and that, if used, the hormones should be taken "at the lowest doses for the shortest duration to reach treatment goals."

The effects of HRT on women who had already had breast cancer had not been studied in a randomized controlled trial, considered the "gold standard" in medical research. Because more than half of breast cancers are fueled by estrogen, some researchers worried that use of the hormone could stimulate recurrence of the disease. However, studies that simply observed breast cancer survivors for several years concluded that the risk of cancer recurring in HRT users was low.

The Study

In 1997, Swedish researchers began a randomized trial to determine whether a two-year course of HRT for menopausal symptoms was safe for women who had been treated for breast cancer. A total of 434 study participants were randomly assigned to receive either HRT or non-hormonal treatment for their menopausal symptoms. The research team was led by Lars Holmberg, M.D., of University Hospital in Uppsala, Sweden.

Results

The researchers intended to follow the women for a median of five years. However, after a median follow-up of just over two years, they found that 26 women in the HRT group—but only seven in the non-HRT group—had had a recurrence of breast cancer. They terminated the study, concluding that even short-term use of HRT posed an "unacceptably high risk" of breast cancer recurrence.

Limitations

The study fell far short of its recruitment goal, enrolling just 434 women instead of 1,300 as originally planned. In addition, the study was not blinded or placebo-controlled, two characteristics that are generally considered to strengthen the findings of a clinical trial.

Comments

"In and of itself, this study would not be strong enough to provide conclusive evidence that breast cancer survivors should avoid HRT," said JoAnne Zujewski, M.D., a medical oncologist who specializes in breast cancer at the National Institutes of Health Clinical Center in Bethesda, Maryland.

"However, these results are consistent with those of other studies, including the Women's Health Initiative study," Zujewski added. "As a practical matter, given what we already know about the serious risks and extremely limited benefits of HRT, these findings can be considered definitive."

Zujewski's comments are supported by an editorial accompanying the study report, which says that the "conclusion that even short-term use of hormone therapy poses an unacceptably high risk of breast cancer can now reasonably guide clinical practice for women with breast cancer." The editorial is written by Rowan T. Chlebowski, M.D., of the Harbor-UCLA Research and Education Institute in Torrance, California, and Nananda Col, M.D. of Brigham and Women's Hospital in Boston.

The study also demonstrates the importance of testing treatments in randomized clinical trials, Zujewski said. "You cannot draw definitive conclusions from observational studies. Definitive conclusions come from randomized studies."

Section 13.5

Cancer Risk Persists after Ending Hormone Therapy

NCI Cancer Bulletin, National Cancer Institute (www.cancer.gov), March 4, 2008.

The increased risk of breast cancer associated with combination hormone therapy (estrogen plus progestin) may not go away once the hormones are stopped. More than two years after discontinuing hormones, women who had used the treatment for five years still had a higher risk of breast cancer than women who never used the hormones, according to an update from the Women's Health Initiative (WHI).

The results, published in the *Journal of the American Medical Association*, confirm the main finding of the WHI's estrogen-plus-progestin trial—that the health risks of this treatment for menopausal symptoms such as hot flashes outweigh the benefits. The trial was halted in 2002 largely because women using hormones had an increased risk of breast cancer and experienced no clear health benefits. (A WHI trial of estrogen-alone therapy did not show increased cancer risks.)

To update the findings, Dr. Gerardo Heiss of the University of North Carolina, Chapel Hill, and his colleagues tracked 95 percent of the original 16,608 trial participants for an additional 2.4 years. In the post-treatment period, women who had stopped taking hormones were 27 percent more likely to develop breast cancer than women who did not take hormones. However, this finding was not statistically significant (79 women in the post-treatment group developed breast cancer compared with 60 in the placebo group).

The risk of any type of cancer was 24 percent higher in women who had stopped taking hormones, and this was statistically significant (281 women in the post-treatment group developed cancer compared with 218 in the placebo group). The reasons for the additional cancers are not yet clear, but the researchers stress the importance of carefully monitoring women for any long-term effects of hormone use in the years ahead.

"When we started the WHI, the prevailing belief was that menopausal hormones were good for women and that we could prevent many major age-related diseases with them," said Dr. Marcia Stefanick of Stanford University, who chaired the WHI steering committee during the trial.

"But we learned during the trial that the risks of combined estrogen-and-progestin therapy, which included increases in breast cancer, heart attacks, stroke, and serious blood clots, clearly outweighed the benefits of fewer fractures and colorectal cancers," Dr. Stefanick continued. "And we now know that the risk of cancer, and in particular, breast cancer, continues years after stopping the hormones, whereas, none of the benefits persist."

The good news is that the cardiovascular risks for the most part disappear after stopping the combined hormone therapy. Still, many experts recommend that women avoid combined hormone therapy or minimize their exposure. Another WHI follow-up study recently showed that combined hormone therapy leads to abnormal mammograms and compromises the ability of mammograms and breast biopsies to detect cancers.

Together, the two reports highlight complementary downsides of this therapy. "Not only does the breast cancer risk not disappear once hormone therapy is stopped, but the sensitivity of mammograms to detect cancer is not as good and women may continue to have abnormal mammograms for at least a year," said Dr. Leslie Ford of NCI's Division of Cancer Prevention and the institute's WHI liaison.

Chapter 14

Environmental Factors and Breast Cancer Risk

For millions of women whose lives have been affected by breast cancer, the 1994 discovery of the first breast cancer gene by researchers from the National Institute of Environmental Health Sciences (NIEHS) was a welcome sign of progress in the fight against this dreaded disease. While this discovery and others like it are certainly encouraging, statistics tell us that breast cancer is still a major health concern for women everywhere. According to the American Cancer Society, more women in the United States are living with breast cancer than with any other non-skin cancer. Breast cancer is the leading cause of cancer death for U.S. women between the ages of 20 and 59, and the leading cause of cancer death for women worldwide.

Gene-Environment Interactions

For years, NIEHS has played a leadership role in funding and conducting studies on the ways in which environmental exposures increase breast cancer risk. These studies have included the use of animal models to understand the role of environmental agents in the initiation and progression of cancer, as well as research on chemical risk factors and genetic susceptibility in human populations.

Although scientists have identified many risk factors that increase a woman's chances of developing breast cancer, they do not yet know how these risk factors work together to cause normal cells to become

---

"Environmental Factors and Breast Cancer Risk," National Institute of Environmental Health Sciences (www.niehs.nih.gov), March 2008.

cancerous. Most experts agree that breast cancer is caused by a combination of genetic, hormonal and environmental factors.

The Sister Study

As new research continues to unravel the mysteries surrounding the causes of breast cancer, NIEHS scientists are laying the groundwork for a landmark study of the possible interplay between genetics and the environment in the development of this disease. The Sister Study is enrolling 50,000 healthy sisters of women diagnosed with breast cancer from across the country. Women of all backgrounds and ethnic groups who are between 35 and 74 years of age are encouraged to participate.

Sisters of breast cancer patients share many of the same genes, are more likely to develop the disease themselves, and are likely to have been exposed to the same environmental risk factors during early childhood.

The researchers will compare the genetic profiles and environmental exposures of sisters who don't develop breast cancer with those who do become cancer patients in order to uncover clues that may ultimately eliminate this dreaded disease.

Study volunteers provide researchers with samples of their blood, urine, toenail clippings, and household dust, each of which will be analyzed for pesticides, heavy metals and other environmental chemicals that may be linked to breast cancer development. The researchers will also look for specific gene variations that may predispose a woman to the effects of cancer-causing agents. Women enrolled in the study also fill out detailed questionnaires about their health history, past environmental exposures, and lifestyle. The participants will be given yearly follow-up questionnaires to account for changes in their health status or environmental exposures.

Discovery of the BRCA1 Gene

The impact of family history on breast cancer risk suggests that genetic factors play an important role in breast cancer susceptibility. Researchers are just beginning to understand how changes in certain genes can impair the gene's ability to control cell growth and division, causing normal breast cells to become cancerous. In 1994, NIEHS scientists collaborated with researchers from the University of Utah Medical Center to identify a gene called BRCA1 that, when defective, can predispose a woman to hereditary breast and ovarian cancer.[1] Diagnostic tests can now identify women who have inherited defective copies of the gene and are more likely to develop breast cancer.

Although genetics is an important contributor to breast cancer development, twin studies conducted by scientists in Scandinavia showed that inherited factors accounted for only 27 percent of breast cancer risk.[2] Another study shows that the breast cancer rates of descendants of Japanese women who migrate account to the United States become similar to the higher breast cancer rates of Western women within one or two generations.[3] These findings point to the significant role played by environmental factors in determining breast cancer susceptibility.

Cancer-Causing Chemicals

Scientists are particularly interested in whether exposure to naturally occurring and synthetic chemicals may influence breast cancer risk. This includes exposure to chemicals in the air we breathe, the food and beverages we consume, and the chemicals that come in contact with our skin. The National Toxicology Program, an interagency testing program headquartered at the NIEHS, has listed more than 40 chemicals in its Report on Carcinogens because they were found to cause tumors laboratory animals. These include pharmaceutical products such as diethylstilbestrol, a synthetic form of estrogen that was used to prevent miscarriages, chemical solvents and flame retardants, and a variety of chemicals used in the manufacturing of dyes, rubber, vinyl, and polyurethane foams.

Breast Cancer and Environment Research Centers

Recent studies suggest that exposures to cancer-causing chemicals during development may affect breast cancer risk later in life. During early childhood and adolescence, the developing breast tissue is composed of rapidly dividing cells. These immature breast cells are much more susceptible to the damaging effects of environmental chemicals. Results from animal studies have shown that early exposures to some chemicals may keep the mammary gland in an immature state for longer periods, increasing its susceptibility to chemical insult.

In an effort to uncover the links between early environmental exposures and cancer risk, NIEHS is partnering with the National Cancer Institute to fund four Breast Cancer and the Environment Research Centers. The purpose of the centers is to investigate the impact of prenatal and childhood exposures on mammary gland development, and the potential of these exposures to alter the risk of breast cancer in later adulthood. The research findings will be developed into public health messages designed to educate young women who are at risk for breast cancer about the roles of environmental agents in breast cancer development, and the importance of reducing their exposures to these agents.

Initiated in 2003, the centers have worked in close collaboration on two different approaches to the early exposure hypothesis. One approach will use basic science techniques in laboratory animals and cell cultures, while the other will use epidemiologic studies in human populations. Each center has a community outreach component to ensure that the views and concerns of the breast cancer advocacy community are heard and that the research findings are disseminated to the public.

Scientists at the University of California, San Francisco have found that GATA-3, a gene that guides the development of stem cells into mature mammary cells, also required for mammary cells to remain in the mature state during adulthood. Experiments with mice reveal that without the critical gene, mature mammary cells revert to a less specialized state that is characteristic of aggressive breast cancer.[4] The results suggest that a defective GATA-3 gene may play a significant role in the development of certain kinds of breast cancer.

At the University of Cincinnati Center, investigators are studying the effect of childhood diet and obesity on the maturation of the developing mammary gland and subsequent risk of cancer later in life. Their preliminary work with animals shows that treatment with soy and other estrogen-like plant compounds may influence not only the rate of mammary gland maturation, but also the susceptibility of the gland to chemical carcinogens. They are also testing the hypothesis that pre-pubertal obesity in young girls may lead to earlier first menstruation and increased susceptibility of the mammary gland to carcinogenic insults. Researchers at Fox Chase Cancer Center are exposing rats to the plasticizers bisphenol A and butyl benzyl phthalate at different times during mammary gland development. The investigators are finding that these endocrine disrupting compounds activate different genes depending on the time of the exposure and the age at which the rats are examined.

Experiments conducted by scientists at Michigan State University are focusing on the role of progesterone, a hormone secreted in the second half of the menstrual cycle, in breast cancer development. The researchers are using animal models to study the influence of progesterone on mammary gland cell growth and maturation. The responses they get from the animal data may shed new light on the role of this female hormone in human breast development.

Chemical Exposures in Human Populations

In some regions of the country, where there is an unusually high incidence of breast cancer, environmental factors have been targeted as a possible cause for this increase. During the 1990's, the NIEHS and the National Cancer Institute co-funded the Long Island Breast Cancer Study Project, one of the largest and most comprehensive studies ever conducted on the environmental causes of breast cancer, to investigate the high rate of breast cancer on Long Island in New York.

The study scientists focused their investigation on three widespread pollutants to which many of the Long Island residents had been exposed—organochlorine pesticides, including DDT (dichlorodiphenyltrichloroethane) and its metabolite DDE (dichlorodiphenyldichloroethylene), polychlorinated biphenyls, toxic compounds used in electrical transformers, and polycyclic aromatic hydrocarbons (PAHs), a primary component of urban air pollution. Although there was some evidence of a modest increase in the risk of breast cancer from PAH exposure, the researchers did not identify any environmental factors that could be responsible for the high incidence of breast cancer in the Long Island area.[5] In a separate study conducted on Long Island women, researchers at Stony Brook University found no association between exposure to electromagnetic fields from residential power use and breast cancer risk.[6]

A similar NIEHS-NCI funded study of environmental exposures and breast cancer incidence, the Northeast Mid-Atlantic Breast Cancer Program, included data from five separate studies—two conducted in New York, one in Connecticut, another in Maryland, and the Nurses' Health Study, a nationwide investigation into the risk factors for major chronic diseases in women. In each of the studies, blood was drawn from both breast cancer patients and healthy controls, and tested for DDT, DDE, and polychlorinated biphenyls. A combined analysis of the data from the five studies revealed no significant association between the subjects' serum concentrations of these compounds and an increased risk of breast cancer.[7]

Pursuing New Leads: Artificial Light

Results from a study conducted by NIEHS-funded researchers in New York are the first experimental evidence that artificial light may play an important role in breast cancer development. The results show that nighttime exposure to artificial light stimulated the growth of human breast tumors by suppressing the levels of a key hormone called melatonin. The study also showed that extended periods of darkness greatly slowed the growth of these tumors.[8] The results provide a possible explanation for the higher rate of breast cancer in female night shift workers and the epidemic rise in breast cancer incidence in industrialized countries like the United States.

While these findings are encouraging, more research is needed to pinpoint the environmental and genetic factors that determine breast cancer susceptibility. Once scientists can identify the elements that are associated with cancer risk, appropriate interventions and precautions can be designed for those who are most likely to develop the disease.

NIEHS Breast Cancer and the Environment Research Centers

- Fox Chase Cancer Center, Philadelphia

- University of California, San Francisco

- Michigan State University, East Lansing

- University of Cincinnati, Cincinnati, Ohio

References

1.   Miki et al. (1994) A Strong Candidate for the Breast and Ovarian Cancer Susceptibility Gene BRCA1. *Science* 266(5182):66–71.

2.   Lichtenstein et al. (2000) Environmental and Heritable Factors in the Causation of Cancer: Analyses of Cohorts of Twins From Sweden, Denmark and Finland. *New England Journal Medicine* 343(2):78–85.

3.   Shimizu et al. (1991) Cancers of the Prostate and Breast Among Japanese and White Immigrants to Los Angeles County. British Journal Cancer 63:963–966.

4.   Kouros-Mehr et al. (2006) GATA-3 Maintains the Differentiation of the Luminal Cell Fate in the Mammary Gland. *Cell* 127:1041–1055.

5.   Gammon et al. (2002) Environmental Toxins and Breast Cancer on Long Island I: Polycyclic Aromatic Hydrocarbon DNA Adducts. *Cancer Epidemiology Biomarkers Prev.* 11:677–685.

6. Schoenfeld et. al. (2003) Electromagnetic Fields and Breast Cancer on Long Island: A Case-Control Study. *American Journal Epidemiology* 158(1):47–58.

7. Laden et al. (2001) 1,1-Dichloro-2,2-bis(p-chlorophenyl)ethylene and Polychlorinated Biphenyls and Breast Cancer: Combined Analysis of Five U.S. Studies. *Journal National Cancer Institute* 93(10):768–775.

8. Blask et al. (2005) Melatonin-Depleted Blood from Premenopausal Women Exposed to Light at Night Stimulates Growth of Human Breast Cancer Xenografts in Nude Rats. *Cancer Research* 65:11174–11184.

Chapter 15

Genes and Breast Cancer Risk

Chapter Contents

Section 15.1

Genes Related to Breast Cancer

Excerpted from "Breast Cancer," Genetics Home Reference,
National Library of Medicine, August 2007.

What genes are related to breast cancer?

Variations of the BRCA1, BRCA2, CDH1, PTEN, STK11, and TP53 genes increase the risk of developing breast cancer.

The AR, ATM, BARD1, BRIP1, CHEK2, DIRAS3, ERBB2, NBN, PALB2, RAD50, and RAD51 genes are associated with breast cancer.

Cancers occur when a buildup of genetic mutations in critical genes—those that control cell growth and division or the repair of damaged DNA—allow cells to grow and divide uncontrollably to form a tumor. In most cases, these genetic changes are acquired during a person's lifetime and are present only in certain cells. These changes, which are called somatic mutations, are not inherited. Less commonly, gene mutations inherited from a parent increase the risk of developing cancer. In people with these inherited genetic changes, additional somatic mutations in other genes must occur for cancer to develop.

In addition to specific genetic changes, researchers have identified many personal and environmental factors that may influence a person's risk of developing breast cancer. These factors include gender, age, ethnic background, a history of previous breast cancer, certain changes in breast tissue, and hormonal factors. A history of breast cancer in closely related family members is also an important risk factor, particularly if the cancer occurred at an early age. Some breast cancers that cluster in families are associated with inherited mutations in particular genes, such as BRCA1 or BRCA2.

BRCA1 and BRCA2 are major genes related to hereditary breast cancer. Women who have inherited certain mutations in these genes have a high risk of developing breast cancer, ovarian cancer, and several other types of cancer during their lifetimes. Men with BRCA1 mutations also have an increased risk of developing breast cancer. Additionally, BRCA1 mutations are associated with an increased risk of pancreatic cancer. Mutations in the BRCA2 gene are associated with an increased chance of developing male breast cancer and cancers of the prostate and pancreas. An aggressive form of skin cancer called melanoma is also more common among people who have BRCA2 mutations.

Inherited changes in several other genes, including CDH1, PTEN, STK11, and TP53, have been found to increase the risk of developing breast cancer. Mutations in these genes cause syndromes that greatly increase the chance of developing several types of cancer over a person's lifetime. Some of these syndromes also include other signs and symptoms, such as the growth of noncancerous (benign) tumors.

Some research suggests that inherited variants of the ATM, BARD1, BRIP1, CHEK2, NBN, PALB2, RAD50, and RAD51 genes, as well as certain versions of the AR gene, may also be associated with breast cancer risk. Not all studies have shown these connections, however. Of these genes, ATM and CHEK2 have the strongest evidence of being related to the risk of developing breast cancer.

Noninherited (somatic) mutations also have been identified in breast tumors. For example, somatic mutations in the ERBB2 (also called HER2/neu), DIRAS3, and TP53 genes have been associated with some cases of breast cancer.

How do people inherit breast cancer?

Most cases of breast cancer are not inherited. These cancers are associated with genetic changes that occur only in breast cancer cells (somatic mutations) and occur during a person's lifetime.

In hereditary breast cancer, the way that cancer risk is inherited depends on the gene involved. For example, mutations in the BRCA1 and BRCA2 genes are inherited in an autosomal dominant pattern, which means one copy of the altered gene in each cell is sufficient to increase a person's chance of developing cancer. In other cases, the inheritance of breast cancer risk is unclear. It is important to note that people inherit an increased risk of cancer, not the disease itself. Not all people who inherit mutations in these genes will develop cancer.

Section 15.2

Small Variations in Estrogen-Receptor Genes Can Determine Risk of Developing Breast Cancer

"Small Variations in Genes Can Determine Risk of Developing Breast Cancer," *NIH News*, National Institutes of Health, news release dated December 15, 2004.

A woman's risk of developing breast cancer is due in part to a group of very small variations in genes which code for a cell's estrogen receptors, according to a collaborative study by scientists at the National Cancer Institute (NCI), part of the National Institutes of Health, Memorial Sloan-Kettering Cancer Center, Celera Diagnostics, SAIC-Frederick Inc., Applied Biosystems, the Massachusetts Institute of Technology and Vanderbilt University School of Medicine. The study appears in the December 15, 2004, issue of *Cancer Research*.

Many breast cancers depend on estrogen and progesterone to grow. Cells in these cancers have proteins called estrogen and progesterone receptors on their surface. Receptors are an outside molecule's gateway to the cell: molecules bind to and sometimes pass through receptors into the cell. In breast cancers dependent on these two steroid hormones to grow, estrogen and progesterone bind to their respective receptors, initiating signaling pathways that cause the cancer cells to multiply.

Researchers led by Bert Gold, Ph.D., a scientist in NCI's Center for Cancer Research, studied the association between breast cancer risk and very small differences in the genes coding for estrogen and progesterone receptors. Called "single nucleotide polymorphisms," these versions of the gene differ by a single nucleotide—the molecular subunit of DNA. Though these differences are small, they can have an impact on how an estrogen receptor performs.

NCI scientists examined connections between an estrogen receptor gene, called ESR1, and breast cancer. Of 17 single nucleotide polymorphisms (variations) of ESR1 under study, there were two polymorphisms associated with breast cancer susceptibility. One was associated with disease only in women over 50; additionally, this polymorphism was very rare in the African-American population. The other polymorphism was associated with disease only in Ashkenazi (Central or Eastern European) Jewish women over 50.

The researchers found that a group of single nucleotide polymorphisms in the third most common ESR2 gene in Ashkenazi women under study was associated with breast cancer susceptibility. This is one of the first studies to examine breast cancer susceptibility and ESR2 polymorphisms since the discovery of ESR2 in 1996. They studied eight other polymorphisms in ESR2 and found no groups of polymorphisms associated with disease in the general population.

Gold and his colleagues also found no association between breast cancer and 13 single nucleotide polymorphisms in the progesterone receptor gene.

The study population included DNA samples from 1,006 women with breast cancer (identities were masked) who were patients at Memorial Sloan-Kettering in New York City and 613 control subjects from 14 sites that are part of the New York Cancer Study. The two groups had similar proportions of women over and under 50 and of women who had menopause before or after age 50. Case and control groups also contained similar proportions of women in six ethnic groups: those of European, African, Asian, Hispanic, Ashkenazi, and unknown descent.

There is good news for some women. "We were pleasantly surprised to discover that some women have some genetic protection from breast cancer," said Gold. Three groups of single nucleotide polymorphisms in the ESR1 gene protected against the risk of the disease across the ethnic and age groups. However, only one of these was protective when NCI scientists examined only European-Americans.

"We know that half of familial breast cancer is due to genetic factors other than BRCA1 and BRCA2," said Kenneth Offit, M.D., a cancer geneticist at Memorial Sloan-Kettering and a co-author of the study. "These findings suggest that genetic variants in estrogen receptor pathways may be one of many such risk factors."

"Hormone receptors are also the target of several anticancer drugs," said Michael Dean, Ph.D., NCI, another co-author of the report. "We hope pharmaceutical developers will take our results into account as they develop new drugs that modulate the effects of estrogen on breast cancer cells."

Section 15.3

CHEK2 Gene Carries Risk of Breast Cancer

National Cancer Institute (www.cancer.gov), September 25, 2006.

Women who carry an abnormal variant of a gene known as CHEK2 are three times more likely to develop breast cancer than women who do not have the genetic mutation, a large study by Danish researchers has found. Along with BRCA1 and BRCA2, the CHEK2 gene is now confirmed as a risk factor for breast cancer.

Some women who have a strong family history of breast cancer have inherited genetic abnormalities, or mutations, that increase their risk for the disease. The so-called BRCA1 and BRCA2 mutations are the most common genetic abnormalities known to be linked to a high risk for breast cancer. However, BRCA1 and BRCA2 mutations account for fewer than one in 10 breast cancer cases. Families in which no one carries a BRCA1 or BRCA2 mutation may still have a strong history of breast cancer. This suggests that other genetic risks for breast cancer have yet to be identified.

In 2002, researchers showed that a mutation in a gene known as CHEK2 increased risk for breast cancer in women from families with a strong history of the disease. CHEK2 normally produces a protein that helps to prevent tumor cells from growing uncontrollably. The mutated form of the CHEK2 gene fails to do its job.

The authors of the 2002 study estimated that women who carried the CHEK2 mutation were at double the risk for breast cancer. Subsequent studies suggested that the CHEK2 mutation might increase risk for prostate and colorectal cancer, as well. However, many of these studies were small and most were retrospective—that is, researchers' conclusions were based on looking back at what happened to patients in the past. This type of study is generally considered less reliable than a prospective study, in which researchers follow patients forward in time to see what happens to them.

The Study

Researchers in Denmark wanted to confirm whether and to what extent the CHEK2 mutation increased risk for breast, colorectal, and

122

prostate cancer in the general population. They studied 9,231 people who had been monitored for cancer development for an average of 34 years.

The study participants had been interviewed and examined periodically since 1976. Their records contained information about their medical histories, families' disease history, and smoking and alcohol habits. For women, the number of pregnancies and births had been recorded. Participants' DNA was analyzed using blood samples they had given between 1991 and 1994. Researchers found out which participants had been diagnosed with cancer by consulting the Danish Cancer Registry, which records 98 percent of all cancers in Denmark.

In addition, the researchers studied 1,101 women with breast cancer who were recruited at a local hospital. The participants gave blood and completed questionnaires that asked about their medical history, family history of breast cancer, pregnancies and births, use of birth control pills or hormone replacement therapy, and alcohol consumption. These women were compared with 4,665 women who were in the same age range but were cancer-free.

Genetic tests were performed on blood samples from all study participants to identify the presence of the CHEK2 mutation. To reduce the chance of incorrect results due to variation in the way the genetic tests were done, all the tests were conducted in the same lab using identical procedures. The researchers then used statistical techniques to estimate cancer risk in both those who had the mutation and those who did not.

The study's senior author is Borge G. Nordestgaard, M.D., of Herlev University Hospital in Herlev, Denmark.

Results

Half of one percent (0.5 percent) of the study participants were found to have the CHEK2 mutation. Women who carried the mutation were 3.2 times more likely to develop breast cancer than those who did not. However, the researchers found no statistically significant increase in risk for colorectal cancer, prostate cancer, or cancer in general among either male or female mutation carriers.

Limitations

Because almost all of the participants in this study were white and of Danish descent, the findings do not shed light on how common the CHEK2 mutation is in people of other races and ethnicities or on whether the mutation confers a similar risk of cancer in other races and ethnic groups.

Comments

This study's results "confirm beyond a doubt" that women who carry the CHEK2 mutation have a two- to threefold elevation in the lifetime risk for breast cancer, says Jeffery P. Struewing, M.D., of the National Cancer Institute's Laboratory of Population Genetics.

The current study is the first prospective study of the cancer risk associated with the CHEK2 mutation, says Struewing. Its findings and those of earlier studies of the association between the CHEK2 mutation and breast cancer have shown "astonishing consistency," he adds.

Studies to date, which have been conducted in predominantly white populations, show that the CHEK2 mutation occurs in roughly one in every 200 people, Struewing says. This makes it about twice as common as the BRCA1 and BRCA2 mutations, but still relatively uncommon.

On average, a woman with a CHEK2 mutation has about a 20 percent to 30 percent lifetime risk of getting breast cancer, according to Struewing. By contrast, the lifetime risk for a woman with a BRCA1 or BRCA2 mutation averages about 60 percent.

Women from families with a strong history of breast cancer may wish to talk to their doctor or to a genetic counselor about the pros and cons of being tested for breast-cancer susceptibility genes, says Struewing. They may also want to talk to their doctor about steps they can consider taking that may reduce their risk of the disease.

Section 15.4

Genetic Testing for Cancer Risk

Excerpted from "Genetic Testing for Breast and Ovarian Cancer Risk:
It's Your Choice," National Cancer Institute (www.cancer.gov), 2006.

It's Your Choice

Some kinds of cancer, such as breast and ovarian cancer, seem to run in families. There is a test that may tell some people if they are at risk for breast, ovarian, and other cancers. Before getting tested, though, there are many factors you should consider.

Who is at higher risk of breast and ovarian cancer?

A woman with a significant family history of breast or ovarian cancer has a higher risk of getting these cancers. You have a significant family history if you have two or more close family members who have had breast and/or ovarian cancer, or the breast cancer in the family members has been found before the age of 50.

Talk with your doctor or other health care professional trained in genetics about your family history. He or she can help you know if you have a significant family history of breast or ovarian cancer. This information may help you learn about your cancer risk and help you decide if genetic testing is right for you.

A Note About Family History: A close family member can be any of the following people:

- Mother
- Father
- Sister
- Brother
- Grandparent (on your mother's or father's side)
- Mother's sister or brother
- Father's sister or brother

Having a family history of cancer does not mean you are going to get cancer. Many things, such as family history and age, may increase a person's chance (or risk) of getting cancer. But family history alone is not the only reason people get cancer. Scientists do not know all the reasons why people get cancer.

Does every woman with an inherited altered BRCA gene get cancer?

A woman with a BRCA1 or BRCA2 alteration is at higher risk for developing breast, ovarian, and other cancers than a woman without an alteration. However, not every woman who has an altered BRCA1 or BRCA2 gene will get cancer, because genes are not the only factor that affects cancer risk.

Most cases of breast cancer do not involve altered genes that are inherited. At most, about one in 10 breast cancer cases can be explained by inherited alterations in BRCA1 and 2 genes.

What about men with an inherited altered BRCA gene?

Although breast cancer in men is rare, men with altered BRCA1 and BRCA2 genes have higher rates of breast cancer than men without an altered gene. Men with an altered BRCA1 or 2 gene may also have a slightly higher risk of other cancers. Even if a man never develops cancer, he can pass the altered gene to his sons and daughters.

What is genetic testing for inherited cancer risk?

Genetic testing is a process that looks for inherited genetic alterations that may increase your risk of certain cancers. This type of testing may show whether the risk in a family is passed through their genes.

Although the lab test itself is quite complex, only a blood sample is needed. For breast and ovarian cancer risk, the testing involves looking for altered genes such as BRCA1 and BRCA2. Finding an altered gene can take several weeks. So your test results may not be ready right away.

The price of testing varies and, in some cases, may not be covered by health insurance. Ask your doctor or other health professionals for more information on genetic testing, privacy issues, and insurance coverage.

What are the limits of the test?

Testing for breast and ovarian cancer risk will not give you a simple "yes" or "no" answer. If a gene alteration is found, this will tell that you have an increased risk of getting cancer, but it will not tell if or when cancer will develop. If an alteration is not found, it still is no guarantee that cancer won't develop.

What are the advantages and disadvantages of testing?

Genetic testing can affect relationships with family members. Think about who in your family might want to know your test results, and who you'd like to tell.

If you are thinking about being tested, you should decide what the advantages and disadvantages of testing are for you. What is right for one person is not always right for another.

What is informed consent?

If you are thinking about genetic testing, you should be informed, both verbally and in writing, about the risks of getting tested, as well as what the test can and cannot tell you. You can decide if testing is or is not right for you. You may also choose to delay the decision, if this is not the best time for you to be tested.

Having a genetic test may help you do the following:

- Make medical and lifestyle choices
- Clarify your cancer risk
- Decide whether or not to have risk-reducing surgery
- Give other family members useful information (if you choose to share your results)
- May explain why you or other family members have developed cancer

The disadvantages to testing include the following:

- There is no guarantee that your test results will remain private
- Although rare, you may face discrimination for health, life, disability, and other insurance
- You may find it harder to cope with your cancer risk when you know your test results

- If you find that you do not have an inherited altered gene, you may think that you have no chance of getting cancer. People who are found not to have an inherited cancer gene can still get cancer.

What can I do if I find out that I have an inherited altered gene?

You can make choices that help lower your risk of getting cancer or help find cancer early. You do not need to be tested to consider these options.

- **Increased monitoring:** You may choose to be watched more closely for any sign of cancer. This can include more frequent breast and pelvic exams, mammograms, breast MRI, breast self-exams, ultrasound of the ovaries and breasts, and blood tests.

- **Risk-reducing surgery:** Called prophylactic surgery, this is when women choose to have healthy ovaries and/or breasts removed to reduce their chance of getting cancer. You may want to talk with your doctor and other health care professionals to learn more about this.

Who can I call?

A person who is considering genetic testing should talk with a professional trained in genetics before deciding whether to be tested. For more information on genetic testing or for a referral to centers that have health care professionals trained in genetics, call the National Cancer Institute's Cancer Information Service toll-free at 800-4-CANCER (800-422-6237), or visit online at http://www.cancer.gov. The Cancer Information Service can also provide information about clinical trials, other research studies, and current risk management information.

If you are thinking about genetic testing, be sure to talk with your doctor, nurse, genetic counselor, or other health professionals, and take some time to answer these questions together. You may want to get more than one opinion. Here are some questions you may want to ask:

- What are the chances that an inherited gene alteration is involved in the cancer in me or my family?

- What are my chances of having an inherited altered gene?

- Besides having altered genes, what are my other risk factors for breast and ovarian cancer?

- Are all genetic tests the same? How much does the test cost? How long will it take to get my results?

- What are the possible results of the test?

- What would a positive result mean for me?

- What would a negative result mean for me?

- How might a positive test result affect my health, life, and disability insurance options?

- How might a positive test result affect my employment?

- Do I want to ask my insurance company to pay for my test?

- Where will my test results be placed/recorded? Who will have access to them?

- Would knowing this information cause me to make changes in my medical care?

- What are my reasons for wanting to be tested?

- What type of cancer screening is recommended if I don't get tested?

Other questions to think about and discuss with your family include the following:

- What effect will the test results have on me and my relationship with my family members if I have an inherited altered gene? If I don't have an altered gene?

- Should I share my test results with my spouse or partner? Parents? Children? Friends? Others? How will they react to the news, which may also affect them?

- Are my children ready to learn new information that may one day affect their own health?

Chapter 16

Can Breast Cancer Be Prevented?

Breast Cancer Prevention

Cancer prevention is action taken to lower the chance of getting cancer. By preventing cancer, the number of new cases of cancer in a group or population is lowered. Hopefully, this will lower the number of deaths caused by cancer.

To prevent new cancers from starting, scientists look at risk factors and protective factors. Anything that increases your chance of developing cancer is called a cancer risk factor; anything that decreases your chance of developing cancer is called a cancer protective factor.

Some risk factors for cancer can be avoided, but many cannot. For example, both smoking and inheriting certain genes are risk factors for some types of cancer, but only smoking can be avoided. Regular exercise and a healthy diet may be protective factors for some types of cancer. Avoiding risk factors and increasing protective factors may lower your risk but it does not mean that you will not get cancer.

Different ways to prevent cancer are being studied, including the following:

- Changing lifestyle or eating habits
- Avoiding things known to cause cancer

Excerpted from PDQ® Cancer Information Summary. National Cancer Institute; Bethesda, MD. Breast Cancer Prevention (PDQ®) - Patient. Updated 02/22/2008. Available at: http://cancer.gov. Accessed March 24, 2008.

- Taking medicines to treat a precancerous condition or to keep cancer from starting

Avoiding risk factors and increasing protective factors may help prevent breast cancer. Most people with a certain risk factor for cancer do not actually get the disease. Doctors cannot always explain why one person gets cancer and another does not. Talk to your doctor or other health care professional about cancer prevention methods that might help you.

Increased Risks

The following risk factors may increase the risk of breast cancer:

Estrogen (endogenous): Endogenous estrogen is a hormone made by the body. It helps the body develop and maintain female sex characteristics. Being exposed to estrogen over a long time may increase the risk of breast cancer. Estrogen levels are highest during the years a woman is menstruating. A woman's exposure to estrogen is increased in the following ways:

- Early menstruation: Beginning to have menstrual periods at age 11 or younger increases the number of years the breast tissue is exposed to estrogen.

- Late menopause: The more years a woman menstruates, the longer her breast tissue is exposed to estrogen.

- Late pregnancy or never being pregnant: Because estrogen levels are lower during pregnancy, breast tissue is exposed to more estrogen in women who become pregnant for the first time after age 35 or who never become pregnant.

Hormone replacement therapy/hormone therapy: Hormones that are made outside the body, in a laboratory, are called exogenous hormones. Estrogen, progestin, or both may be given to replace the estrogen no longer produced by the ovaries in postmenopausal women or women who have had their ovaries removed. This is called hormone replacement therapy (HRT) or hormone therapy (HT) and may be given in one of the following ways:

- Combination HRT/HT is estrogen combined with progesterone or progestin. This type of HRT/HT increases the risk of developing breast cancer.

- Estrogen-only therapy may be given to women who have had a hysterectomy. It is not known if this type of HRT/HT increases the risk of breast cancer.

Exposure to radiation: Radiation therapy to the chest for the treatment of cancers increases the risk of breast cancer, starting 10 years after treatment and lasting for a lifetime. The risk of developing breast cancer depends on the dose of radiation and the age at which it is given. The risk is highest if radiation treatment was used during puberty. For example, radiation therapy used to treat Hodgkin disease by age 16, especially radiation to the chest and neck, increases the risk of breast cancer.

Radiation therapy to treat cancer in one breast does not appear to increase the risk of developing cancer in the other breast.

For women who are at risk of breast cancer due to inherited changes in the BRCA1 and BRCA2 genes, exposure to radiation, such as that from chest x-rays, may further increase the risk of breast cancer, especially in women who were x-rayed before 20 years of age.

Obesity: Obesity increases the risk of breast cancer in postmenopausal women who have not used hormone replacement therapy.

Alcohol: Drinking alcohol increases the risk of breast cancer. The level of risk rises as the amount of alcohol consumed rises.

Inherited risk: Women who have inherited certain changes in the BRCA1 and BRCA2 genes have a higher risk of breast cancer, and the breast cancer may develop at a younger age.

Decreased Risks

The following protective factors may decrease the risk of breast cancer:

Exercise: Exercising four or more hours a week may decrease hormone levels and help lower breast cancer risk. The effect of exercise on breast cancer risk may be greatest in premenopausal women of normal or low weight. Care should be taken to exercise safely, because exercise carries the risk of injury to bones and muscles.

Estrogen (decreased exposure): Decreasing the length of time a woman's breast tissue is exposed to estrogen may help prevent breast cancer. Exposure to estrogen is reduced in the following ways:

- Pregnancy: Estrogen levels are lower during pregnancy. The risk of breast cancer appears to be lower if a woman has her first full-term pregnancy before she is 20 years old.

- Breast-feeding: Estrogen levels may remain lower while a woman is breast-feeding.

- Ovarian ablation: The amount of estrogen made by the body can be greatly reduced by removing one or both ovaries, which make estrogen. Also, drugs may be taken to lower the amount of estrogen made by the ovaries.

- Late menstruation: Beginning to have menstrual periods at age 14 or older decreases the number of years the breast tissue is exposed to estrogen.

- Early menopause: The fewer years a woman menstruates, the shorter the time her breast tissue is exposed to estrogen.

Selective estrogen receptor modulators: Selective estrogen receptor modulators (SERMs) are drugs that act like estrogen on some tissues in the body, but block the effect of estrogen on other tissues. Tamoxifen is a SERM that belongs to the family of drugs called antiestrogens. Antiestrogens block the effects of the hormone estrogen in the body. Tamoxifen lowers the risk of breast cancer in women who are at high risk for the disease. This effect lasts for several years after drug treatment is stopped.

Taking tamoxifen increases the risk of developing other serious conditions, including endometrial cancer, stroke, cataracts, and blood clots, especially in the lungs and legs. The risk of developing these conditions increases with age. Women younger than 50 years who have a high risk of breast cancer may benefit the most from taking tamoxifen. Talk with your doctor about the risks and benefits of taking this drug.

Raloxifene is another SERM that helps prevent breast cancer. In postmenopausal women with osteoporosis (decreased bone density), raloxifene lowers the risk of breast cancer for women at both high risk and low risk of developing the disease. It is not known if raloxifene would have the same effect in women who do not have osteoporosis. Like tamoxifen, raloxifene may increase the risk of blood clots, especially in the lungs and legs, but does not appear to increase the risk of endometrial cancer.

Other SERMs are being studied in clinical trials.

Aromatase inhibitors: Aromatase inhibitors lower the risk of new breast cancers in postmenopausal women with a history of breast cancer. In postmenopausal women, taking aromatase inhibitors decreases the amount of estrogen made by the body. Before menopause, estrogen is made by the ovaries and other tissues in a woman's body, including the brain, fat tissue, and skin. After menopause, the ovaries stop making estrogen, but the other tissues do not. Aromatase inhibitors block the action of an enzyme called aromatase, which is used to make all of the body's estrogen. Possible harms from taking aromatase inhibitors include osteoporosis and effects on brain function (such as talking, learning, and memory).

Prophylactic mastectomy: Some women who have a high risk of breast cancer may choose to have a prophylactic mastectomy (the removal of both breasts when there are no signs of cancer). The risk of breast cancer is lowered in these women. However, it is very important to have a cancer risk assessment and counseling about all options for possible prevention before making this decision. In some women, prophylactic mastectomy may cause anxiety, depression, and concerns about body image.

Prophylactic oophorectomy: Some women who have a high risk of breast cancer may choose to have a prophylactic oophorectomy (the removal of both ovaries when there are no signs of cancer). This decreases the amount of estrogen made by the body and lowers the risk of breast cancer. However, it is very important to have a cancer risk assessment and counseling before making this decision. The sudden drop in estrogen levels may cause the onset of symptoms of menopause, including hot flashes, trouble sleeping, anxiety, and depression. Long-term effects include decreased sex drive, vaginal dryness, and decreased bone density. These symptoms vary greatly among women.

Fenretinide: Fenretinide is a type of vitamin A called a retinoid. When given to premenopausal women who have a history of breast cancer, fenretinide may lower the risk of forming a new breast cancer. Taken over time, fenretinide may cause night blindness and skin disorders. Women must avoid pregnancy while taking this drug because it could harm a developing fetus.

Unknown and Unproven Risk Factors

The following have been proven not to be risk factors for breast cancer or their effects on breast cancer risk are not known:

Abortion: There does not appear to be a link between abortion and breast cancer.

Oral contraceptives: Taking oral contraceptives ("the pill") may slightly increase the risk of breast cancer in current users. This risk decreases over time. The most commonly used oral contraceptive contains estrogen.

Progestin-only contraceptives that are injected or implanted do not appear to increase the risk of breast cancer.

Environment: Studies have not proven that being exposed to certain substances in the environment (such as chemicals, metals, dust, and pollution) increases the risk of breast cancer.

Diet: Diet is being studied as a risk factor for breast cancer. It is not proven that a diet low in fat or high in fruits and vegetables will prevent breast cancer.

Active and passive cigarette smoking: It has not been proven that either active cigarette smoking or passive smoking (inhaling secondhand smoke) increases the risk of developing breast cancer.

Statins: Studies have not found that taking statins (cholesterol-lowering drugs) affects the risk of breast cancer.

Cancer Prevention Trials

Cancer prevention clinical trials are used to study ways to lower the risk of developing certain types of cancer. Some cancer prevention trials are conducted with healthy people who have not had cancer but who have an increased risk for cancer. Other prevention trials are conducted with people who have had cancer and are trying to prevent another cancer of the same type or to lower their chance of developing a new type of cancer. Other trials are done with healthy volunteers who are not known to have any risk factors for cancer.

The purpose of some cancer prevention clinical trials is to find out whether actions people take can prevent cancer. These may include exercising more or quitting smoking or taking certain medicines, vitamins, minerals, or food supplements.

Chapter 17

Preventive Mastectomy: Questions, Answers, and Concerns

Preventive Mastectomy: Questions and Answers

What is preventive mastectomy, and what types of procedures are used in preventive mastectomy?

Preventive mastectomy (also called prophylactic or risk-reducing mastectomy) is the surgical removal of one or both breasts in an effort to prevent or reduce the risk of breast cancer.[1] Preventive mastectomy involves one of two basic procedures: total mastectomy and subcutaneous mastectomy. In a total mastectomy, the doctor removes the entire breast and nipple. In a subcutaneous mastectomy, the doctor removes the breast tissue but leaves the nipple intact. Doctors most often recommend a total mastectomy because it removes more tissue than a subcutaneous mastectomy. A total mastectomy provides the greatest protection against cancer developing in any remaining breast tissue.

Why would a woman consider undergoing preventive mastectomy?

Women who are at high risk of developing breast cancer may consider preventive mastectomy as a way of decreasing their risk of this

This chapter includes "Preventive Mastectomy: Questions and Answers," National Cancer Institute (www.cancer.gov), July 27, 2006; and, "Preventive Double Mastectomies Increasing Despite Some Concerns," NCI, November 1, 2007.

disease. Some of the factors that increase a woman's chance of developing breast cancer include the following:[2, 3, 4, 5, 6]

- **Previous breast cancer:** A woman who has had cancer in one breast is more likely to develop a new cancer in the opposite breast. Occasionally, such women may consider preventive mastectomy to decrease the chance of developing a new breast cancer.

- **Family history of breast cancer:** Preventive mastectomy may be an option for a woman whose mother, sister, or daughter had breast cancer, especially if they were diagnosed before age 50. If multiple family members have breast or ovarian cancer, then a woman's risk of breast cancer may be even higher.

- **Breast cancer-causing gene alteration:** A woman who tests positive for changes, or mutations, in certain genes that increase the risk of breast cancer (such as the BRCA1 or BRCA2 gene) may consider preventive mastectomy.

- **Lobular carcinoma in situ:** Preventive mastectomy is sometimes considered for a woman with lobular carcinoma in situ, a condition that increases the risk of developing breast cancer in either breast.

- **Diffuse and indeterminate breast microcalcifications or dense breasts:** Rarely, preventive mastectomy may be considered for a woman who has diffuse and indeterminate breast microcalcifications (tiny deposits of calcium in the breast) or for a woman whose breast tissue is very dense. Dense breast tissue is linked to an increased risk of breast cancer and also makes diagnosing breast abnormalities difficult. Multiple biopsies, which may be necessary for diagnosing abnormalities in dense breasts, cause scarring and further complicate examination of the breast tissue, by both physical examination and mammography.

- **Radiation therapy:** A woman who had radiation therapy to the chest (including the breasts) before age 30 is at an increased risk of developing breast cancer throughout her life. This includes women treated for Hodgkin's lymphoma.

It is important for a woman who is considering preventive mastectomy to talk with a doctor about her risk of developing breast cancer (with or without a mastectomy), the surgical procedure, and potential complications. All women are different, so preventive mastectomy should be considered in the context of each woman's unique risk factors and her level of concern.

How effective is preventive mastectomy in preventing or reducing the risk of breast cancer?

Existing data suggest that preventive mastectomy may significantly reduce (by about 90 percent) the chance of developing breast cancer in moderate- and high-risk women.[2, 6, 7] However, no one can be certain that this procedure will protect an individual woman from breast cancer. Breast tissue is widely distributed on the chest wall, and can sometimes be found in the armpit, above the collarbone, and as far down as the abdomen. Because it is impossible for a surgeon to remove all breast tissue, breast cancer can still develop in the small amount of remaining tissue.

What are the possible drawbacks of preventive mastectomy?

Like any other surgery, complications such as bleeding or infection can occur.[1] Preventive mastectomy is irreversible and can have psychological effects on a woman due to a change in body image and loss of normal breast functions.[3, 4, 5, 7, 8, 9] A woman should discuss her feelings about mastectomy, as well as alternatives to surgery, with her health care providers. Some women obtain a second medical opinion to help with the decision.

What alternatives to surgery exist for preventing or reducing the risk of breast cancer?

Doctors do not always agree on the most effective way to manage the care of women who have a strong family history of breast cancer and/or have other risk factors for the disease. Some doctors may advise very close monitoring (periodic mammograms, regular checkups that include a clinical breast examination performed by a health care professional, and monthly breast self-examinations) to increase the chance of detecting breast cancer at an early stage.[2, 4] Some doctors may recommend preventive mastectomy, while others may prescribe tamoxifen or raloxifene, medications that have been shown to decrease the chances of getting breast cancer in women at high risk of the disease.[2, 4, 8, 10, 11] (More information about tamoxifen and raloxifene is available in the National Cancer Institute's fact sheets, "Tamoxifen:

Questions and Answers," which can be found at http://www.cancer.gov/ cancertopics/factsheet/Therapy/tamoxifen on the internet, and "The Study of Tamoxifen and Raloxifene (STAR): Questions and Answers," which can be found at http://www.cancer.gov/newscenter/pressreleases/ STARresultsQandA on the internet.)

Doctors may also encourage women at high risk to limit their consumption of alcohol, eat a low-fat diet, engage in regular exercise, and avoid menopausal hormone use.[8] Although these lifestyle recommendations make sense and are part of an overall healthy way of living, we do not yet have clear and convincing proof that they specifically reduce the risk of developing breast cancer.

What is breast reconstruction?

Breast reconstruction is a plastic surgery procedure in which the shape of the breast is rebuilt. Many women who choose to have preventive mastectomy also decide to have breast reconstruction, either at the time of the mastectomy or at some later time.

Before performing breast reconstruction, the plastic surgeon carefully examines the breasts and discusses the reconstruction options. In one type of reconstructive procedure, the surgeon inserts an implant (a balloon-like device filled with saline or silicone) under the skin and the chest muscles. Another procedure, called tissue flap reconstruction, uses skin, fat, and muscle from the woman's abdomen, back, or buttocks to create the breast shape. The surgeon will discuss with the patient any limitations on exercise or arm motion that might result from these operations.

What type of follow-up care is needed after reconstructive surgery?

Women who have reconstructive surgery are monitored carefully to detect and treat complications, such as infection, movement of the implant, or contracture (the formation of a firm, fibrous shell or scar tissue around the implant caused by the body's reaction to the implant). Women who have tissue flap reconstruction may want to ask their surgeon about physical therapy, which can help them adjust to limitations in activity and exercise after surgery.[12] Routine screening for breast cancer is also part of the postoperative follow-up, because the risk of cancer cannot be completely eliminated. When women with breast implants have mammograms, they should tell the radiology technician about the implant. Special procedures may be necessary to improve the accuracy of the mammogram and to avoid damaging the implant. However, women who have had reconstructive surgery on both breasts should ask their doctors whether mammograms are still necessary.

Where can a person find more information about breast implants?

The U.S. Food and Drug Administration (FDA) regulates the use of breast implants and can supply detailed information about these devices. To listen to recorded information or request free printed material on breast implants, consumers can contact the FDA Center for Devices and Radiological Health (CDRH) at:

Address: Consumer Staff
CDRH/FDA
HFZ–210
1350 Piccard Drive
Rockville, MD 20580
Toll-Free: 301-827-3990 (Call between 8:00 a.m. and 4:30 p.m., Eastern Standard Time, for either number.)
Phone: 888-INFO-FDA (888-463-6332)
Website: http://www.fda.gov/cdrh/consumer/index.html; or
http://www.fda.gov/cdrh/breastimplants (Breast Implants Home Page)
E-mail: dsma@cdrh.fda.gov

Selected References

1. Singletary SE. Techniques in surgery: Therapeutic and prophylactic mastectomy. In: Harris JR, Lippman ME, Morrow M, Osborn CK, editors. *Diseases of the Breast*. 3rd ed. Philadelphia: Lippincott Williams and Wilkins, 2004.

2. Sherry RM. Cancer prevention: Role of surgery in cancer prevention. In: DeVita VT Jr., Hellman S, Rosenberg SA, editors. *Cancer: Principles and Practice of Oncology*. Vol. 1 and 2. 6th ed. Philadelphia: Lippincott Williams and Wilkins, 2001.

3. Dickson RB, Lippman ME. Cancer of the breast. In: DeVita VT Jr., Hellman S, Rosenberg SA, editors. *Cancer: Principles and Practice of Oncology*. Vol. 1 and 2. 6th ed. Philadelphia: Lippincott Williams and Wilkins, 2001.

4.   Sakorafas GH. Women at high risk for breast cancer: Preventive strategies. *The Mount Sinai Journal of Medicine* 2002; 69(4):264–266.

5.   Taucher S, Gnant M, Jakesz R. Preventive mastectomy in patients at breast cancer risk due to genetic alterations in the BRCA1 and BRCA2 gene. *Langenbeck's Archives of Surgery* 2003; 388(1):3–8.

6.   Anderson BO. Prophylactic surgery to reduce breast cancer risk: A brief literature review. *The Breast Journal* 2001; 7(5):321–330.

7.   Hartmann LC, Schaid DJ, Woods JE, et al. Efficacy of bilateral prophylactic mastectomy in women with a family history of breast cancer. *The New England Journal of Medicine* 1999; 340(2):77–84.

8.   Keefe KA, Meyskens FL Jr. Cancer prevention. In: Abeloff MD, Armitage JO, Lichter AS, Niederhuber JE, editors. *Clinical Oncology*. 2nd ed. London: Churchill Livingstone, 2000.

9.   Levine DA, Gemignani ML. Prophylactic surgery in hereditary breast/ovarian cancer syndrome. *Oncology* 2003; 17(7):932–941.

10.   Fisher B, Costantino JP, Wickerham DL, et al. Tamoxifen for the prevention of breast cancer: Current status of the National Surgical Adjuvant Breast and Bowel Project P-1 Study. *Journal of the National Cancer Institute* 2005; 97(22):1652–1662.

11.   Vogel VG, Costantino JP, Wickerham DL, et al. Effects of tamoxifen vs raloxifene on the risk of developing invasive breast cancer and other disease outcomes: The NSABP Study of Tamoxifen and Raloxifene (STAR) P-2 Trial. *Journal of the American Medical Association* 2006; 295(23):2727–2741.

12.   Monteiro M. Physical therapy implications following the TRAM procedure. *Physical Therapy* 1997; 77(7):765–770.

Preventive Double Mastectomies Increasing Despite Some Concerns

Rates of surgical removal of both breasts as a preventive measure in women diagnosed with cancer in only one breast have more than doubled in the United States within a recent six-year period, according to a study published online October 22, 2007, in the *Journal of Clinical Oncology*. This trend has occurred even though in many cases the aggressive treatment may be unnecessary and other, less invasive preventive options are available, the scientists cautioned.

The annual incidence of contralateral breast cancer is about 0.5 percent to 0.75 percent and does not change with time. Some patients with cancer in a single breast (unilateral breast cancer) choose to have the other (contralateral) breast removed to prevent cancer in the opposite breast. The procedure is called a contralateral prophylactic mastectomy (CPM). In the first national study of trends in CPM use in the United States, researchers from the University of Minnesota analyzed data from NCI's Surveillance, Epidemiology, and End Results (SEER) database to review the treatment of patients with unilateral breast cancer diagnosed from 1998 through 2003. They determined the rate of CPM as a proportion of all surgically treated patients and as a proportion of all mastectomies.

The investigators identified 152,755 patients, of whom 4,969 chose CPM. The rate for CPM was 3.3 percent for all surgically treated patients and 7.7 percent for those undergoing mastectomy. The overall rate significantly increased from 1.8 percent in 1998 to 4.5 percent in 2003. Likewise, the CPM rate for patients undergoing mastectomy significantly increased from 4.2 percent in 1998 to 11.0 percent in 2003. These increased rates applied to all cancer stages and continued to the end of the study period.

CPM significantly reduces the risk of contralateral breast cancer, the scientists acknowledged, but the procedure is more aggressive and irreversible and "it is also unnecessary for preventing contralateral breast cancer in most patients." In addition, since the risk of systemic metastases from unilateral disease often exceeds the risk of contralateral breast cancer, most patients will not experience any survival benefit from CPM.

"Although breast cancer is now often diagnosed at earlier stages, we're seeing more women having CPM, even though there are very little data showing that this irreversible procedure improves overall survival," explained lead author Dr. Todd M. Tuttle. "We need to determine why this is occurring and use this information to help counsel women about the potential for less invasive options."

Dr. Larissa Korde, staff clinician with NCI's Division of Cancer Epidemiology and Genetics (DCEG) noted of the study's findings, "Interestingly, during this same time period the rate of breast-conserving lumpectomies also increased, leading the authors to conclude that patients are either choosing less aggressive (lumpectomy) or more aggressive (CPM) surgical treatment rather than unilateral mastectomy."

Dr. Tuttle proposed several potential reasons for the increase in the rate of CPM. There is more public awareness of the genetics of breast cancer and more frequent testing for mutations in BRCA genes, which increase contralateral breast cancer risk (this study, though, did not examine patients' BRCA status). Less invasive mastectomy approaches and improved breast reconstruction techniques may also persuade more women to have both breasts removed at the same time, he suggested.

Dr. Korde pointed out the study also found that patients diagnosed at a young age and those diagnosed with lobular carcinoma were more likely to opt for CPM. "This is not surprising, since both these factors have been shown to be associated with an increased risk of contralateral breast cancer," she said. "It would have been very helpful to have some information on family history in this study, since women with a strong family history and particularly those with known BRCA1 and BRCA2 mutations have a very significant risk of contralateral breast cancer. However, this information is not available in the SEER database."

Patients with unilateral breast cancer have options that are "less extreme" than CPM, the researchers contended. Those include surveillance with clinical breast examination, mammography, and newer imaging modalities such as breast magnetic resonance imaging that may detect cancers at earlier stages.

Dr. Korde noted that research done in women who undergo genetic risk assessment suggests that those with more cancer-related distress are more likely to choose CPM. Additional research will be necessary to fully understand this decision making process.

Part Three

Breast Cancer Screening and Diagnosis

Chapter 18

Screening for Breast Cancer

What Is Screening?

Screening is looking for cancer before a person has any symptoms. This can help find cancer at an early stage. When abnormal tissue or cancer is found early, it may be easier to treat. By the time symptoms appear, cancer may have begun to spread.

Scientists are trying to better understand which people are more likely to get certain types of cancer. They also study the things we do and the things around us to see if they cause cancer. This information helps doctors recommend who should be screened for cancer, which screening tests should be used, and how often the tests should be done.

It is important to remember that your doctor does not necessarily think you have cancer if he or she suggests a screening test. Screening tests are given when you have no cancer symptoms.

If a screening test result is abnormal, you may need to have more tests done to find out if you have cancer. These are called diagnostic tests.

Breast Cancer Screening

Different tests are used to screen for cancer. Some screening tests are used because they have been shown to be helpful both in finding cancers early and in decreasing the chance of dying from these cancers.

Excerpted from PDQ® Cancer Information Summary. National Cancer Institute; Bethesda, MD. Breast Cancer Screening (PDQ®) - Patient. Updated 06/2007. Available at: http://cancer.gov. Accessed March 24, 2008.

Other tests are used because they have been shown to find cancer in some people; however, it has not been proven in clinical trials that use of these tests will decrease the risk of dying from cancer.

Scientists study screening tests to find those with the fewest risks and most benefits. Cancer screening trials also are meant to show whether early detection (finding cancer before it causes symptoms) decreases a person's chance of dying from the disease. For some types of cancer, finding and treating the disease at an early stage may result in a better chance of recovery.

Clinical trials that study cancer screening methods are taking place in many parts of the country. Information about ongoing clinical trials is available from the National Cancer Institute's (NCI) website, available online at http://www.cancer.gov/clinicaltrials.

Three tests are commonly used to screen for breast cancer:

Mammogram: A mammogram is an x-ray of the breast. This test may find tumors that are too small to feel. A mammogram may also find ductal carcinoma in situ, abnormal cells in the lining of a breast duct, which may become invasive cancer in some women. The ability of a mammogram to find breast cancer may depend on the size of the tumor, the density of the breast tissue, and the skill of the radiologist.

Clinical breast exam (CBE): A clinical breast exam is an exam of the breast by a doctor or other health professional. The doctor will carefully feel the breasts and under the arms for lumps or anything else that seems unusual.

Breast self-exam (BSE): Breast self-exam is an exam to check your own breasts for lumps or anything else that seems unusual.

If a lump or other abnormality is found using one of these three tests, ultrasound may be used to learn more. It is not used by itself as a screening test for breast cancer. Ultrasound is a procedure in which high-energy sound waves (ultrasound) are bounced off internal tissues or organs and make echoes. The echoes form a picture of body tissues called a sonogram.

New Screening Tests Being Studied in Clinical Trials

Magnetic resonance imaging (MRI): MRI is a procedure that uses a magnet, radio waves, and a computer to make a series of detailed pictures of areas inside the body. This procedure is also called nuclear magnetic resonance imaging (NMRI). Screening trials of MRI in women with a high genetic risk of breast cancer have shown that MRI is more sensitive than mammography for finding breast tumors.

MRI scans are used to make decisions about breast masses that have been found by a clinical breast exam or a breast self-exam. MRIs also help show the difference between cancer and scar tissue. MRI does not use any x-rays.

Tissue sampling: Breast tissue sampling is taking cells from breast tissue to examine under a microscope. Abnormal cells in breast fluid have been linked to an increased risk of breast cancer in some studies. Scientists are studying whether breast tissue sampling can be used to find breast cancer at an early stage or predict the risk of developing breast cancer. Three methods of tissue sampling are under study:

- Fine-needle aspiration: A thin needle is inserted into the breast tissue around the areola (darkened area around the nipple) to withdraw cells and fluid.

- Nipple aspiration: The use of gentle suction to collect fluid through the nipple. This is done with a device similar to the breast pumps used by nursing women.

- Ductal lavage: A hair-size catheter (tube) is inserted into the nipple and a small amount of salt water is released into the duct. The water picks up breast cells and is removed.

Risks of Breast Cancer Screening

Decisions about screening tests can be difficult. Not all screening tests are helpful and most have risks. Before having any screening test, you may want to discuss the test with your doctor. It is important to know the risks of the test and whether it has been proven to reduce the risk of dying from cancer.

The risks of breast cancer screening tests include the following:

Finding breast cancer may not improve health or help a woman live longer. Screening may not help you if you have fast-growing breast cancer or if it has already spread to other places in your body. Also, some breast cancers found on a screening mammogram may never cause symptoms or become life-threatening. When such cancers are found, treatment would not help you live longer and may instead cause serious treatment-related side effects. At this time, it is not possible to be sure which breast cancers found by screening will cause symptoms and which breast cancers will not.

False-negative test results can occur. Screening test results may appear to be normal even though breast cancer is present. A woman who receives a false-negative test result (one that shows there is no cancer when there really is) may delay seeking medical care even if she has symptoms.

One in five cancers may be missed by mammography. False-negatives occur more often in younger women than in older women because the breast tissue of younger women is more dense. The size of the tumor, the rate of tumor growth, the level of hormones, such as estrogen and progesterone, in the woman's body, and the skill of the radiologist can also affect the chance of a false-negative result.

False-positive test results can occur. Screening test results may appear to be abnormal even though no cancer is present. A false-positive test result (one that shows there is cancer when there really isn't) can cause anxiety and is usually followed by more tests (such as biopsy), which also have risks.

Most abnormal test results turn out not to be cancer. False-positives are more common in younger women, women who have had previous breast biopsies, women with a family history of breast cancer, and women who take hormones, such as estrogen and progesterone. The skill of the doctor also can affect the chance of a false-positive result.

Mammograms expose the breast to radiation. Being exposed to radiation is a risk factor for breast cancer. The risk of developing breast cancer from radiation exposure, such as screening mammograms or x-rays, is greater with higher doses of radiation and in younger women. For women older than 40 years, the benefits of an annual screening mammogram may be greater than the risks from radiation exposure.

The risks and benefits of screening for breast cancer may be different for different groups of people. The benefits of breast cancer screening may vary among age groups:

- In women who have a life expectancy of five years or less, finding and treating early stage breast cancer may reduce their quality of life without helping them live longer.

- In women older than 65 years, the results of a screening test may lead to more diagnostic tests and anxiety while waiting for the test results. Also, the breast cancers found are usually not life-threatening.

- In women 35 years or younger who go to the doctor for breast symptoms, mammogram results may not be helpful in managing their care.

Routine breast cancer screening is advised for women who have had radiation treatment to the chest, especially at a young age. The benefits and risks of mammograms and MRIs for these women are not known. There is no information on the benefits or risks of breast cancer screening in men.

No matter how old you are, if you have risk factors for breast cancer you should ask for medical advice about when to begin having mammograms and how often to be screened.

Chapter 19

Understanding Mammography

Chapter Contents

Section 19.1

What You Should Know about Screening and Diagnostic Mammograms

Excerpted from "Mammograms and Breast Health: An Information Guide for Women," Centers for Disease Control and Prevention (CDC), March 2006.

Understanding Mammograms

Why should I get a mammogram?

A mammogram can show early signs of cancer long before you or your doctor can feel or see changes. When breast cancer is found and treated early, many women go on to live a long and healthy life.

What is a mammogram and how is it done?

Regular mammograms are the best tool doctors have to find breast cancer early. A mammogram is a low-dose x-ray picture of the breast. A woman stands in front of a mammography machine, and one of her breasts is placed on a clear plastic plate and gently, but firmly, pressed from another plate above her breast. The plates flatten the breast and keep it still, which helps produce a better mammogram image. The pressure lasts a few seconds and

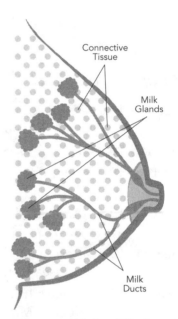

Figure 19.1. What are breasts made of? The breast is made up of three main parts: glands that produce milk; ducts, or passages, that carry milk to the nipple; and connective tissue (which consists of fibrous and fatty tissue) that connects and holds everything together. Most breast cancers occur in the glands and ducts.

does not harm the breast. The same steps are repeated with the other breast. The plates of the machine are then tilted to take a side view of each breast. When done, a woman will have had two different x-rays, or views of each breast, for a total of four x-rays.

Will the mammogram hurt?

Most women say that getting a mammogram is uncomfortable. A few women say that it is painful, although the pain doesn't last long. What you experience will depend upon the size of your breasts, how much your breasts need to be pressed, the skill of the technologist, and where you are in your monthly menstrual cycle.

How does mammography work?

The mammography machine produces a mammogram, or a black-and-white x-ray of the breast on a large sheet of film. A doctor, usually a specialist called a radiologist, then views the film carefully. Radiologists are medical doctors who have special training in diagnosing diseases by examining x-rays. The radiologist will carefully look at or "read" your mammogram, interpreting it for signs of cancer or other problems. The breast image on a mammogram varies a great deal from woman to woman, and there is a wide range in what is considered normal. That is why radiologists prefer to compare your mammogram with any previous ones you have had. This makes it easier to find small changes and detect cancer as early as possible.

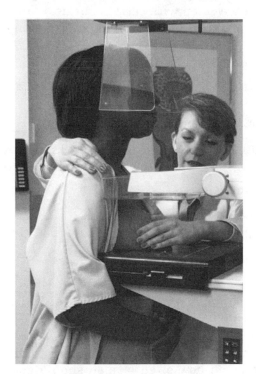

Figure 19.2. *A women getting a mammogram.*

When do I get the results?

The way you get the results of your mammogram varies by facility. At many facilities, the radiologist reads the mammogram in a few days to a few weeks and sends the results to you and your doctor. Some facilities ask you to wait several hours while the radiologist reads it that day.

Almost all facilities ask you to wait until the mammogram film is developed and checked to make sure it is clear and doesn't need to be redone. Keep in mind that the technologist can only say if the film is of good quality. She cannot read the film or tell you the results of your mammogram.

Before you get your mammogram, ask when and how you will get the results. All facilities are required by law to give you a written report of your mammogram results within 30 days—sooner if your results are abnormal. If you do not receive a report of your results within 30 days, contact your health professional or the mammography facility.

What can affect my mammogram?

Surgery and major injuries can affect your mammogram. Be sure to tell your health care team if you have had breast reduction, breast reconstruction, or breast implants. Women with certain surgical procedures may need additional x-ray pictures taken during their mammogram.

What questions should I ask my doctor or mammogram facility?

When getting a mammogram, consider asking:

- What's involved in getting a mammogram? How long will I be there?
- Do you have my previous mammograms?
- When will my doctor get the results?
- When and how will I learn about the results?
- When will I need to schedule my next mammogram?

When should I get a mammogram?

Most medical experts agree that women who have no previous breast symptoms or problems should begin getting mammograms at age 40. (They no longer recommend getting a baseline mammogram at age 35.) Experts' opinions vary on how often women should get mammograms, but most recommend that a woman get a mammogram every one or two years. Talk to your doctor if you have any breast symptoms or a family history of breast cancer. You may need to get tested earlier or more frequently.

What is the difference between screening and diagnostic mammograms?

Mammograms are used for two main reasons: screening and diagnosis. Screening mammograms are used to check women who have no signs or symptoms of breast cancer. It usually involves two x-rays of each breast. The goal of a screening mammogram is to find cancer early, when it is too small to be felt by a woman or her doctor. Finding breast cancer early greatly increases a woman's chance for successful treatment.

Diagnostic mammograms are used when a woman has breast symptoms or an abnormal mammogram. During a diagnostic mammogram, different pictures are taken to carefully study the breast. In most cases, special images magnify a small area of the breast, making it easier to read. Sometimes a woman will receive a diagnostic mammogram shortly after her screening mammogram. It is used to examine abnormalities found on the first mammogram.

What are some tips for getting a mammogram?

- When possible, try to avoid scheduling your mammogram when your breasts are tender or swollen, such as the week before or during your period.

- On the day of the exam, don't wear deodorant, perfume, or talcum powder. Sometimes ingredients in these products can show up as white spots on a mammogram.

- You may find it more comfortable to wear a top with a skirt or pants, instead of a dress. This way you'll only have to remove your top during the mammogram.

- Be prepared to describe any breast symptoms, changes, or problems to your health care team. They may also ask you about your medical history, such as prior surgeries or injuries, hormone use, and family or personal history of breast cancer.

- If you are changing mammogram facilities or seeing a new doctor, try to arrange for your previous mammograms to be sent to the facility before your appointment. This will help the radiologist check for changes in your breasts.

How accurate is a mammogram?

Getting regular mammograms is the most effective way to detect changes in the breast, but the test is not perfect. Sometimes a woman's mammogram will show signs of abnormalities, but further testing will show that there is no cancer. Other times, a woman's mammogram will appear to be normal, when she actually had signs of cancer. Not all cancers show up on a mammogram, or they can be difficult to see. Before menopause, women tend to have dense breast tissue that is harder to read on a mammogram. As women age and go through menopause, their breasts change and signs of breast cancer are easier to detect.

If 1,000 women over age 40 get a mammogram 920 will have a normal mammogram (although a small number of these women will have a cancer that was missed by the mammogram), and 80 will have an abnormal mammogram and require further tests. After further testing, results will show 76 do not have breast cancer and four have cancer.

Is there any new technology?

Research is being done to study new ways of taking images of the breast and detecting cancer early. They include MRI (magnetic resonance imaging), CAT (computerized axial tomography scans), and PET (positron emission tomography scans). These tests may help make a diagnosis after a woman has had an abnormal mammogram. The effectiveness of these new techniques in screening large numbers of women without signs or symptoms of breast cancer is uncertain.

After the Mammogram

What if my mammogram is normal?

Ask your health professional when you should get your next one and continue to get mammograms on a regular basis. Also, find out how often your health plan covers them. Some plans pay for screening mammograms once a year; others pay for them every two years.

What if my mammogram is abnormal?

Do not panic. Mammograms find many conditions that are not cancer. Most women who need further exams or testing do not have cancer. Some of the usual follow-up exams and tests are described below. The tests your doctor recommends will depend on what showed up on your mammogram.

Additional diagnostic mammograms: A doctor may ask for additional diagnostic mammograms to get different or bigger views of a particular area of a breast. These views supplement what a doctor sees on a regular mammogram, letting him or her examine an area more carefully.

Ultrasound: An ultrasound is a test that can be used to supplement (not replace) a mammogram. It uses sound waves to make pictures of the breast. This test is more commonly used in younger women or women with dense breast tissue. The doctor or technician views the picture on a monitor.

Exams by specialists: Your doctor may send you to a specialist, such as a breast specialist or surgeon, for a physical exam or other tests. It does not necessarily mean you have cancer or need surgery. Breast specialists are experienced in conducting physical exams of the breasts, diagnosing breast problems, and performing biopsies.

Biopsy: A biopsy involves removal of small samples of breast tissue, which can be done with a needle or through surgery. A needle biopsy is usually performed in the doctor's office. A woman receives a shot in the breast to numb the area, and the doctor inserts a needle to withdraw some tissue. A surgical biopsy is usually performed at a surgical center, the doctor's office, or a hospital. Typically, a woman will receive sedation (medication to help her feel relaxed and drowsy) before the surgeon makes a small cut in the skin of the breast. He or she removes a small piece of breast tissue in the suspicious area and sends it to a laboratory. A pathologist (a doctor who specializes in diagnosing diseases) examines the sample under a microscope to see if cancer cells are present.

What happens if they find breast cancer?

For many women, treatment for breast cancer begins within a few weeks after the diagnosis. Usually, a woman has time to learn about her options and doesn't have to make an immediate decision. She can discuss her treatment choices with her doctor, get a second opinion, talk to friends, or learn from other women with cancer. Not all breast cancers are treated the same way, and different treatments have different advantages and disadvantages. It is normal to feel some shock and stress, making it hard to process information at first or even to ask questions. Some women find it helps to make a list of questions, take notes, or have a family member or friend with them when they talk to the doctor. The most important thing is that a woman feels informed of her options and comfortable with her decision.

Resources

Where can I get a mammogram?

If you have a regular doctor, talk to him or her about getting a mammogram. Most private health insurance companies, HMOs, Medicaid, and Medicare pay for part or all of the cost of mammograms. Check with your plan for details or if you have any questions about your coverage. If you don't have health insurance and need help finding a low-cost or free mammogram, check with your local hospital, health department, women's center, or other community groups. The Centers for Disease Control and Prevention (CDC) also has a program called the National Breast and Cervical Cancer Early Detection Program. It works with health departments and other groups across the country to provide free or low-cost mammograms for women who qualify. To find out more about this program, please call your local health department or the numbers below.

Who can I talk to if I have additional questions?

Talk to your health professional. You can also call the National Cancer Institute's Cancer Information Service (CIS) at 800-4CANCER (800-422-6237). CIS Information Specialists can answer your questions about mammograms, breast cancer, and other issues in English or Spanish from 9:00 a.m. to 4:30 p.m. in your time zone. If you have TTY equipment, the number is 800-332-8615. Information about CDC programs and services is also available at 800-CDC-INFO (800-232-4636). Call 800-MEDICARE (800-633-4227) for information about Medicare.

Section 19.2

Digital vs. Film Mammography

Excerpted from "Digital vs. Film Mammography in the Digital Mammographic Imaging Screening Trial (DMIST): Questions and Answers," National Cancer Institute (www.cancer.gov), September 16, 2005.

Study Background

How is digital mammography different from film mammography?

Both digital and film mammography use x-rays to produce an image of the breast.

In film mammography, which has been used for over 35 years, the image is created directly on a film. While standard film mammography is very good, it is less sensitive for women who have dense breasts. Prior studies have suggested that approximately 10 percent to 20 percent of breast cancers that were detected by breast self-examination or physical examination are not visible on film mammography. A major limitation of film mammography is the film itself. Once a film mammogram is obtained, it cannot be significantly altered; if the film is underexposed, for example, contrast is lost and cannot be regained.

Digital mammography takes an electronic image of the breast and stores it directly in a computer. Digital mammography uses less radiation than film mammography. Digital mammography allows improvement in image storage and transmission because images can be stored and sent electronically. Radiologists also can use software to help interpret digital mammograms. One of the obstacles to greater use of digital mammography is its cost, with digital systems currently costing approximately 1.5 to 4 times more than film systems.

How was DMIST conducted?

The Digital Mammographic Imaging Screening Trial (DMIST), begun in October 2001, enrolled 49,528 women, who had no signs of breast cancer, at 33 sites in the United States. On the appointment day, women provided background health information and filled out brief questionnaires. They also had both digital and film mammograms taken on that day, each with a minimum of two views of each breast. Two different certified radiologists interpreted the conventional and digital mammogram exams for each individual patient. All radiologists who participated read both types of mammograms, and each radiologist read approximately an equal number of mammograms of each type.

Participants were asked to return in one year for their annual mammogram. At that time, a mammogram was performed as part of routine health care. Women who were not able to return to the same site as in year one were asked to submit films from another institution for review by study radiologists.

Why was DMIST important?

For women, breast cancer is the most common non-skin cancer and the second leading cause of cancer-related death in the United States. Death rates from breast cancer have been declining since 1990, and these decreases are believed to be the result, in part, of earlier detection and improved treatment.

DMIST was performed to measure relatively small, but potentially clinically important, differences in diagnostic accuracy between digital and film mammography. While any differences that were detected might be relatively small, they could improve breast cancer detection for all or some groups of women.

Digital mammography is a newer technology that is becoming more common. Currently, approximately eight percent of breast imaging units provide digital mammography. Past trials of digital mammography have shown no difference in diagnostic accuracy between digital and film mammography. The U.S. Food and Drug Administration (FDA) trials and three smaller screening trials showed no significant difference in the performance of digital mammography vs. film mammography. These studies were limited, however, because they each included only one type of digital detector and had relatively small numbers of patients, perhaps limiting their ability to detect small differences in diagnostic accuracy.

Who were the women who enrolled in DMIST?

Over 49,500 women who were requesting their usual breast cancer screening mammogram were recruited at 33 sites in the United States and Canada. The women had no breast cancer symptoms, and they agreed to undergo a follow-up mammogram at the same participating site or provide their mammograms from another institution for review one year from study entry. All women reviewed and signed the study consent form.

The following women were ineligible:

- Pregnant women

- Women with breast implants

- Women who had undergone a screening mammogram in the past 11 months

- Women with a focal dominant lump, which is defined as a single lump felt by a woman or her doctor

- Women with a bloody or clear nipple discharge

- Women with a history of breast cancer treated with lumpectomy

Breast cancer status for DMIST participants was determined through available breast biopsy information within 15 months of study entry or through follow-up mammography ten months or later after study entry.

Study Results

What were the main results of DMIST?

DMIST showed that, for the entire population of women studied, digital and film mammography had very similar screening accuracy. Digital mammography was significantly better in screening women who fit any of these three categories:

- Under age 50 (no matter what level of breast tissue density they had)

- Of any age with heterogeneously (very dense) or extremely dense breasts

- Pre- or perimenopausal women of any age (defined as women who had a last menstrual period within 12 months of their mammograms)

There is no apparent benefit of digital over film mammography for women who fit all of the following three categories:

- Over age 50

- Those who do not have dense or heterogeneously dense (very dense) breast tissue

- Those who are not still menstruating

In addition, there was no statistically significant difference in the accuracy of digital mammography compared to film according to digital mammography machine type, race, or breast cancer risk.

These results suggest that for women who fall into three subgroups (women under age 50, women with heterogeneously dense or extremely dense breasts, and pre- and perimenopausal women), digital mammography may be better at detecting breast cancer than traditional film mammography. Approximately 65 percent of the women in DMIST fit into one of the three subsets that showed a benefit with digital mammography.

Some earlier studies had suggested that digital mammography would result in fewer false positives than film mammography, but the rates of false positives for digital mammography and traditional mammography were the same in DMIST.

How many of the study participants were diagnosed with cancer?

During the course of the study, including initial screening and follow-up, 335 women were diagnosed with cancer. In general, cancers detected by either film or digital mammography were similar in histology (microscopic structure) and stage (how advanced they were).

However, lesions detected by digital mammography and missed by film in women under age 50, in women with heterogeneously dense or extremely dense breasts, and in pre- and perimenopausal women, included many invasive cancers and medium and high grade in situ lesions. Many of these cancers were confined to the breast at diagnosis; that is, they had not yet spread to the lymph nodes under the arm. These are precisely the lesions that must be detected early to save more lives through screening. In situ lesions in the breast are those confined to the breast duct without invading the surrounding breast tissue and are known as DCIS, or ductal carcinoma in situ.

Neither digital nor film mammography found all the breast cancers in the study population. Women who develop lumps, breast changes, or symptoms after screening mammography should report them to their physician even if their mammogram showed no signs of breast cancer.

What were the secondary goals of this trial and what were those results?

Secondary goals included measurement of the relative cost-effectiveness of both digital and film technologies, as digital mammography costs one and a half to four times more than film mammography and the measurement of the effect on participant quality of life due to the expected reduction of false positives.

The results of these parts of the study are still under analysis and will be presented at a later date. In fact, even though a reduction in false positives with digital mammography was expected, none was found in DMIST. The effect of false positive results on quality of life will be reported at a later date.

Information for Women

How can women obtain digital mammograms?

Film mammography is still much more common that digital mammography. Women who would like to have digital mammograms can ask their doctors or contact local hospitals or imaging centers to find out if digital mammography is available in their area.

Should women who live in communities that don't have digital mammography facilities, or don't have enough available machines, delay their next mammograms until they can have digital mammograms? Should women in the affected categories try to get digital mammograms before they are scheduled for their next mammogram?

Women should have their next mammogram when they are scheduled for it. It would be better to have a film mammogram when a woman is supposed to have her next mammogram than for her to delay her screening in order to get a digital mammogram. Women should not defer screening with mammography just because of a lack of access to digital mammography. Film mammography has been successfully used as a screening tool for breast cancer for over 35 years.

Women should not receive an extra mammogram because of these trial results. That is, if a woman has had a mammogram in the last year, and she has no breast signs or symptoms, she should undergo her next screening mammogram only when she is due for one, not earlier than she would ordinarily be scheduled.

How does a postmenopausal woman over age 50 determine if she has extremely dense or heterogeneously dense breasts?

At present, this can only be determined by a prior mammogram. Usually the density rating on mammography should be noted in the written report from the interpreting radiologist who reads the mammogram. If it is not included in the mammography report, it can be determined by a radiologist or qualified mammography technologist by viewing a prior mammogram. Women who are uncertain about their density status should inquire about it at the time of their next mammography visit.

If a woman has dense breasts, will she have dense breasts for the rest of her life?

Breast density can change over time. Most frequently, breast tissue becomes less dense with age. Estrogen replacement therapy, menopause, and weight loss or gain can change a woman's breast density. If a woman has questions about her breast density, she can discuss it with her primary care physician or the staff at the clinic where she receives her mammograms.

Does getting a digital mammogram feel similar to getting a film mammogram?

From a woman's perspective, a digital mammography examination is similar to a traditional mammography examination. Positioning and compression of the breast are identical.

What other breast imaging techniques might be useful for breast cancer screening?

In addition to mammography, ultrasound and magnetic resonance imaging (MRI) are both sometimes used to screen for breast cancer. ACRIN is currently conducting another trial of breast cancer screening, which compares ultrasound vs. mammography in high-risk women. MRI has shown promise for women at high-risk for breast cancer. DMIST did not study either of these other technologies. In fact, women who participated in DMIST were not permitted to participate in other screening trials during the one year immediately before and after their entry into DMIST.

There are no multicenter clinical trials investigating the use of either MRI or ultrasound in place of mammography as screening tools for breast cancer for the general population of women over age 40.

Section 19.3

Computer-Aided Detection Reduces Accuracy of Mammograms

National Cancer Institute (www.cancer.gov), April 4, 2007.

Computer-aided detection (CAD) that uses software designed to improve how radiologists interpret mammograms may instead make readings less accurate, according to new research. Use of CAD did not clearly improve the detection of breast cancer. The research was conducted by investigators at the University of California Davis Health System, Sacramento, California, and colleagues in the Breast Cancer Surveillance Consortium, which is sponsored by the National Cancer Institute (NCI), part of the National Institutes of Health.

The results of the study show that women who got screening mammograms at centers using CAD devices were more likely to be told their mammogram was abnormal and thus undergo a biopsy to rule out breast cancer. Findings appear in the April 5, 2007 issue of the *New England Journal of Medicine* and were funded by NCI, the Agency for Healthcare Research and Quality, and the American Cancer Society.

CAD software analyzes the mammogram image and marks suspicious areas for radiologists to review, thus assisting them in determining which images could lead to invasive tumors. CAD was approved by the U.S. Food and Drug Administration in 1998 and has been incorporated into many mammography imaging practices, but its effect on the accuracy of interpretation has been unclear.

"This study points out the need for the use of other techniques to find cancer at its earliest stages. NCI is incorporating techniques for imaging at the molecular level into many of its studies and is also conducting studies to improve the use of CAD and conventional mammography," said John E. Niederhuber, M.D., NCI Director. "In the end, technology facilitates screening. Ultimately, treatment requires radiologists working with the examining physician and the responsible surgeon to put everything together. We worry about false positives, but we certainly don't want to miss any cancers, either."

Investigators looked at the use of screening mammography in 222,135 women who had 429,345 mammograms. The period of observation was from 1998 through 2002 and took place at 43 facilities in Colorado, New Hampshire, and Washington states. The study included 2,351 women who received a diagnosis of breast cancer within one year after screening and also received a mammogram that did or did not use CAD.

"Within three years of FDA approval, 10 percent of the mammography facilities in the country were using CAD," said lead researcher Joshua J. Fenton, M.D., UC Davis Health System. "There had been no large-scale community-based review of CAD efficacy despite the rapid adoption of this technology so we did this study to see if CAD was proving to be beneficial."

Seven facilities, representing 16 percent of the study sites, implemented computer-aided detection during the study period. With the use of CAD, 32 percent more women were recalled for more tests and 20 percent more women had a breast biopsy. Use of the software had no clear impact on the early detection of breast cancer. The study suggests that, if anything, the software may promote the detection of the least dangerous breast cancers, such as localized, in situ breast cancers. The effect of in situ cancers on breast cancer mortality remains unknown and some evidence suggests that not all develop into invasive cancers.

Every time the CAD software marks a real cancer, a radiologist has to consider about 2,000 additional false-positive marks, making it very difficult to distinguish between real cancers and those that are not cancer. The authors estimate that for every additional woman diagnosed with breast cancer on the basis of CAD, 156 women are falsely recalled for more tests and 14 had unnecessary biopsies to exclude cancer.

"It's unfortunate that the use of the software has proliferated so widely before we are certain of its benefits," said Fenton. "We need studies to determine if the benefits of the software outweigh its harms and costs. There is also the potential for new studies to improve the performance of CAD software."

The authors estimate that if all mammography facilities adopt CAD, the annual cost of mammograms in the United States could increase 18 percent, or an additional $550 million nationwide.

Section 19.4

Annual Mammography Reduces Mortality in Older Breast Cancer Survivors

National Cancer Institute (www.cancer.gov), July 18, 2007.

Annual mammography surveillance for breast cancer survivors older than 65 is associated with a dramatically reduced risk of death from breast cancer, whether by recurrence or another primary tumor.

Results from a study to be published in the July 20, 2007, *Journal of Clinical Oncology* showed that each successive annual mammogram lowered a woman's breast cancer mortality risk by about 31 percent. Compounding this benefit over a period of four years would cut a woman's cumulative risk of breast cancer death by 88 percent.

Dr. Timothy L. Lash of Boston University was the lead author of the cohort study, which identified 1,846 breast cancer patients from six Cancer Research Network (CRN) sites chosen to maximize ethnic and geographic diversity.

All women were diagnosed with stage I or II breast cancer between 1990 and 1994, and were designated as "survivors" for the purposes of the study 90 days after finishing their initial breast cancer treatment. The 178 women who died of breast cancer within five years were closely matched to 634 control subjects who were followed at least as long as the women who died. Protective effects of annual mammography were found to be the strongest among women with stage I disease, those who had received mastectomy, and those older than 79.

In an editorial, Dr. Jeanne Mandelblatt from the Lombardi Comprehensive Cancer Center in Washington, DC, commended "this high-quality observational research" that emerged from CRN, a National Cancer Institute–funded collaboration between 12 large managed care systems. The large cohort study provides the best data likely to be developed on this question, because a clinical trial that randomized women to "no mammography" would disregard current guidelines, which recommend that survivors receive annual surveillance mammograms.

169

Section 19.5

Recent Drop in Mammography Rates Causes Concern

From "Cancer Research Highlights," *NCI Cancer Bulletin*, National Cancer Institute (www.cancer.gov), May 15, 2007.

The drop in mammography rates in the United States in recent years is cause for concern because it could contribute to a future rise in breast cancer deaths, according to an analysis of data from representative national surveys published early online in *Cancer*.

Scientists from NCI's Division of Cancer Control and Population Sciences (DCCPS), led by Dr. Nancy Breen, examined data from the Centers for Disease Control and Prevention's National Health Interview Surveys (NHIS) and found a decline in mammography screening in 2005 compared with 2000—from 70 percent to 66 percent. After many years of increases in mammography use, "[t]his report establishes for the nation what has already been observed in some local data. It confirms that use of mammography may be falling. Although small, this decline is cause for concern, as it signals a change in direction."

Mammography screening rates were lower in 2005 than in 2000 for nearly all the groups of women examined. "The largest significant declines were among women who have traditionally used mammography at high rates, including the 50–64 age group, those with higher incomes, and women aged 40–64 with private, non-HMO insurance coverage," the DCCPS investigators noted.

When screening rates drop, women with breast cancer will be diagnosed later, resulting in a short-term drop in incidence, they add. "Consequently, we are concerned that some of the observed decline in incidence may be due in part to the leveling off and reduction in mammography rates." The trend "may presage a future increase in mortality from breast cancer" from later detection of more advanced disease. "If future NHIS data continue to show a decline in mammography use, then we as a nation need to be prepared to address it," the NCI scientists concluded.

The recent decline in breast cancer incidence rates was examined in a separate study published May 3, 2007 in *Breast Cancer Research*.

Scientists from the American Cancer Society, led by Dr. Ahmedin Jemal, examined data from NCI's Surveillance, Epidemiology, and End Results (SEER) program.

"Two distinct patterns are observed in breast cancer trends," they reported. The downturn in incidence rates in all age groups above 45 years coincides with a plateau in mammography use, which typically reduces incidence rates "due to a reduced pool of undiagnosed cases." The sharp decrease in incidence from 2002 to 2003 that occurred in women 50 to 69 years old who predominantly, but not exclusively, had ER-positive tumors may reflect the early benefit of the reduced use of hormone replacement therapy. A number of investigators within NCI-funded initiatives are now examining the contribution of recent changes in screening and hormone therapy to breast cancer trends.

Section 19.6

Breast Implant Adverse Events during Mammography

Center for Devices and Radiological Health,
U.S. Food and Drug Administrations, April 23, 2004.

A U.S. Food and Drug Administration (FDA) study on problems with mammography for women with breast implants was published in the *Journal of Women's Health* in May, 2004. The preliminary results of this study were presented at the FDA Science Forum in April 2003.

The study was a review of adverse event reports from the FDA's Manufacturer and User Facility Device Experience (MAUDE) database (http://www.fda.gov/cdrh/databases.html). Researchers found 66 reports that mentioned problems with mammography for women with breast implants. The majority (62.1%) of problems reported were for breast implant rupture that was suspected to occur during mammography. Rupture during compression for mammography was reported for both silicone gel-filled and saline-filled breast implants. Other adverse events reported to FDA included implants crushed by mammographic compression, pain during mammography attributed to the implants, inability to perform mammography because of capsular contracture or because of fear of implant rupture, and delayed detection of cancer attributed to the breast implants. It is unknown how often these problems occur because the MAUDE database cannot be used to determine rates of problems occurring.

FDA researchers also reviewed published medical literature on mammography for women with breast implants. Their review found medical reports describing the following:

- An additional 17 reported cases of breast implant rupture during mammographic compression

- Breast implant interference with imaging breast tissue, with between 22% and 83% of mammographically visible breast tissue obscured by breast implants

- Special techniques needed to maximize breast tissue visualization for women with breast implants

- A delay in breast cancer detection in women with implants, but without increased mortality to women with implants

The risk for breast cancer does not differ in women with breast implants compared to other women. Recommendations for breast cancer screening also apply to women with breast implants. Women considering breast implants should be aware of potential issues with mammography in order to make an informed decision. Women who already have breast implants should always inform the mammography center that they have breast implants when they make an appointment and always remind the mammography technician that they have breast implants when they go for their exam.

Chapter 20

Using Magnetic Resonance Imaging (MRI) to Detect Breast Cancer

A new study has demonstrated a significant benefit of adding a magnetic resonance imaging (MRI) study to the standard diagnostic workup following a new diagnosis of breast cancer in one breast.

By using MRI to examine the opposite breast in a population of 969 women with newly diagnosed breast cancer, researchers from the National Cancer Institute (NCI)-funded American College of Radiology Imaging Network (ACRIN) discovered 3.1 percent of the patients had cancers in the contralateral breast that were missed by standard practice mammography and clinical breast exam. A negative result on the MRI exam of the contralateral breast nearly eliminated the likelihood (0.3 percent) of cancer being found in that breast over the next year, they reported in the March 29 *New England Journal of Medicine.*

MRI demonstrated a 91-percent sensitivity (percentage of true cancers detected) and 88-percent specificity (percentage of true negatives), and MRI efficacy was not affected by patients' cancer type, age, or breast density.

"We can now identify the vast majority of contralateral cancers at the time of a woman's initial breast cancer diagnosis," said the study's principal investigator, Dr. Constance Lehman, professor of radiology and director of breast imaging at the University of Washington and Seattle Cancer Care Alliance.

Finding cancer in the opposite breast at this juncture will help avoid the cost, morbidity, and stress of multiple or delayed treatments,

"MRI Detects Nearly All Contralateral Breast Cancers," *NCI Cancer Bulletin,* National Cancer Institute, April 3, 2007.

173

Dr. Lehman said. And a negative result on the opposite breast with mammography, clinical exam, and MRI also may allow women to forego prophylactic bilateral mastectomies, "a potential outcome that we would be delighted to see," she added.

The NCI-funded trial is the first of this size on the topic, with more than 1,000 patients enrolled, including those being treated at academic medical centers, community hospitals, and private practices. Adding a contemporaneous MRI to the diagnostic workup effectively doubled the number of contralateral cancers typically found. In 121 cases, MRI findings led to biopsies, 30 of which resulted in cancer diagnoses. Of these, 60 percent were invasive cancers, while the remainder were ductal carcinoma in situ (DCIS), abnormal cell clusters in the lining of the breast duct that have not invaded other tissue but that can progress to full-blown invasive tumors.

Three additional tumors—all DCIS less than five mm in size—were diagnosed upon analyses of mastectomy tissue samples.

That one of every four cases referred for biopsy based on the MRI turned out to be cancerous is an important finding, according to Dr. Carl Jaffe, chief of the NCI Cancer Imaging Program's Diagnostic Imaging Branch. With conventional mammography, that ratio is generally closer to one in six.

"So, relative to mammography, MRI was far more specific," Dr. Jaffe said. "These contralateral breasts would have been considered negative based on mammography and a clinical exam. This is important because treatment planning for these women would have been based on incomplete information on the full extent of the disease. That's why these results are so striking."

Dr. Christy A. Russell, co-director of the University of Southern California/Norris Comprehensive Cancer Center's Lee Breast Center, suggested that this study and others should be considered in the development of consensus guidelines related to the diagnostic evaluation of a woman with newly diagnosed breast cancer.

"What we're seeing in this study and our new ACS [American Cancer Society] guidelines is that the use of MRI is evolving to better meet the needs of subgroups of women, either women at very high risk and for whom mammography may be less effective, or in women with a newly diagnosed breast cancer, where MRI can identify cancers in the same breast or contralateral breast that were missed by mammography," continued Dr. Russell, who chaired the American Cancer Society panel that released new recommendations last week on breast screening in high risk individuals using MRI.

Because the use and practice of breast MRI is still evolving in the United States and is not available in all clinical settings, Drs. Jaffe and Russell indicated that some obstacles still remain to its wider adoption.

Although its use for breast screening has increased—for example, as a follow-up to an abnormal mammogram—insurers generally do not cover MRI for screening the opposite breast. That could change, however, based on these study results.

And, as Dr. Jaffe pointed out, MRI machines specifically set up to do breast screenings—those that have a breast "coil" and in settings with the ability to perform biopsy—need to become more widely available.

To ensure the highest quality scan, Dr. Russell advised that women undergoing a diagnostic MRI go to a center that has an MRI machine appropriately equipped for breast imaging. She also advised having the screening procedure done at a facility with biopsy capability and experience.

If a suspicious lesion is found on the MRI, but the center is not equipped to do a biopsy, she explained, then the woman will have to be referred to another center and repeat the entire imaging procedure to guide the biopsy.

Guidelines Recommend Annual MRI Breast Screening for High-Risk Women

New guidelines from the American Cancer Society (ACS) released last week recommend that some women at high risk of developing breast cancer should undergo annual screenings with both mammography and magnetic resonance imaging (MRI). In certain groups of women, the recommendations explain, conducting both tests annually increases the likelihood of early detection. The guidelines were published in the March 2007 issue of *CA: A Cancer Journal for Clinicians*.

To minimize the risk of avoidable biopsies, fear, anxiety, and adverse health effects, explained Dr. Christy Russell, who chaired the ACS expert advisory group that developed the recommendations, it is "imperative to carefully select those women who should be screened using this technology."

The guidelines advise that women should receive an annual MRI screening and mammogram if they have or have had: a BRCA1 or BRCA2 mutation or a first-degree relative with a BRCA1 or BRCA2 mutation; a lifetime breast cancer risk of 20 to 25 percent or greater based on one of several accepted risk assessment tools; radiation to the chest between the ages of 10 and 30; or Li-Fraumeni syndrome, Cowden syndrome, Bannayan-Riley-Ruvalcaba syndrome, or a history of these syndromes in a first-degree relative.

The recommendations state that MRI breast screenings should be conducted on machines equipped with a breast coil and that meet certain performance parameters. They also state that "the ability to perform MRI-guided biopsy is absolutely essential to offering screening MRI."

Chapter 21

Evaluating a Breast Lump

The discovery of a breast lump—whether by chance, during a routine breast self-exam, or during a clinical breast exam—can be stressful for a woman. Because a lump can be a symptom of breast cancer, all persistent breast lumps should be evaluated by a physician. However, the majority of breast lumps (approximately 80%) are due to non-cancerous causes.

What should a woman do if she finds a breast lump?

First, it is important for all women to practice monthly breast self-exams beginning at age 20. These self-exams allow women to become familiar with how their breasts look and feel so they can more readily detect any changes that may occur. Many women naturally have some lumpiness and asymmetry (differences between the right and left breast). The key to the breast self-exam is to learn to find changes in the breast(s) that persist over time. If a new lump is found and does not disappear after the menstrual cycle, then it should be reported to a physician for clinical evaluation.

All persistent breast lumps should be evaluated by a physician. Practicing monthly breast self-exams helps women get to know their breasts and more easily detect changes.

What signs suggest a lump is likely to be cancerous?

It is not possible for a woman or a physician to know for certain whether a breast lump indicates breast cancer until imaging exams (such as mammography and ultrasound) and/or biopsy are performed. A breast biopsy involves taking a sample of breast tissue and examining it under a microscope to determine whether it contains cancer cells. However, there are certain characteristics associated with lumps that can suggest whether they are more likely to be cancer or benign (non-cancerous).

Signs that suggest a lump is more likely to be cancerous:

- The lump is firm and hard
- The lump is not discrete; it is not easily distinguishable
- The lump is fixed in the breast; it does not move
- There is only one lump
- There is not an identical lump in the opposite breast
- The skin of breast is dimpled
- The lump is accompanied by bloody nipple discharge

Signs that suggest a lump is less likely to be cancerous:

- The lump is soft
- The lump is discrete; it is easily distinguishable
- The lump moves in the breast
- There are multiple breast lumps
- There is an identical lump in the opposite breast
- The lump disappears after the menstrual cycle

While the above signs can help suggest whether a lump is more likely or less likely to be cancerous, having one or more of these characteristics does not guarantee or eliminate the possibility of having breast cancer. These characteristics merely provide clues for the physician when evaluating a lump. Some breast cancers can have characteristics found in the "less likely to be cancerous" category. Therefore, all persistent breast lumps need to be presented to a physician.

Fibrocystic breasts: Fibrocystic breast condition is a common, non-cancerous condition that affects more than 50% of women at some point in their lives. In fact, the condition is so common that many physicians refrain from using the term "fibrocystic" and simply tell their patients that their breasts are lumpier than average but are still normal.

The most common signs of fibrocystic breasts include: lumpiness, tenderness, cysts, areas of thickening, fibrosis, and breast pain. Having fibrocystic breasts, in and of itself, is not a risk factor for breast cancer. However, fibrocystic breast condition can sometimes make it more difficult to detect a hidden breast cancer with standard examination and imaging techniques. Therefore, it is important that women with fibrocystic breasts practice monthly breast self-exams, receive regular clinical breast exams, and have yearly screening mammograms (the latter beginning at age 40).

Symptoms of fibrocystic breasts:

- Cysts (fluid-filled sacs)
- Fibrosis (scar-like connective tissue)
- Lumpiness
- Areas of thickening
- Tenderness
- Pain

The degree to which women experience symptoms of fibrocystic breast condition varies considerably. Some women with fibrocystic breasts have only mild breast pain and may not be able to feel any breast lumps when performing breast self-exams. Other women with fibrocystic breasts may experience more severe breast pain or tenderness and may feel multiple lumps in their breasts. Most fibrocystic breast lumps are found in the upper, outer quadrant of the breasts (near the armpit), although these lumps can occur anywhere in the breasts. Fibrocystic breast lumps tend to be smooth, rounded, and mobile (not attached to other breast tissue), though some fibrocystic tissue may have a thickened, irregular feel. The lumps or irregularities associated with fibrocystic breasts are often tender to touch and may increase or decrease in size during the menstrual cycle.

How are breast lumps evaluated by physicians?

Whether a breast lump is first detected by a physician during a clinical breast exam or by the woman herself, the process of evaluation usually begins with a detailed patient history. The physician will ask the patient specific questions about the lump and her medical history to help identify the cause of the lump. Sample questions may include:

- How long have you had the lump?
- Does the lump change in size with your menstrual cycle?
- How long has it been since your last menstrual period?
- Have you recently been pregnant or are you breast-feeding?
- Have you experienced discharge from the nipple?
- Do you use hormone replacement therapy?
- Have you experienced any recent trauma to the breast?
- Have you had any previous breast biopsies? If yes, what were the diagnoses?
- Do you have a history of cancer?
- Do you have a history of other medical conditions?
- Have you had a mammogram or other breast imaging test before?

These questions can provide important information as to what is causing the lump. For example, a woman who has recently been pregnant and who is breast-feeding may have a galactocele (milk-filled cyst). A woman who is taking hormone replacement therapy (HRT) may have more nodules in her breast due to the therapy. Trauma to the breast may cause a hematoma (a blood-filled packet), fat necrosis (swelling of fatty breast tissue), or a ruptured cyst (fluid-filled packet).

Learning the patient's family and personal medical history can also be helpful. A family history of breast cancer can increase a woman's chances of developing breast cancer herself. A personal history of non-cancerous conditions such as atypical hyperplasia (an abnormal increase in breast cells) or lobular carcinoma in situ (LCIS) can also increase the risk of breast cancer.

Once a thorough patient history is taken, the physician will perform a thorough clinical breast exam to investigate the lump and other areas of the breast and axilla (armpit). In addition to feeling for breast masses, the physician will check for any skin dimpling, nipple retraction, or other visual changes. The clinical breast exam typically lasts several minutes and the patient will usually need to raise her arms, place her hands on her hips and exert pressure, and lie down during the exam so the breasts can be examined from different angles.

After the clinical breast exam, the evaluation of a breast lump will differ depending on the woman's age, history, and characteristics of the lump. The following descriptions provide information on how women in different age groups are typically evaluated:

- **Women age 30 or older:** A diagnostic mammogram is usually ordered. A diagnostic mammogram differs from the routine screening mammogram in that it involves additional x-ray views from different angles and/or special magnification. A diagnostic mammogram is used instead of a screening mammogram when a breast abnormality is present. Depending on the results of the mammogram, additional breast imaging (such as ultrasound) may be ordered. In many cases, further breast imaging will be ordered even if a mammogram does not show a suspicious abnormality. This is because a small percentage of breast cancers can be missed with mammography. Depending on the results of the mammogram and additional imaging tests, a breast biopsy may be performed. A biopsy involves removing a sample of breast tissue and examining it under a microscope to determine whether cancer cells are present. Sometimes, a biopsy (or fine needle aspiration—sampling of a few breast cells) will be performed even if breast imaging tests are normal. This usually happens when the physician suspects that the breast lump is suspicious regardless of the results of the imaging tests.

- **Women under age 30:** In this group of women, a mammogram may or may not be the first test ordered. This is because mammography is not always beneficial in younger women who tend to have dense breast tissue which can mask breast cancer and other abnormalities on a mammogram film. In some cases, ultrasound or other tests may be performed. However, mammography can still be beneficial in some women younger than 30. If the breast imaging tests reveal a suspicious abnormality, a biopsy may be ordered to examine a sample of breast tissue. As with women over age 30, a biopsy (or fine needle aspiration—sampling a few breast cells) may be performed even if breast imaging tests are normal. Again, this usually happens when the physician suspects that the breast lump is suspicious regardless of the results of the imaging tests.

In approximately 80% of cases, breast lumps are benign (noncancerous). Benign conditions that can cause breast lumps include:

- Fibrocystic breasts
- Cysts
- Fibroadenomas
- Papillomas

- Phyllodes tumors (usually benign)
- Galactoceles
- Granular cell tumors
- Duct ectasia
- Fat necrosis

If a biopsy reveals breast cancer, then the woman and her cancer team will discuss treatment options. Treatment options include surgery (lumpectomy or mastectomy), radiation, chemotherapy, and/or other drug therapies, such as tamoxifen. Practicing monthly breast self exams, receiving regular clinical breast exams, and yearly screening mammograms (the latter beginning at age 40) can help detect breast cancer early when the chances of successful treatment and survival are the greatest.

Breast Lumps during Pregnancy

Breast cancer during pregnancy can be difficult to diagnose because the breasts naturally undergo several changes. During pregnancy, the breasts increase in size and become more tender, especially during the first half of pregnancy. The most rapid period of breast growth is during the first eight weeks of pregnancy. As the pregnancy progresses, the breasts become firmer and more nodular to prepare for lactation (breast-feeding). It is very important for women to continue to perform monthly breast self-exams during pregnancy and receive monthly physician-performed clinical breast exams so as not to delay the possible diagnosis of breast cancer.

As in non-pregnant women, the majority of breast lumps found during pregnancy are benign (non-cancerous). However, because a lump can signal breast cancer, all persistent lumps should be evaluated by a physician. Approximately one in 3,000 (0.03%) to one in 10,000 (0.01%) women are diagnosed with breast cancer during pregnancy. Breast cancer itself does not appear to harm a fetus.

If a lump is detected during pregnancy, an ultrasound exam and/ or mammogram will typically be performed. Ultrasound is excellent at distinguishing cysts (packets of fluid) and is routinely used for fetal imaging because it does not harm the fetus. Mammography is also considered safe for pregnant women and the fetus because it uses a very low dose of radiation. In many cases, a biopsy will be performed if a suspicious breast lump is detected in a pregnant woman. A biopsy confirms or denies the presence of breast cancer.

Non-cancerous conditions that are common during pregnancy include:

- Cysts (collections of fluid)
- Galactoceles (milk-filled cysts)
- Fibroadenomas (tumors; existing ones may enlarge during pregnancy)

If breast cancer is detected during pregnancy, it is not necessary to terminate the pregnancy. Treatment options should be discussed with the patient's cancer team. Surgery, such as lumpectomy and mastectomy, can be performed safely during pregnancy. Radiation, chemotherapy, and drug therapies (such as tamoxifen) are usually delayed until after childbirth.

Additional Resources and References

- O'Grady, Lois et al, *A Practical Approach to Breast Disease*, Boston: Little Brown and Company, 1995.
- The National Cancer Institute provides information on breast lumps at http://www.cancer.gov.

Chapter 22

Breast Biopsies

Breast Biopsy: Indications and Methods

It is estimated that over 48 million mammograms are performed each year and that less than one million of them (less than 5%) are recalled to undergo a biopsy (in some instances the number of cases requiring biopsy can be as low as 2%, depending on population demographics and methods of care). Fortunately, 65% to 80% of breast biopsies result in benign (non-cancerous) diagnosis.

However, if cancer is found to be present after pathological analysis of the biopsy sample(s), it is critical that the type and stage of the cancer be identified as soon as possible. Generally, the earlier breast cancer is diagnosed, the greater a patient's chances of survival.

There are several different methods of breast biopsy, many of which are discussed in detail herein. These types include:

- Fine needle aspiration (FNA)

- Core needle biopsy

- Vacuum-assisted biopsy (Mammotome or minimally invasive breast biopsy)

- Large core surgical (ABBI [advanced breast biopsy instrumentation])
- Open surgical (excisional or incisional)

One method of biopsy will likely be most favorable depending on a number of factors, including how suspicious the abnormality appears; the size, shape, and location of the abnormality; the number of abnormalities present; the patient's medical history; the patient's preference; the training of the radiologist or surgeon who is performing the biopsy; and the breast imaging center or surgical center where the biopsy is performed.

The side effects and risks of biopsy vary depending on the type of biopsy performed. Women are strongly encouraged to discuss the advantages and disadvantages of the different biopsy methods with their physician(s) prior to undergoing the procedure.

Fine Needle Aspiration Biopsy (FNA)

What is FNA?

Fine needle aspiration (FNA) is a percutaneous ("through the skin") procedure that uses a fine gauge needle (22 or 25 gauge) and a syringe to sample fluid from a breast cyst or remove clusters of cells from a solid mass. With FNA, the cellular material taken from the breast is usually sent to the pathology laboratory for analysis. The needle used during FNA is smaller than a needle that is normally used to draw blood. If the radiologist or surgeon just drains fluid from a cyst and does not send the sample to the pathology laboratory for analysis, the procedure is simply called cyst aspiration.

How is FNA performed?

First, the skin of the breast is cleaned. If a breast lump can be felt, the radiologist or surgeon will guide a needle into the area of concern by palpating (feeling) the lump. If the lump is non-palpable (cannot be felt), the FNA procedure will be done under image-guidance using either stereotactic mammography or ultrasound with the patient in either the upright or prone (face down) position. Stereotactic mammography involves using computers to pinpoint the exact location of a breast mass based on mammograms (x-rays) taken from two different angles. The computer coordinates will help the physician to guide the needle to the correct area in the breast. With ultrasound, the radiologist or surgeon will watch the needle on the ultrasound monitor to help guide it to the area of concern. FNA is usually performed under ultrasound image guidance.

After the needle is placed into the breast in the region of the lesion (abnormality), a vacuum is created and multiple in and out needle motions are performed. Several needle insertions are usually required to ensure that an adequate tissue sample is taken. The samples are then smeared on a microscope slide and are: 1) allowed to dry in air, 2) are "fixed" by spraying, or 3) are immersed in a liquid. The fixed smears are then stained and examined by a pathologist under the microscope.

FNA does not require stitches and can usually be performed on an outpatient basis. A very small bandage is placed over the area after the procedure. Many patients resume their normal lifestyle and routine the same day of the FNA procedure.

Note: The effectiveness of FNA is largely operator-dependent; it requires a skilled radiologist or surgeon who has gained experience by performing several cases.

How do FNA samples appear?

Fluid extracted from the breast lump may be clear, straw-colored, green or brown tinged, white, yellow, or more rarely, bloody. In most cases, these fluids are benign (non-cancerous). If the fluid is not bloody, it is usually simply discarded because there is not typically any benefit gained from microscopic examination by a pathologist. However, bloody fluid may indicate cancer and is usually sent to the laboratory for analysis.

How should patients prepare for FNA?

Prior to FNA, the skin of the breast is cleansed and then may be anesthetized with a small hypodermic needle. Many times, the breast is not anesthetized for FNA because administering the anesthesia tends to cause more pain for the patient than the procedure itself. Also, lidocaine (an anesthesia) may cause artifacts to appear in the cytology sample when examined under the microscope.

Patients may eat a light meal prior to the procedure. A comfortable two piece garment should be worn. Women should not wear talcum powder, deodorant, lotion, or perfume under their arms or on their breasts on the day of the procedure (since these may cause image artifacts or other problems). Patients who take blood thinners or aspirin should talk to their physicians about whether they should discontinue using them prior to FNA. Any jewelry worn (especially earrings or necklaces) should be easily and quickly removable.

What are the advantages and disadvantages to FNA?

FNA is the fastest and easiest method of breast biopsy, and the results are rapidly available. FNA is excellent for confirming breast cysts, and since the procedure does not require stitches, patients are usually able to resume normal activity almost immediately after the procedure.

One disadvantage of FNA is that the procedure only removes very small samples of tissue or cells from the breast. If the sample is benign fluid (for example, a cyst), then the procedure is ideal. However, if the tissue is solid or if a sample of cloudy, suspicious-looking fluid is obtained, the small number of cells removed by FNA only allow for a cytologic (cell) diagnosis. This can be an incomplete assessment because the cells cannot be evaluated in relation to the surrounding tissue.

For example, a pathologist may diagnose ductal carcinoma in situ (DCIS), a non-invasive breast cancer, based on the FNA breast sample obtained when in fact, the patient has infiltrating ductal carcinoma (IDC), in a nearby area. IDC is an invasive and potentially more serious breast cancer. A larger sample (such as that obtained with core needle or vacuum-assisted biopsy) can help the pathologist determine the extent of the cancer.

Core Needle Biopsy

What is core needle biopsy?

A core needle biopsy is a percutaneous ("through the skin") procedure that involves removing small samples of breast tissue using a hollow "core" needle. For palpable (able to be felt) lesions, this is accomplished by fixing the lesion with one hand and performing a freehand needle biopsy with the other. In the case of non-palpable lesions (those unable to be felt), stereotactic mammography or ultrasound image guidance is used. Stereotactic mammography uses computers to pinpoint the exact location of a breast mass based on mammograms (x-rays) taken from two different angles. The computer coordinates will help the physician to guide the needle to the correct area in the breast. With ultrasound, the radiologist or surgeon will watch the needle on the ultrasound monitor to help guide it to the area of concern.

The needle used during core needle biopsy is larger than the needle used with FNA (usually a 16, 14, or 11 gauge needle is used with the core needle biopsy procedure). The core needle biopsy needle also has a special cutting edge.

How is core needle biopsy performed?

First, the breast area is anesthetized with an injection of lidocaine. Then, the needle is placed into the breast with the patient position in either the upright or prone (face down) position. As with FNA, the radiologist or surgeon will guide the needle into the area of concern by palpating (feeling) the lump. If the lump is non-palpable (cannot be felt), the core needle biopsy is performed under image-guidance using either stereotactic mammography or ultrasound.

Three to six separate core needle insertions are typically needed to obtain a sufficient sample of breast tissue. Patients may experience a slight pressure during core needle biopsy but should not experience any significant pain. As tissue samples are taken, clicks may be heard from the needle and sampling instrument. Typically, samples approximately 0.75 inches long (approximately 2.0 centimeters) and 0.0625 inches (approximately 0.16 centimeters) in diameter are removed. The samples are then sent to the pathology laboratory for diagnosis.

The core needle biopsy procedure typically only takes a few minutes, and most patients are able to resume normal activity almost immediately afterwards. Core needle biopsy may cause some bruising but does not usually leave an external scar or an internal scar that is seen on later mammograms (which can obscure future mammogram interpretations). However, core needle biopsy may not be suitable for patients who have very small or very hard breast lumps.

How should patients prepare for core needle biopsy?

To prepare for a core needle biopsy, patients may eat a light meal prior to the exam and biopsy procedure. A comfortable two piece garment should be worn. Women should not wear talcum powder, deodorant, lotion, or perfume under their arms or on their breasts on the day of the procedure (since these may cause image artifacts or other problems). Patients who take blood thinners or aspirin should talk to their physicians about whether they should discontinue using them prior to core needle biopsy. Any jewelry worn (especially earrings or necklaces) should be easily and quickly removable.

What are the advantages and disadvantages to core needle biopsy?

Core needle biopsy usually allows for a more accurate assessment of a breast mass than fine needle aspiration (if the sample is found to be solid or cloudy, suspicious-looking fluid) because the larger core needle usually removes enough tissue for the pathologist to evaluate abnormal cells in relation to the surrounding small sample of breast tissue taken in the specimen.

Nevertheless, core needle biopsy, like fine needle aspiration, only removes samples of a mass and not the entire area of concern. Therefore, it is possible that a more serious diagnosis may be missed by limiting the sampling of a lesion (abnormality).

A relatively new biopsy procedure called vacuum-assisted breast biopsy is able to remove approximately twice the amount of breast tissue compared with core needle biopsy while still offering the patient a minimally invasive breast biopsy procedure.

Vacuum-Assisted Biopsy

What is vacuum-assisted biopsy?

The relatively new vacuum-assisted breast biopsy is a percutaneous ("through the skin") procedure that relies on stereotactic mammography or ultrasound imaging. Stereotactic mammography uses computers to pinpoint the exact location of a breast mass based on mammograms (x-rays) taken from two different angles. The computer coordinates will help the physician to guide the needle to the correct area in the breast. With ultrasound, the radiologist or surgeon will watch the needle on the ultrasound monitor to help guide it to the area of concern. The patient will either by positioned in the upright or prone (face down) position for a vacuum-assisted biopsy.

Vacuum-assisted biopsy is a minimally invasive procedure that allows for the removal of multiple tissue samples. However, unlike core needle biopsy, which involves several separate needle insertions to acquire multiple samples, the special biopsy probe used during vacuum-assisted biopsy is inserted only once into the breast through a small skin nick made in the skin of the patient's breast.

Two companies currently manufacturer vacuum-assisted breast biopsy systems, and often, vacuum-assisted biopsy will be referred to by the brand name: either Mammotome made by Johnson & Johnson Ethicon Endo-Surgery or MIBB (which stands for minimally invasive breast biopsy) made by Tyco/United States Surgical Corporation. In 1999, a hand-held version of the Mammotome was also approved by the U.S. Food and Drug Administration (FDA).

How is vacuum-assisted biopsy performed?

First, the skin of the breast is cleaned. Then, a small amount of local anesthetic (lidocaine), similar to what one might have at a dentist's office, is injected into the skin and deeper tissues of the breast using a small hypodermic needle. Under stereotactic or ultrasound guidance, the radiologist or breast surgeon positions the special breast probe into the area of the breast where the lesion (abnormality) is located.

After the probe has been properly positioned, a vacuum line draws the breast tissue through the aperture of the probe into the sampling chamber of the device. Once the tissue is in the sampling chamber, the rotating cutting device is advanced and a tissue sample is captured. The tissue sample is then carried through the probe to the tissue collection area (a standard pathology tissue cassette).

After a tissue sample is captured, the radiologist or surgeon then rotates the thumbwheel of the probe, moving the sampling chamber approximately 30 degrees to new position. The entire cycle is repeated, until all desired areas have been sampled (typically, eight to 10 samples of breast tissue are taken 360 degrees around the lesion).

When a sufficient number of tissue samples have been collected, the radiologist or surgeon will remove the probe and apply pressure to the biopsy site. An adhesive bandage will be applied to the skin nick. In some cases, a small sterile clip will be placed into the biopsy site of the breast to mark the location in case a future biopsy is needed. This microclip is left inside the breast and causes no pain, disfigurement, or harm to the patient. After the biopsy is complete, the tissue samples will be sent to the pathology laboratory for diagnosis.

How should patients prepare for vacuum-assisted biopsy?

To prepare for a vacuum-assisted biopsy, patients may eat a light meal prior to the exam and biopsy procedure. A comfortable two-piece garment should be worn. Women should not wear talcum powder, deodorant, lotion, or perfume under their arms or on their breasts on the day of the procedure (since these may cause image artifacts or other problems). Patients who take blood thinners or aspirin should talk to their physicians about whether they should discontinue using them prior to vacuum-assisted biopsy. Any jewelry worn (especially earrings or necklaces) should be easily and quickly removable.

What should patients expect after vacuum-assisted biopsy?

An adhesive bandage is applied to the biopsy site after the procedure is complete. A cold pack may also be used to relieve swelling and reduce bruising. Patients may be instructed to take Tylenol or other pain relievers for discomfort if needed. Some bruising of the breast may occur during the first five to seven days after the biopsy (or longer if the initial bleeding during the biopsy was greater than usual). Temporary bruising of the breast after biopsy is normal and is usually not a medical concern.

Patients should contact their physicians if they experience any excessive swelling, bleeding, drainage, redness, or heat in the area of the biopsy or breast. Patients should also discuss the final results of the biopsy procedure with their referring physician within a few days of the procedure.

What are the advantages and disadvantages to vacuum-assisted biopsy?

Vacuum-assisted breast biopsy is becoming more common but requires a highly skilled radiologist or surgeon who is experienced in performing the procedure. Some patients are not good candidates for vacuum-assisted biopsy or may have lesions (breast abnormalities) that are difficult to locate with minimally-invasive equipment.

However, many breast lesions (abnormalities) are able to be biopsied using the vacuum-assisted method, and if a patient is a candidate for vacuum-assisted biopsy, there are several advantages over the traditional open surgical biopsy.

Table 22.1. Vacuum-assisted biopsy vs. surgical biopsy

Vacuum-Assisted Biopsy	Open Surgical Biopsy
Minimally invasive, requires 0.25 inch incision (approximately 0.6 cm)	Requires 1.5 to 2 inch incision (approximately 3.8 cm to 5.1 cm)
Usually no significant scarring	May potentially cause substantial scarring
Performed under local anesthesia	Performed under local or general anesthesia
Does not require stitches	Requires stitches
Procedure takes less than one hour	Procedure takes longer than one hour
Patients can usually return to normal activity shortly after procedure	Requires at least one full day of recovery after the procedure
Typically costs significantly less than open surgical biopsy	Typically costs more than vacuum-assisted biopsy and is usually the most expensive method of biopsy
Usually provides a definitive diagnosis based on tissue samples	Provides a definitive diagnosis based on tissue samples

Open Surgical Biopsy (Excisional and Incisional)

What is open surgical biopsy?

Traditional open surgical biopsy is the gold standard to which other methods of breast biopsies are compared. Surgical biopsy requires a 1.5 to 2.0 inch incision (approximately 3.8 centimeters to 5.1 centimeters) in the breast. Until about a decade ago, most breast biopsies were open surgical procedures. However today, many patients are candidates for less invasive biopsy procedures such as vacuum-assisted biopsy (Mammotome or MIBB) or core needle biopsy.

How is open surgical biopsy performed?

First, the breast is cleaned and covered with special surgical drapes. Often, surgical biopsy does not require general anesthesia. Instead, the patient will be given a local anesthetic (to the breast only), or a combination of intravenous (through the vein) sedation with local anesthetic.

During an excisional surgical biopsy, the surgeon will attempt to completely remove the area of concern (lesion), often along with a surrounding margin of normal breast tissue. If the lesion is palpable (can be felt by examination), excisional biopsy is generally a brief, straightforward surgery performed in an operating room.

An incisional surgical biopsy is similar to an excisional biopsy except that the surgeon only removes part of the breast lesion. Incisional breast biopsy is usually only performed on large lesions.

In some cases, the surgeon will use mammography (x-rays) to help locate the area of concern and then mark the area with a wire marker, visible dye, carbon particles, or several of these methods. This technique is referred to as "needle" or "wire" localization and is necessary when the abnormality can only be seen on imaging tests, such as a mammogram or ultrasound, and cannot be felt by routine examination. With "needle" or "wire" localization, the radiologist will localize (identify) the abnormality seen on a mammogram or ultrasound using a thin, hollow needle. He or she will then insert a thin wire through the center of the hollow needle to indicate the exact area of removal. A hook at the end of the wire keeps it from slipping from the soft breast tissue. The radiologist will then remove the hollow needle, and the wire will be used as a guide to located the lesion (breast abnormality). A second mammogram is taken to ensure the wire is positioned in the correct area of the breast.

The woman is then taken to the operating room where the surgeon will remove the wire (which indicates the area of the breast abnormality) and a surrounding margin of breast tissue. One set of x-rays will be taken of the removed specimen with the wire. Another set of x-rays will be taken of the breast to confirm that the area in question has in fact been removed. When this is completed, the entire specimen will then be sent to the laboratory for examination by a pathologist.

The incision will be closed with suture material. If the suture material is absorbable, the stitches will usually dissolve on their own. However, if non-absorbable suture material is used, patients will need to have the stitches removed during a follow-up office visit.

How should patients prepare for open surgical biopsy?

Patients are typically given detailed instructions by their physician and anesthesiologist in advance of the day of their surgical biopsy. Patients should avoid eating or drinking anything after midnight if they are scheduled for a surgical biopsy the next morning or afternoon. There are exceptions when patients may be instructed to take certain regular medications, such as blood pressure medications or diabetes medication, by their physician or anesthesiologist.

Women should not wear talcum powder, deodorant, lotion, or perfume under their arms or on their breasts on the day of the biopsy (as these may cause image artifacts or other problems). Patients who take blood thinners or aspirin should ask their physician about discontinuing them prior to surgery (typically three days for Coumadin or other blood thinners, seven days for aspirin or ibuprofen).

What should patients expect after open surgical biopsy?

Open surgical biopsy requires stitches and a longer period of recovery than percutaneous ("through the skin") breast biopsy procedures (such as fine needle aspiration (FNA), core needle biopsy, or vacuum-assisted biopsy). Usually, at least one full day of recovery is required.

The scar from a surgical biopsy is typically small. However, whether or not surgery will change the shape of a woman's breast depends on a number of factors, including:

- The size of the breast lesion
- The location of the breast lesion
- The amount of surrounding breast tissue that is removed in addition to the lesion

What are the advantages and disadvantages to open surgical biopsy?

Surgical biopsy yields the largest breast tissue sample of all the breast biopsy methods, and the accuracy of a diagnosis using the open surgical method is close to 100%, making it the "gold standard" of breast biopsy methods.

Nevertheless, while surgical biopsy may be the best choice for some patients, it does have disadvantages, especially if the breast lesion is found to be benign (non-cancerous):

- It requires stitches and can leave a scar
- Scar formation within the breast may persist for 12 months or longer and may complicate the interpretation of follow up mammograms

Other, more rare complications may include:

- Chances of bleeding, infection, or problems with wound healing
- Mortality risks associated with the use of anesthesia
- The chance of having a piece of the localizing wire break off deep within the breast (though this is not usually a serious problem even if it does occur)

Women are strongly encouraged to discuss all aspects of their biopsy with their surgeon prior to undergoing the procedure. Surgical biopsy usually requires at least one day of recuperation at home after surgery. Women should also discuss possible alternatives to surgical breast biopsy with their physician, such as vacuum-assisted biopsy and core needle biopsy.

Chapter 23

Sentinel Lymph Node Biopsy

What is a lymph node?

A lymph node is part of the body's lymphatic system. In the lymphatic system, a network of lymph vessels carries clear fluid called lymph. Lymph vessels lead to lymph nodes, which are small, round organs that trap cancer cells, bacteria, or other harmful substances that may be in the lymph. Groups of lymph nodes are found in the neck, underarms, chest, abdomen, and groin.

What is a sentinel lymph node (SLN)?

The sentinel lymph node is the first lymph node to which cancer is likely to spread from the primary tumor. Cancer cells may appear in the sentinel node before spreading to other lymph nodes. In some cases, there can be more than one sentinel lymph node.

What is SLN biopsy?

SLN biopsy is a procedure in which the sentinel lymph node is removed and examined under a microscope to determine whether cancer cells are present. SLN biopsy is based on the idea that cancer cells spread (metastasize) in an orderly way from the primary tumor to the sentinel lymph node(s), then to other nearby lymph nodes.[1, 2]

"Sentinel Lymph Node Biopsy: Questions and Answers," National Cancer Institute (www.cancer.gov), April 27, 2005.

197

A negative SLN biopsy result suggests that cancer has not spread to the lymph nodes. A positive result indicates that cancer is present in the SLN and may be present in other lymph nodes in the same area (regional lymph nodes). This information may help the doctor determine the stage of cancer (extent of the disease within the body) and develop an appropriate treatment plan.[2]

What happens during the SLN biopsy procedure?

In SLN biopsy, one or a few lymph nodes (the sentinel node or nodes) are removed. To identify the sentinel lymph node(s), the surgeon injects a radioactive substance, blue dye, or both near the tumor. The surgeon then uses a scanner to find the sentinel lymph nodes(s) containing the radioactive substance or looks for the lymph node(s) stained with dye. Once the SLN is located, the surgeon makes a small incision (about ½ inch) in the skin overlying the SLN and removes the lymph node(s).

The sentinel node(s) is/are checked for the presence of cancer cells by a pathologist (a doctor who identifies diseases by studying cells and tissue under a microscope). If cancer is found, the surgeon will usually remove more lymph nodes during the biopsy procedure or during a follow-up surgical procedure. SLN biopsy may be done on an outpatient basis or require a short stay in the hospital.

What are the possible benefits of SLN biopsy?

To understand the possible benefits of SLN biopsy, it helps to know about standard lymph node removal. Standard lymph node removal involves surgery to remove most of the lymph nodes in the area of the tumor (regional lymph nodes). For example, breast cancer surgery may include removing most of the axillary lymph nodes, the group of lymph nodes under the arm. This is called axillary lymph node dissection (ALND).

If SLN biopsy is done and the sentinel node does not contain cancer cells, the rest of the regional lymph nodes may not need to be removed. Because fewer lymph nodes are removed, there may be fewer side effects. When multiple regional lymph nodes are removed, the patient may experience side effects such as lymphedema (swelling caused by excess fluid build-up), numbness, a persistent burning sensation, infection, and difficulty moving the affected body area.[1, 3]

What are the side effects and disadvantages of SLN biopsy?

Side effects of SLN biopsy can include pain or bruising at the biopsy site and the rare possibility of an allergic reaction to the blue dye used to find the sentinel node. Patients may find that their urine is discolored or that their skin has been stained the same color as the dye. These problems are temporary.[2]

Although some surgeons consider SLN biopsy to be the standard of care for some cancers, its role and benefit are yet to be determined.[2] We do not know whether SLN biopsy improves a patient's survival or reduces the chance that the cancer will recur (come back). That is why studies are being conducted to compare SLN biopsy with standard lymph node dissection.

What research has been done with SLN biopsy?

The concept of mapping (finding) the SLN was first reported in 1977 by a researcher studying cancer of the penis.[2, 3, 4] In the 1980s, researchers at the University of California, Los Angeles (UCLA) developed the technique of lymphatic mapping to identify the SLN in patients with melanoma.[3] SLN mapping for breast cancer was first reported in 1994.[1, 3] Since then, researchers have improved methods for finding the SLN. Several studies have shown that when the sentinel node is negative, the remaining nodes are usually negative.[1, 3] However, these studies were done in a small number of centers and overall survival was not examined.

Other research has focused on the identification of the SLN in patients with cancer of the vulva, cervix, prostate, bladder, thyroid, head and neck, colon, rectum, stomach, as well as non-small-cell lung cancer and Merkel cell cancer.[2, 3, 4, 5] Clinical studies continue to examine the accuracy of SLN biopsy and its effect on survival of people with various cancers.

What clinical trials (research studies) are being conducted with SLN biopsy?

The National Cancer Institute (NCI) recently sponsored two large randomized clinical trials (research studies) for breast cancer comparing SLN biopsy with conventional axillary lymph node dissection. The trials were conducted by the National Surgical Adjuvant Breast and Bowel Project (NSABP) and the American College of Surgeons Oncology Group (ACOSOG). NSABP and ACOSOG are both NCI-sponsored Clinical Trials Cooperative Groups, which are networks of institutions and physicians across the country who jointly conduct trials. Although several studies have examined the correlation between the sentinel node and the remaining axillary nodes, these are the first two randomized trials that will compare the long-term results of SLN removal with full axillary node dissection. Both of these large trials are now closed.

Where can people find more information about clinical trials with SLN biopsy?

The NCI's website provides general information about clinical trials at http://www.cancer.gov/clinicaltrials on the internet. It also links to PDQ®, the NCI's cancer information database. PDQ contains detailed information about specific ongoing clinical trials in the United States, Europe, and elsewhere.

Information about clinical trials with SLN biopsy is also available from the NCI's Cancer Information Service (CIS). The CIS, a national information and education network, is a free public service of the NCI, the Nation's primary agency for cancer research. The toll-free phone number for the CIS is 800-4-CANCER (800-422-6237). For callers with TTY equipment, the number is 800-332-8615. The CIS also offers online assistance through the Help link at http://www.cancer.gov on the internet.

Selected References

1. Harris JR, Lippman ME, Morrow M, Osborne CK, editors. *Diseases of the Breast*. 3rd ed. Philadelphia: Lippincott Williams & Wilkins, 2004.

2. DeVita VT Jr., Hellman S, Rosenberg SA, editors. *Cancer: Principles and Practice of Oncology*. Vol. 1 and 2. 6th ed. Philadelphia: Lippincott Williams and Wilkins, 2001.

3. Cochran AJ, Roberts AA, Saida T. The place of lymphatic mapping and sentinel node biopsy in oncology. *International Journal of Clinical Oncology* 2003; 8:139–150.

4. Gipponi M, Solari N, Di Somma FC, Bertoglio S, Cafiero F. New fields of application of the sentinel lymph node biopsy in the pathologic staging of solid neoplasms: Review of literature and surgical perspectives. *Journal of Surgical Oncology* 2004; 85:171–179.

5. Ota DM. What's new in general surgery: Surgical oncology. *Journal of the American College of Surgeons* 2003; 196(6):926–932.

Chapter 24

Questions and Answers about Your Pathology Report

What is a pathology report?

A pathology report is a document that contains the diagnosis determined by examining cells and tissues under a microscope. The report may also contain information about the size, shape, and appearance of a specimen as it looks to the naked eye. This information is known as the gross description.

A pathologist is a doctor who does this examination and writes the pathology report. Pathology reports play an important role in cancer diagnosis and staging (describing the extent of cancer within the body, especially whether it has spread), which helps determine treatment options.

How is tissue obtained for examination by the pathologist?

In most cases, a doctor needs to do a biopsy or surgery to remove cells or tissues for examination under a microscope.

Some common ways a biopsy can be done are as follows:

- A needle is used to withdraw tissue or fluid.

- An endoscope (a thin, lighted tube) is used to look at areas inside the body and remove cells or tissues.

"Pathology Reports: Questions and Answers," National Cancer Institute (www.cancer.gov), December 6, 2007.

- Surgery is used to remove part of the tumor or the entire tumor. If the entire tumor is removed, typically some normal tissue around the tumor is also removed.

Tissue removed during a biopsy is sent to a pathology laboratory, where it is sliced into thin sections for viewing under a microscope. This is known as histologic (tissue) examination and is usually the best way to tell if cancer is present. The pathologist may also examine cytologic (cell) material. Cytologic material is present in urine, cerebrospinal fluid (the fluid around the brain and spinal cord), sputum (mucus from the lungs), peritoneal (abdominal cavity) fluid, pleural (chest cavity) fluid, cervical/vaginal smears, and in fluid removed during a biopsy.

How is tissue processed after a biopsy or surgery? What is a frozen section?

The tissue removed during a biopsy or surgery must be cut into thin sections, placed on slides, and stained with dyes before it can be examined under a microscope. Two methods are used to make the tissue firm enough to cut into thin sections: frozen sections and paraffin-embedded (permanent) sections. All tissue samples are prepared as permanent sections, but sometimes frozen sections are also prepared.

Permanent sections are prepared by placing the tissue in fixative (usually formalin) to preserve the tissue, processing it through additional solutions, and then placing it in paraffin wax. After the wax has hardened, the tissue is cut into very thin slices, which are placed on slides and stained. The process normally takes several days. A permanent section provides the best quality for examination by the pathologist and produces more accurate results than a frozen section.[1]

Frozen sections are prepared by freezing and slicing the tissue sample. They can be done in about 15 to 20 minutes while the patient is in the operating room.[1] Frozen sections are done when an immediate answer is needed; for example, to determine whether the tissue is cancerous so as to guide the surgeon during the course of an operation.

How long after the tissue sample is taken will the pathology report be ready?

The pathologist sends a pathology report to the doctor within 10 days after the biopsy or surgery is performed. Pathology reports are written in technical medical language. Patients may want to ask their doctors to give them a copy of the pathology report and to explain the report to them. Patients also may wish to keep a copy of their pathology report in their own records.[1]

What information does a pathology report usually include?

The pathology report may include the following information:[1]

- **Patient information:** Name, birth date, biopsy date

- **Gross description:** Color, weight, and size of tissue as seen by the naked eye

- **Microscopic description:** How the sample looks under the microscope and how it compares with normal cells

- **Diagnosis:** Type of tumor/cancer and grade (how abnormal the cells look under the microscope and how quickly the tumor is likely to grow and spread)

- **Tumor size:** Measured in centimeters

- **Tumor margins:** There are three possible findings when the biopsy sample is the entire tumor:
  - Positive margins mean that cancer cells are found at the edge of the material removed
  - Negative, not involved, clear, or free margins mean that no cancer cells are found at the outer edge
  - Close margins are neither negative nor positive

- **Other information:** Usually notes about samples that have been sent for other tests or a second opinion

- **Pathologist's signature** and name and address of the laboratory

What might the pathology report say about the physical and chemical characteristics of the tissue?

After identifying the tissue as cancerous, the pathologist may perform additional tests to get more information about the tumor that cannot be determined by looking at the tissue with routine stains, such as hematoxylin and eosin (also known as H&E), under a microscope.[2] The pathology report will include the results of these tests. For example, the pathology report may include information obtained from immunochemical stains (IHC). IHC uses antibodies to identify specific antigens on the surface of cancer cells. IHC can often be used for the following:

- Determine where the cancer started

- Distinguish among different cancer types: for example, carcinoma, melanoma, and lymphoma

- Help diagnose and classify leukemias and lymphomas[3]

The pathology report may also include the results of flow cytometry. Flow cytometry is a method of measuring properties of cells in a sample, including the number of cells, percentage of live cells, cell size and shape, and presence of tumor markers on the cell surface. (Tumor markers are substances produced by tumor cells or by other cells in the body in response to cancer or certain noncancerous conditions.) Flow cytometry can be used in the diagnosis, classification, and management of cancers such as acute leukemia, chronic lymphoproliferative disorders, and non-Hodgkin lymphoma.[2]

Finally, the pathology report may include the results of molecular diagnostic and cytogenetic studies. Such studies investigate the presence or absence of malignant cells, and genetic or molecular abnormalities in specimens.

What information about the genetics of the cells might be included in the pathology report?

Cytogenetics uses tissue culture and specialized techniques to provide genetic information about cells, particularly genetic alterations. Some genetic alterations are markers or indicators of a specific cancer. For example, the Philadelphia chromosome is associated with chronic myelogenous leukemia (CML). Some alterations can provide information about prognosis, which helps the doctor make treatment recommendations.[3] Some tests that might be performed on a tissue sample include the following:

- Fluorescence in situ hybridization (FISH) determines the positions of particular genes. It can be used to identify chromosomal abnormalities and to map genes.

- Polymerase chain reaction (PCR) is a method of making many copies of particular DNA sequences of relevance to the diagnosis.

- Real-time PCR or quantitative PCR is a method of measuring how many copies of a particular DNA sequence are present.

- Reverse-transcriptase polymerase chain reaction (RT-PCR) is a method of making many copies of a specific RNA sequence.

- Southern blot hybridization detects specific DNA fragments.

- Western blot hybridization identifies and analyzes proteins or peptides.

Can individuals get a second opinion about their pathology results?

Although most cancers can be easily diagnosed, sometimes patients or their doctors may want to get a second opinion about the pathology results.[1] Patients interested in getting a second opinion should talk with their doctor. They will need to obtain the slides and/or paraffin block from the pathologist who examined the sample or from the hospital where the biopsy or surgery was done.

Some cancer centers and other facilities, such as the Armed Forces Institute of Pathology (AFIP), provide second opinions on pathology specimens. Patients should contact the facility in advance to determine if this service is available, the cost, and shipping instructions. Contact information for National Cancer Institute (NCI)-designated cancer centers can be found in the NCI-Designated Cancer Centers database available at http://www.cancer.gov/cancertopics/factsheet/NCI/cancer-centers on the internet. Additional information about the AFIP is available on their website at http://www.afip.org on the internet.

What research is being done to improve the diagnosis of cancer?

NCI, a component of the National Institutes of Health, is sponsoring clinical trials that are designed to improve the accuracy and specificity of cancer diagnoses. Before any new method can be recommended for general use, doctors conduct clinical trials to find out whether it is safe and effective.

People interested in taking part in a clinical trial should talk with their doctor. Information about clinical trials is available from the NCI's Cancer Information Service (CIS) at 800-4-CANCER and in the NCI fact sheet "Clinical Trials: Questions and Answers," which is available at http://www.cancer.gov/cancertopics/factsheet/Information/clinical-trials on the internet. This fact sheet includes information about types of clinical trials, who sponsors them, how they are conducted, how participants are protected, and who pays for the patient care costs associated with a clinical trial. Further information about clinical trials is available at http://www.cancer.gov/clinicaltrials on the NCI's website. The website offers detailed information about specific ongoing studies by linking to PDQ®, the NCI's comprehensive cancer information database. The CIS also provides information from PDQ.

Selected References

1. Morra M, Potts E. *Choices*. 4th ed. New York: HarperResource, 2003.

2. Borowitz M, Westra W, Cooley LD, et al. Pathology and laboratory medicine. In: Abeloff MD, Armitage JO, Niederhuber JE, Kastan MB, McKenna WG, editors. *Clinical Oncology*. 3rd ed. London: Churchill Livingstone, 2004.

3. Connolly JL, Schnitt SJ, Wang HH, et al. Principles of cancer pathology. In: Bast RC Jr., Kufe DW, Pollock RE, et al., editors. *Cancer Medicine*. 6th ed. Hamilton, Ontario, Canada: BC Decker Inc., 2003.

Chapter 25

Hormone Receptor Status Testing

At a Glance

Why get tested?

To determine whether a breast cancer tumor is positive for estrogen and/or progesterone receptors, which helps to guide treatment and determine prognosis.

When to get tested?

If you have been diagnosed with breast cancer and your doctor wants to determine whether the tumor's growth is influenced by the hormones estrogen and/or progesterone.

Sample required?

A sample of breast cancer tissue obtained during a biopsy or a tumor removed surgically during a lumpectomy or mastectomy.

The Test Sample

What is being tested?

Estrogen receptors (ER) and progesterone receptors (PR) are specialized proteins found within certain cells throughout the body. These

---

receptors bind to estrogen and progesterone, female hormones that circulate in the blood, and promote new cell growth and division.

Many breast cancer tumors have receptors for estrogen and/or progesterone, often in large numbers. These tumors are said to be hormone-dependent, and estrogen and/or progesterone feed their growth. Breast cancer tissue can be tested to see if it is positive for these receptors.

How is the sample collected for testing?

A sample of breast cancer tissue is obtained (such as by doing a fine needle aspiration, needle biopsy, or surgical biopsy) or a tumor removed surgically during a lumpectomy or mastectomy is tested.

The Test

How is it used?

Hormone receptor status is used as a prognostic marker. Those with ER-positive and PR-positive tumors tend to have a better prognosis than those with ER-negative or PR-negative tumors.

The hormone receptor status test is also used to help determine treatment options, including endocrine therapy (anti-hormone treatments, such as tamoxifen), when a primary tumor has been removed or to help guide treatment decisions when a tumor recurs.

When is it ordered?

Hormone receptor status testing is recommended as part of an initial workup of invasive breast cancer. It is not diagnostic but helps the doctor to determine treatment options and to understand more about the tumor's characteristics.

What does the test result mean?

In general, if a patient's cancer is ER-positive and PR-positive, the patient will have a better-than-average prognosis, and their cancer is likely to respond to endocrine therapy (anti-hormone treatments). The more receptors present and the more intense their reaction, the more likely the response. However, an individual's response depends on a variety of factors.

If a patient's cancer is ER-negative but PR-positive, the patient may still benefit from endocrine therapy but may have a diminished response.

If the cancer is both ER-negative and PR-negative, then the patient will probably not benefit from endocrine therapy.

Is there anything else I should know?

HER2/neu testing may be done at the same time as hormone receptor status testing. A patient with a positive estrogen and/or progesterone receptor status may find their response to endocrine therapy diminished if they are also HER2/neu-positive.

Hormone receptor status testing is not available in every laboratory. It requires experience and special training to perform and interpret. Your doctor will probably send your sample to a reference laboratory and it may take several weeks before your results are available.

It takes a small amount of cancer tissue to perform the hormone receptor status testing. If a sufficient sample is not available, your doctor may make an assumption that your cancer is ER-positive and PR-positive in order to broaden your treatment options.

Common Question

Is there a blood test that can be done to check my hormone receptor status?

No. The cancer cells do not "shed" the receptors, so they are not detectable in the blood. They must be evaluated in the cancer tissue itself.

Chapter 26

Human Epidermal Growth Factor Receptor (HER2/neu) Testing

At a Glance

Why get tested?

To determine whether a breast cancer tumor is positive for HER2/ neu, which helps to guide treatment and determine prognosis.

When to get tested?

If you have been diagnosed with invasive breast cancer and your doctor wants to determine whether the HER2/neu gene is being over-expressed in the tumor.

Sample required?

A sample of breast cancer tissue obtained during a biopsy; some-times a blood sample, drawn from a vein in your arm, is also required.

The Test Sample

What is being tested?

HER2/neu is an oncogene. It codes for a receptor for a particular growth factor that causes cells to grow. Normal epithelial cells contain two copies of the HER2/neu gene and produce low levels of the HER2 protein on the surface of their cells. In about 20–30% of invasive breast cancers (and some other cancers, such as ovarian and bladder cancer), the HER2/neu gene is amplified and its protein is over-expressed. Tumors that have this over-expression tend to grow more aggressively and resist hormonal therapy and some chemotherapies, and patients generally have a poorer prognosis.

There are two main ways to test HER2/neu status: immunohistochemistry (IHC) and fluorescent in situ hybridization (FISH). IHC measures the amount of HER2/neu protein present. FISH looks at the genetic level for actual gene amplification—the number of copies of the gene present. IHC is currently the most widely used initial testing method; however, if it is indeterminate or negative, then the FISH method is often done as a follow-up test.

How is the sample collected for testing?

A sample of breast cancer tissue is obtained by doing a fine needle aspiration, needle biopsy, or surgical biopsy. HER2/neu protein sometimes is measured in a blood sample, drawn from a vein in the arm. The amount of HER2/neu protein present in serum is loosely associated with the amount of cancer present; however it will not be positive until the tumor is fairly big and is not widely used for determining HER2/neu status.

The Test

How is it used?

HER2/neu testing is used as a prognostic marker to help determine how aggressive a breast cancer tumor is likely to be.

It is also used as a predictor of response to therapy, such as hormone therapy and chemotherapy.

The serum HER2/neu test is sometimes used to monitor cancer therapy. If the level is initially elevated then falls, it is likely that treatment is working; if it stays elevated, treatment is not working; and if the level falls then rises, the cancer may be recurring.

When is it ordered?

HER2/neu testing is recommended as part of an initial workup of invasive breast cancer and is sometimes done with recurrent breast cancer. It is not diagnostic but helps the doctor determine treatment options and understand more about the tumor's characteristics.

Serum HER2/neu is sometimes ordered initially to establish a baseline and then, if elevated, used to monitor cancer treatment. However, this method is not widely used because levels are only elevated when a large amount of cancer is present so early cancers are likely to be negative for serum HER2/neu.

What does the test result mean?

If an IHC HER2/neu test is positive, it means that the HER2/neu gene is over-expressing the HER2/neu protein. If a FISH test is done, then amplification of the HER2/neu gene can be detected. If either of these is positive, then the patient is likely to have a tumor that is aggressive, that will respond poorly to hormone treatment, and that will be resistant to chemotherapy. These patients may be considered candidates for Herceptin therapy.

If the IHC is negative but the FISH is positive, the patient still may benefit from Herceptin, but if both are negative the treatment will not be useful.

Is there anything else I should know?

HER2/neu-positive tumors are susceptible to Herceptin (trastuzumab), a drug therapy that was created to target HER2/neu protein. Herceptin attaches itself to the excess protein molecules and inhibits the growth of the cancer. The development of this specialized therapy has increased the use of HER2/neu testing. Herceptin may be used alone or with some chemotherapy agents but is only useful in those who have HER2/neu amplification and protein over-expression.

HER2/neu testing is not available in every laboratory. Both IHC and FISH require experience and special training to perform and interpret. Your doctor will probably send your sample to a reference laboratory and the results may take several weeks to return.

It takes a small amount of cancer tissue to perform the HER2/neu test. If a sufficient sample is not available, your doctor may try running a serum HER2/neu test and/or make an assumption that you are HER2/neu-positive in order to broaden your treatment options.

Common Questions

Besides HER2/neu, what other laboratory tests may my doctor be ordering on my breast cancer tissue?

During an initial workup of invasive breast cancer, your doctor will likely do a tissue test for hormone receptor status. A patient with a positive estrogen and/or progesterone receptor status may find their response to endocrine/hormone therapy diminished if they are also HER2/neu-positive, limiting that treatment option.

Does Herceptin work for everyone who is HER2/neu positive?

Unfortunately, no. Only about one-third of patients who are positive for HER2/neu will respond to Herceptin therapy. There are other cellular factors involved that are not well understood yet. Herceptin is sometimes combined with other chemotherapy agents to make it more effective.

Chapter 27

Cancer Antigen (CA) 15-3 Testing

At a Glance

Why get tested?

To monitor the response to treatment of invasive breast cancer and to watch for recurrence of the disease.

When to get tested?

When you have been or are being treated for invasive breast cancer.

Sample required?

A blood sample drawn from a vein in your arm.

The Test Sample

What is being tested?

Cancer antigen 15-3 (CA 15-3) is a normal product of breast cells; it is produced by a gene that is often over-expressed (that is, the body makes too many copies) in cancerous breast tumors, leading to an increased production of CA 15-3 and the related cancer antigen 27.29

(which measures the same marker but in a different way). CA 15-3 does not cause cancer; rather, it is a protein that is shed by the tumor cells, making it useful as a tumor marker to follow the course of the cancer.

CA 15-3 is elevated in about 30% of women with localized breast cancer and in about 75% of those with metastatic breast cancer (cancer that has spread to other organs). CA 15-3 also may be elevated in healthy people and in individuals with other cancers, conditions, or diseases, such as colorectal cancer, lung cancer, cirrhosis, hepatitis, and benign breast disease.

How is the sample collected for testing?

A blood sample is obtained by inserting a needle into a vein in the arm.

The Test

How is it used?

CA 15-3 is not sensitive or specific enough to be considered useful as a tool for cancer screening. Its main use is as a tumor marker to monitor a patient's response to breast cancer treatment and to watch for breast cancer recurrence. CA 15-3 can only be used as a marker if the cancer is producing elevated amounts of it; however, since only a small percent of women with localized breast cancer have increased CA 15-3, it may still be able to be used later as a marker. CA 15-3 sometimes may also be used to give a doctor a general sense of how much cancer may be present.

When is it ordered?

CA 15-3 may be ordered along with other tests, such as estrogen and progesterone receptors, HER2/neu, and BRCA-1 and BRCA-2 genetic testing, when advanced breast cancer is first diagnosed to help determine cancer characteristics and treatment options.

If CA 15-3 is initially elevated, then it may be used to monitor treatment and, if repeated on a regular basis, to detect recurrence. CA 15-3 is usually not done when breast cancer is detected early, before it has metastasized, because levels will not be elevated in the majority of early cancers.

What does the test result mean?

In general, the higher the CA 15-3 level the more advanced the breast cancer and the larger the tumor burden (amount of tumor present). The level tends to increase as the cancer grows. In metastatic breast cancer, the highest levels of CA 15-3 often are seen when the cancer has spread to the bones and/or the liver.

Mild to moderate elevations of CA 15-3 also are seen in a variety of conditions, including liver and pancreatic cancer, cirrhosis, and benign breast disorders as well as in a certain percentage of apparently healthy individuals. The CA 15-3 elevations seen in these non-cancerous conditions tend to be stable over time.

Negative CA 15-3 levels do not ensure that a patient does not have cancer. It may be too soon in the disease for elevated levels to be detected. In addition, 25% to 30% of individuals with advanced breast cancer have tumors that do not shed CA 15-3.

Is there anything else I should know?

Levels of CA 15-3 are not usually taken immediately after breast cancer treatment begins. There have been instances of transient (temporary) increases and decreases in CA 15-3 that do not correlate with the patient's progress. Usually, your doctor will wait a few weeks after starting treatment to begin monitoring CA 15-3 levels.

Common Questions

Should I have a test for CA 27.29 in addition to the CA 15-3 test?

CA 27.29 is protein that is produced by the same gene (MUC1) as CA 15-3 and is used in the same way. It is newer than CA 15-3, but most doctors consider it essentially equivalent to CA 15-3. It can be used instead of CA 15-3, but you usually wouldn't have both tests.

I have a strong family history of breast cancer. Shouldn't I be screened for CA 15-3?

CA 15-3 is not recommended as a screening tool. It is not specific or sensitive enough to detect early breast cancer. Any CA 15-3 elevations seen may be due to other causes, and negative results do not ensure that you do not have cancer. It should only be used after breast cancer has been diagnosed.

What can I do to lower my CA 15-3?

There is nothing you can do directly to lower your CA 15-3 level. It is not a risk factor like cholesterol that can be lowered through dietary restrictions and exercise. It is a reflection of what is going on in your body. CA 15-3 may rise with tumor growth and fall with treatment, or it may be mildly elevated and stable in a benign condition.

Part Four

Breast Cancer Treatment

Chapter 28

Treatment Options for Breast Cancer Patients

Treatment Option Overview

Different types of treatment are available for patients with breast cancer. Some treatments are standard (the currently used treatment), and some are being tested in clinical trials. Before starting treatment, patients may want to think about taking part in a clinical trial. A treatment clinical trial is a research study meant to help improve current treatments or obtain information on new treatments for patients with cancer. When clinical trials show that a new treatment is better than the standard treatment, the new treatment may become the standard treatment.

Clinical trials are taking place in many parts of the country. Information about ongoing clinical trials is available from the National Cancer Institute (NCI) website (available online at http://www.cancer.gov/clinicaltrials). Choosing the most appropriate cancer treatment is a decision that ideally involves the patient, family, and health care team.

Four types of standard treatment are used:

Surgery

Most patients with breast cancer have surgery to remove the cancer from the breast. Some of the lymph nodes under the arm are usually

Excerpted from PDQ® Cancer Information Summary. National Cancer Institute; Bethesda, MD. Breast Cancer (PDQ®): Treatment - Patient. Updated 02/07/2008. Available at: http://cancer.gov. Accessed March 24, 2008.

taken out and looked at under a microscope to see if they contain cancer cells.

Breast-conserving surgery, an operation to remove the cancer but not the breast itself, includes the following:

- **Lumpectomy:** Surgery to remove a tumor (lump) and a small amount of normal tissue around it.

- **Partial mastectomy:** Surgery to remove the part of the breast that has cancer and some normal tissue around it. This procedure is also called a segmental mastectomy.

Patients who are treated with breast-conserving surgery may also have some of the lymph nodes under the arm removed for biopsy. This procedure is called lymph node dissection. It may be done at the same time as the breast-conserving surgery or after. Lymph node dissection is done through a separate incision.

Other types of surgery include the following:

- **Total mastectomy:** Surgery to remove the whole breast that has cancer. This procedure is also called a simple mastectomy. Some of the lymph nodes under the arm may be removed for biopsy at the same time as the breast surgery or after. This is done through a separate incision.

- **Modified radical mastectomy:** Surgery to remove the whole breast that has cancer, many of the lymph nodes under the arm, the lining over the chest muscles, and sometimes, part of the chest wall muscles.

- **Radical mastectomy:** Surgery to remove the breast that has cancer, chest wall muscles under the breast, and all of the lymph nodes under the arm. This procedure is sometimes called a Halsted radical mastectomy.

Even if the doctor removes all the cancer that can be seen at the time of the surgery, some patients may be given radiation therapy, chemotherapy, or hormone therapy after surgery to kill any cancer cells that are left. Treatment given after the surgery, to increase the chances of a cure, is called adjuvant therapy.

If a patient is going to have a mastectomy, breast reconstruction (surgery to rebuild a breast's shape after a mastectomy) may be considered. Breast reconstruction may be done at the time of the mastectomy or at a future time. The reconstructed breast may be made with the patient's own (nonbreast) tissue or by using implants filled with saline or silicone gel. Before the decision to get an implant is made, patients can call the Food and Drug Administration's (FDA) Center for Devices and Radiologic Health at 888-INFO-FDA (888-463-6332) or visit the FDA's website (http://www.fda.gov/cdrh/breastimplants) for more information on breast implants.

Radiation therapy

Radiation therapy is a cancer treatment that uses high-energy x-rays or other types of radiation to kill cancer cells or keep them from growing. There are two types of radiation therapy. External radiation therapy uses a machine outside the body to send radiation toward the cancer. Internal radiation therapy uses a radioactive substance sealed in needles, seeds, wires, or catheters that are placed directly into or near the cancer. The way the radiation therapy is given depends on the type and stage of the cancer being treated.

Chemotherapy

Chemotherapy is a cancer treatment that uses drugs to stop the growth of cancer cells, either by killing the cells or by stopping them from dividing. When chemotherapy is taken by mouth or injected into a vein or muscle, the drugs enter the bloodstream and can reach cancer cells throughout the body (systemic chemotherapy). When chemotherapy is placed directly into the spinal column, an organ, or a body cavity such as the abdomen, the drugs mainly affect cancer cells in those areas (regional chemotherapy). The way the chemotherapy is given depends on the type and stage of the cancer being treated.

Hormone Therapy

Hormone therapy is a cancer treatment that removes hormones or blocks their action and stops cancer cells from growing. Hormones are substances produced by glands in the body and circulated in the bloodstream. Some hormones can cause certain cancers to grow. If tests show that the cancer cells have places where hormones can attach (receptors), drugs, surgery, or radiation therapy are used to reduce the production of hormones or block them from working.

Hormone therapy with tamoxifen is often given to patients with early stages of breast cancer and those with metastatic breast cancer (cancer that has spread to other parts of the body). Hormone therapy with tamoxifen or estrogens can act on cells all over the body and may increase the chance of developing endometrial cancer. Women taking tamoxifen should have a pelvic exam every year to look for any signs of cancer. Any vaginal bleeding, other than menstrual bleeding, should be reported to a doctor as soon as possible.

Hormone therapy with an aromatase inhibitor is given to some postmenopausal women who have hormone-dependent breast cancer. Hormone-dependent breast cancer needs the hormone estrogen to grow. Aromatase inhibitors decrease the body's estrogen by blocking an enzyme called aromatase from turning androgen into estrogen.

For the treatment of early stage breast cancer, certain aromatase inhibitors may be used as adjuvant therapy instead of tamoxifen or after two or more years of tamoxifen. For the treatment of metastatic breast cancer, aromatase inhibitors are being tested in clinical trials to compare them to hormone therapy with tamoxifen.

New Treatments

New types of treatment are being tested in clinical trials. These include the following:

Sentinel lymph node biopsy followed by surgery: Sentinel lymph node biopsy is the removal of the sentinel lymph node during surgery. The sentinel lymph node is the first lymph node to receive lymphatic drainage from a tumor. It is the first lymph node the cancer is likely to spread to from the tumor. A radioactive substance or blue dye is injected near the tumor. The substance or dye flows through the lymph ducts to the lymph nodes. The first lymph node to receive the substance or dye is removed. A pathologist views the tissue under a microscope to look for cancer cells. If cancer cells are not found, it may not be necessary to remove more lymph nodes. After the sentinel lymph node biopsy, the surgeon removes the tumor (breast-conserving surgery or mastectomy).

High-dose chemotherapy with stem cell transplant: High-dose chemotherapy with stem cell transplant is a way of giving high doses of chemotherapy and replacing blood-forming cells destroyed by the cancer treatment. Stem cells (immature blood cells) are removed from the blood or bone marrow of the patient or a donor and are frozen and stored. After the chemotherapy is completed, the stored stem cells are thawed and given back to the patient through an infusion. These re-infused stem cells grow into (and restore) the body's blood cells.

Studies have shown that high-dose chemotherapy followed by stem cell transplant does not work better than standard chemotherapy in the treatment of breast cancer. Doctors have decided that, for now, high-dose chemotherapy should be tested only in clinical trials. Before taking part in such a trial, women should talk with their doctors about the serious side effects, including death, that may be caused by high-dose chemotherapy.

Monoclonal antibodies as adjuvant therapy: Monoclonal antibody therapy is a cancer treatment that uses antibodies made in the laboratory, from a single type of immune system cell. These antibodies can identify substances on cancer cells or normal substances that may help cancer cells grow. The antibodies attach to the substances and kill the cancer cells, block their growth, or keep them from spreading. Monoclonal antibodies are given by infusion. They may be used alone or to carry drugs, toxins, or radioactive material directly to cancer cells. Monoclonal antibodies are also used in combination with chemotherapy as adjuvant therapy.

Trastuzumab (Herceptin) is a monoclonal antibody that blocks the effects of the growth factor protein HER2, which transmits growth signals to breast cancer cells. About one-fourth of patients with breast cancer have tumors that may be treated with trastuzumab combined with chemotherapy.

Tyrosine kinase inhibitors as adjuvant therapy: Tyrosine kinase inhibitors are targeted therapy drugs that block signals needed for tumors to grow. Tyrosine kinase inhibitors may be used in combination with other anticancer drugs as adjuvant therapy.

Lapatinib is a tyrosine kinase inhibitor that blocks the effects of the HER2 protein and other proteins inside tumor cells. It may be used to treat patients with HER2-positive breast cancer that has progressed following treatment with trastuzumab.

Treatment Options by Stage

Ductal Carcinoma in Situ (DCIS)

Treatment of ductal carcinoma in situ (DCIS) may include the following:

- Breast-conserving surgery and radiation therapy with or without tamoxifen

- Total mastectomy with or without tamoxifen

- Breast-conserving surgery without radiation therapy

- Clinical trials testing breast-conserving surgery and tamoxifen with or without radiation therapy

Check for clinical trials from NCI's PDQ Cancer Clinical Trials Registry (http://www.cancer.gov/search/ResultsClinicalTrials.aspx?protocolsearchid=4557704) that are now accepting patients with ductal breast carcinoma in situ.

Lobular Carcinoma in Situ (LCIS)

Treatment of lobular carcinoma in situ (LCIS) may include the following:

- Biopsy to diagnose the LCIS followed by regular examinations and regular mammograms to find any changes as early as possible. This is referred to as observation.
- Tamoxifen to reduce the risk of developing breast cancer
- Bilateral prophylactic mastectomy: This treatment choice is sometimes used in women who have a high risk of getting breast cancer. Most surgeons believe that this is a more aggressive treatment than is needed.
- Clinical trials testing cancer prevention drugs

Check for clinical trials from NCI's PDQ Cancer Clinical Trials Registry (http://www.cancer.gov/search/ResultsClinicalTrials.aspx?protocolsearchid=4555487) that are now accepting patients with lobular breast carcinoma in situ.

Stage I, Stage II, Stage IIIA, and Operable Stage IIIC Breast Cancer

Treatment of stage I, stage II, stage IIIA, and operable stage IIIC breast cancer may include the following:

- Breast-conserving surgery to remove only the cancer and some surrounding breast tissue, followed by lymph node dissection and radiation therapy
- Modified radical mastectomy with or without breast reconstruction surgery
- A clinical trial evaluating sentinel lymph node biopsy followed by surgery

Adjuvant therapy (treatment given after surgery to increase the chances of a cure) may include the following:

- Radiation therapy to the lymph nodes near the breast and to the chest wall after a modified radical mastectomy
- Systemic chemotherapy with or without hormone therapy
- Hormone therapy
- A clinical trial of trastuzumab (Herceptin) combined with systemic chemotherapy

Check for clinical trials from NCI's PDQ Cancer Clinical Trials Registry that are now accepting patients with:

- Stage I breast cancer (http:// www.cancer.gov/search/ ResultsClinicalTrials.aspx?protocolsearchid= 4556563);
- Stage II breast cancer (http://www.cancer.gov/search/ ResultsClinicalTrials.aspx?protocolsearchid=4556819);
- Stage IIIA breast cancer (http://www.cancer.gov/search/ ResultsClinicalTrials.aspx?protocolsearchid=4556836);
- Stage IIIC breast cancer (http://www.cancer.gov/search/ ResultsClinicalTrials.aspx?protocolsearchid=4558881).

Stage IIIB, Inoperable Stage IIIC, Stage IV, and Metastatic Breast Cancer

Stage IIIB and Inoperable Stage IIIC Breast Cancer

Treatment of stage IIIB and inoperable stage IIIC breast cancer may include the following:

- Systemic chemotherapy
- Systemic chemotherapy followed by surgery (breast-conserving surgery or total mastectomy), with lymph node dissection followed by radiation therapy. Additional systemic therapy (chemotherapy, hormone therapy, or both) may be given.
- Clinical trials testing new anticancer drugs, new drug combinations, and new ways of giving treatment

Stage IV and Metastatic Breast Cancer

Treatment of stage IV or metastatic breast cancer may include the following:

- Hormone therapy and/or systemic chemotherapy with or without trastuzumab (Herceptin)

- Tyrosine kinase inhibitor therapy with lapatinib combined with capecitabine

- Radiation therapy and/or surgery for relief of pain and other symptoms

- Clinical trials testing new systemic chemotherapy and/or hormone therapy

- Clinical trials of new combinations of trastuzumab (Herceptin) with anticancer drugs

- Clinical trials of new combinations of lapatinib with anticancer drugs

- Clinical trials testing other approaches, including high-dose chemotherapy with stem cell transplant

- Bisphosphonate drugs to reduce bone disease and pain when cancer has spread to the bone

Check for clinical trials from NCI's PDQ Cancer Clinical Trials Registry that are now accepting patients with:

- Stage IIIB breast cancer (http://www.cancer.gov/search/ ResultsClinicalTrials.aspx ?protocolsearchid=4556838);

- Stage IIIC breast cancer (http://www .cancer.gov/search/ ResultsClinicalTrials.aspx?protocolsearchid =4558881);

- Stage IV breast cancer (http://www.cancer.gov/search/ ResultsClinicalTrials.aspx?protocolsearchid=4557988).

Treatment Options for Inflammatory Breast Cancer

Treatment of inflammatory breast cancer may include the following:

- Systemic chemotherapy

- Systemic chemotherapy followed by surgery (breast-conserving surgery or total mastectomy), with lymph node dissection followed by radiation therapy. Additional systemic therapy (chemotherapy, hormone therapy, or both) may be given.

- Clinical trials testing new anticancer drugs, new drug combinations, and new ways of giving treatment

Check for clinical trials from NCI's PDQ Cancer Clinical Trials Registry (http://www.cancer.gov/search/ResultsClinicalTrials.aspx?protocolsearchid=4495565) that are now accepting patients with inflammatory breast cancer.

Treatment Options for Recurrent Breast Cancer

Treatment of recurrent breast cancer (cancer that has come back after treatment) in the breast or chest wall may include the following:

- Surgery (radical or modified radical mastectomy), radiation therapy, or both
- Systemic chemotherapy or hormone therapy
- A clinical trial of trastuzumab (Herceptin) combined with systemic chemotherapy

Check for clinical trials from NCI's PDQ Cancer Clinical Trials Registry (http://www.cancer.gov/search/ResultsClinicalTrials.aspx?protocolsearchid=4556753) that are now accepting patients with recurrent breast cancer.

Chapter 29

A Guide to Making Breast Cancer Treatment Choices

If you have just been diagnosed with breast cancer or have a strong suspicion that you might be, you are probably feeling overwhelmed, anxious, and powerless... all normal feelings when confronted with a disease that effects one in eight women in the United States. All too often women travel blindly through the health care system not knowing if they are in the best of hands that they could be.... and should be. For treatment of the common cold and other common disorders it is fine to seek out care from local physicians who would normally provide you primary care. When dealing with a life threatening situation like breast cancer however, choosing the wrong doctor or the wrong breast center can be fatal. You must choose carefully and wisely. After all, we are talking about your life.

I am a breast cancer survivor. I am also a nurse. I have been where you are right now and know the anxiousness that you feel. For more than a decade I was the director of quality of care and utilization management at Johns Hopkins Hospital, striving every day to measure and assess quality of care and work with the health care professionals here to continuously improve the care we provide. I joined the team of the Johns Hopkins Breast Center to further accomplish this goal, but have chosen to channel all my energies and expertise into the area of breast cancer. My goal is to make it easier for women like you who come behind me to also become one of the survivors like myself.

There have been many women who come to the Johns Hopkins Breast Center who have been seen by physicians elsewhere who did not provide them the ideal care and treatment they needed, this resulted in major medical problems for them long term—wrong diagnosis, incomplete or inaccurate information, misleading information, confusing information. As an institution committed to patient care and teaching, we want to provide you some guidelines as to how to go about choosing a physician and facility that is right for you. We want you to know how to choose who will take good care of you and give you your best opportunity to defeat this disease. The best answer is not always the same for each person. We want you to have the tools needed to make the very best choices for you and your family in the battle against this disease.

Though a diagnosis of breast cancer is devastating to hear, it is not something that requires emergency treatment. This is often a misleading piece of information for women. They assume that because they now have breast cancer that it must be treated immediately. Not true. Though delaying for a prolonged time period (more than a couple of months) is not advisable, in most cases, you do not have to rush into making decisions. More importantly, if a doctor tells you that you must have surgery immediately take caution. If your cancer was diagnosed with either a mammogram or because you or a physician felt a lump, the cancer has probably been growing for five to eight years. It took a long time for a few tiny cells to mature enough to become a tumor which could be seen on x-ray or felt. So you don't have to have surgery right away. You don't have to make hurried decisions without adequate information about your treatment options and about what is really best for you. You have time to gather information. You have time to gather your family and friends for support. You have time to seek out the best doctors and facilities to take of you.

At a time when you feel powerless having heard the verdict of breast cancer, it is important to seek out constructive ways to empower yourself once again and gain some stability over your life and the situation placed before you. The breast cancer specialists of the Johns Hopkins Breast Center are strong believers in the value of providing women with information about their disease and its treatment options. An informed patient is a patient who will do well psychologically. An informed patient is someone who can participate in the decision making about her care and feel confident in the choices made. An informed patient knows what to expect along each step of the way from point of diagnosis through to completion of treatment and beyond so that she is actually a member of her own health care team... an equal partner with the breast cancer specialists who have her best interest in mind—survival, good quality of life, confidence in the choices made about her health and well-being.

We have spoken to patients who have been to other physicians elsewhere and made them feel pressured to proceed quickly with treatment before they've had time to think things through and really participate in the decision making about what is best for them. If you are confronted with a doctor who is pressuring you to have surgery "right away" or who is not informing you about what all your options are, you need to seek care elsewhere. In the same light, if you are being told by a doctor information that sounds "too good to be true" compared to opinions you have gotten elsewhere (for example, if you have been told that you probably have a large tumor and/or positive lymph nodes based on physical exam, biopsy results, and mammography which would definitely require chemotherapy as part of your treatment don't be fooled by a doctor who tells you "if you have your treatment here you won't need chemotherapy." It simply isn't true... and isn't logical.) Though getting good news like this from another physician can at first sound great, if you have done your homework and study up on your clinical situation, you would know that this doesn't sound right. Don't be fooled by such an opinion. Get a third opinion if you need it. You are far better off with a breast cancer specialist who tells you frankly and honestly what your situation is than to have someone paint a rosy picture which in the end isn't so rosy.

The decisions you make can and will effect the rest of your life. That's why it is so important that you empower yourself with information so that you can determine for yourself if you are in good hands. It doesn't mean that you have to have a medical degree either. It does mean that you need to take some time and read about breast cancer, the various treatments that are available to treat this disease, and how to best determine for you personally what will be the right choices for your situation. You have time to gather information too through reading literature. Many sources are helpful in explaining in laymen's terms what the nature of this disease is all about, what are the types of surgery done and types of adjuvant therapy (chemotherapy and radiation therapy) are available to eradicate this disease and have you become a long term survivor.

So how do I start?—by taking a deep breath, sitting down, talking with family and friends who can offer you emotional support, and tackling this new crisis one step at a time. Below is a guide to help you become an empowered, informed woman who will have the knowledge and resources needed to make decisions confidently about her breast cancer treatment.

Choosing a doctor: Once you have been told that you do have breast cancer or might have breast cancer, you will be referred to a surgeon. There are many doctors who perform breast cancer surgery but not that many who are truly breast surgeons. Breast surgery, whether it be in the form of a lumpectomy or mastectomy has historically been thought to be a "simple" surgical procedure to do. Well, if it is your breast it might not sound so simple. There are many general surgeons who perform breast cancer surgery. They might do one case a year or perhaps as many as twenty. You want to go and be seen by a surgeon who is a breast surgeon... who has chosen this to be his or her surgical specialty and who does a lot of breast surgeries every year. These are physicians with the surgical experience you are seeking. They have chosen this as their field of specialty and will be probably more up to date on the latest surgical techniques. High volume surgeons tend to have better results and are more attuned to subtle differences in individual cases. Seek out a physician who does fifty or more breast cancer operations a year. (For example in Maryland during 1996, there were 287 surgeons who only performed one inpatient breast cancer surgery. There were an additional 94 physicians who only did two such operations. Of all the women having breast cancer surgery in Maryland during this period, only 8.6 % of them were treated by a surgeon who had done more than 50 breast surgical procedures that year. Additionally, of the 647 surgeons who did inpatient breast cancer surgery, only 1.5% of them had done more than 30 inpatient operations in 1996.) You can find out this kind of information from several sources: call the hospital where the doctor is in practice and ask for information about case volume. His or her office should be more than willing to provide this type of information to you. Call your state board of quality assurance and ask for information on file about the physician you are considering seeing. They will also have information about any malpractice cases he has had and other quality of care complaints that have been filed against him. This information isn't published data but is available by making a simple call. (Keep in mind however that physicians who treat large numbers of women with breast cancer may have some information on file where as a physician who only treats a handful of patients a year may have nothing on file.) You also want to know about the credentialing of the physicians you choose; this includes your breast surgeon, medical oncologist, radiation oncologist, radiologist, and others involved in your care. Your wisest choice is to choose a physician board certified by The American Board of Surgery as your breast surgeon. He or she had to be trained in a recognized approved training program and pass rigorous exams after training. The American Board of Medical Specialists can be reached by calling 847-491-9091. They can provide you information regarding who in your region meets this criteria. Surgeons of this specialty also frequently are members of the American College of Surgeons. This distinction comes only after having become board certified and practicing in a community for greater than three years. These surgeons are considered by their peers to be above average in the care of surgical patients. Finally, most true breast surgeons are also members of The Society of Surgical Oncology. This society only accepts as members those with substantially greater training and/or experience in the management of cancer. Most of the latest developments in the surgical management of breast cancer are presented at annual educational meetings of this society. The standards for the surgical care of breast cancer patients are developed by the American College of Surgeons and The Society of Surgical Oncology jointly. Not all breast surgeons do breast cancer surgeries 100% of the time. But consider this—some full time breast surgeons do surgery on only 25–30 new cancer cases each year but others who do only 75% breast surgery treat over 200 new cases a year!

The same criteria applies for each other specialty physicians who will be providing your care. They should be board certified for their specialty with a subspecialty in breast cancer. There are lots of physicians for example who are medical oncologists and provide treatment to cancer patients. You want to receive your care however from someone whose specialty or major interest is "breast cancer."

The American Board of Medical Specialties provides services for finding doctors in your area and checking upon their credentials.

Physician attitude: Seek out someone who is going to be very frank and honest with you. This is not a time to have a sugared version of what your situation is. You need the facts and you want them presented to you candidly. This can be emotionally difficult for some physicians so you never really end up with the whole unvarnished truth. Seek out a physician who is willing to spend time with you and answer all your questions. No physician knows all—they should be willing to discuss the uncertainties in treatment and results. Beware of the omniscient doctor. That person may not be able to recognize their shortcomings or see alternatives in treatment that may not be the usual local treatment policy.

Seek a physician who wants to help educate you about this disease and your treatment options and not someone who wants to make the decisions for you. You need to be part of your own treatment team remember. That is important. It can be tempting to just have the doctor tell you what to do but that really isn't in your best interest. There are critical choices that you must make which need to be your decision alone. An example is whether to have mastectomy or breast conservation surgery (lumpectomy with lymph node removal). Depending on your clinical condition and the size of the tumor along with some other factors, it may very well be that from a survival perspective, you will be given the choice of having one type of surgery or the other, both having equal outcomes regarding your survival rate. This is a decision that should be left for you to decide based on many factors including your emotional well being and the feelings you have about your self image. You, not the doctor, will face the consequences of these decisions for the rest of your life. Make sure these decisions and treatments have your seal of approval.

Talk with other survivors: Getting information from other women who are breast cancer survivors can be very valuable. Also take comfort in knowing that there are many of us who have survived this disease (there are 1.3 million breast cancer survivors in the U.S. today). These women can give you candid information about their own experiences with physicians who provided them care and treatment when they were diagnosed. It is best to talk with someone who has been treated fairly recently though because treatment modalities change. For example if you spoke to someone who had a mastectomy seven years ago she would tell you that she spent several days in the hospital and suffered with nausea and vomiting and a lot of pain. Physicians who have chosen to continuously improve care for women battling breast cancer will make changes in their surgical care to prevent the side effects that women in the past had to overcome. There are various types of surgical treatments for breast cancer too and you will find that the experiences women share with you based on the type of surgery they had will also vary. The results also vary dramatically between hospitals and individual doctors. Do not expect the good results from one hospital to translate into similar results at others.

For example, women having mastectomies or lumpectomies with lymph node removal and not having reconstruction at the same time should describe an experience free of severe pain and absence of nausea and vomiting. However the reported rates of nausea and vomiting in most hospitals in the country exceed 85%. Several years ago, we at Johns Hopkins pioneered improvements in anesthesia management and other perioperative surgical care so that the majority of our women patients can awaken from this type of surgery and feel relatively normal from a physical perspective. I know our own experience here at Hopkins since 1995 has been that women undergoing one of these two procedures without reconstruction feel well enough to go home the same day. The emotional aspects of this disease and its treatment cannot be underplayed. We want patients to focus on addressing their emotional needs as a priority and not have to worry with feeling ill from surgery. If you find that previous patients you speak to are describing unpleasant experiences from their surgical event, then you might want to get more information before selecting the same doctor that they chose to see. There will be other important services to ask former patients about too which will be described in more detail below such as the ease of reaching a health care professional in an urgent way after you go home.

Multidisciplinary care: Lots of facilities boast that they offer this. What does it really mean though? Multidisciplinary means that you are being seen and cared for by a team of breast cancer specialists with expertise in breast surgery, medical oncology, radiation oncology, plastic surgery, cytopathology, and mammography with diagnostic imaging. Some hospitals or breast centers have such a team. This team may be however the only team, meaning that they only have one medical oncologist or one breast surgeon. Ideally you want to go to a place where there are several physicians of each specialty and where your specific case gets discussed and reviewed by the specific team caring for you as well as well by the other physicians there who can offer second opinions on an ongoing basis. In most cases the types of facilities that offer this level of faculty staffing are at larger teaching hospitals. It is important to have this type of specialized care and expertise however. Each step of the care of you is too important to delegate to a single individual—only through open review and debate of each step in the treatment process, can the ideal treatment and management be certain.

Skill, knowledge, and technology: The effective treatment of your breast cancer is critical for you. You deserve to receive your care in the most up to date facility where the latest and newest technology for diagnosing and treating breast cancer is available. The physicians and nurses who care for you should be specialized in the diagnosis and treatment of breast cancer. There is always new research and innovative treatments being developed for this disease. Having your care at a facility that can offer state of the art diagnostic evaluation and treatments should be your priority. Being able to have access to the latest treatment modalities including clinical trials for treatment of breast cancer will be valuable for you. Don't settle for a program that is limiting in its offerings as to what it can provide to you. Facilities for example that offer state of the art biopsies in the form of "percutaneous biopsies" means that you can be biopsied in mammography by a radiologist who has been specially trained and credentialed to perform such a procedure. The physician can remove tissue for further examination by a pathologist without having to make an incision in the breast or having to put you to sleep. Doing the procedure this way is less painful, allows most women to do it on their lunch hour and get the results within 24 hours. If the facility you have chosen doesn't have such equipment or professional expertise then you expose yourself to having procedures done the old fashioned way which may limit some of the future treatment options.

Features of a Breast Center

You will note that I chose to say "breast center." I guess that is my own bias. I believe that you have a better opportunity of having a truly integrated and comprehensive program for diagnosing and treating breast cancer if the facility has chosen to invest in developing a "center" for breast health and treatment of breast cancer. Tagging the word "center" onto a title though doesn't mean it is one. There are certain features of a breast center that you should expect to be offered as part of their program if they are in fact truly a comprehensive breast center. I've listed some of them below for you.

Easy access: If you have been advised to see a surgeon due to an abnormal mammogram or lump discovered on examination you will want an appointment as soon as possible. Until you are seen by a surgeon and answers known about your clinical situation, your anxiety and stress level will remain high. Most breast centers, in acknowledgment of this, will (and should) schedule you for an appointment within 48 hours of your call or doctor's referral. Fear of the unknown is the worst fear of all. Even if the news you receive is bad you can take comfort in knowing that now you can begin working with the doctors to plan what will be the best treatment choices for you.

Patient empowerment: It is important that you be given the knowledge you need to enable you to actively participate in decisions about your care and treatment. Some physicians are reluctant to empower women in this way. It is a patient's right and should be a key factor in deciding where you want to receive your treatment.

Patient education: Not only do you need to be educated about breast cancer, the treatment options, and what to expect each step along the way but so do important members of your family. This requires an investment of time and resources by the health care professionals taking care of you. You want to receive and be educated about your treatment plans as thoroughly as possible. You need to have easy access to someone in the breast center who you can ask questions of and feel confident in the responses as well as comfortable asking the question. By doing so you will come to understand what is happening to your body and what needs to be done to get you well again. Your family members who love you and need to support you benefit from this education too because they worried about you. They need to understand what is happening so they can devote their time and energy in emotionally supporting you.

Multidisciplinary case conferences: A key advantage to having a multidisciplinary team approach is the special expertise each health care professional offers to each patient's unique situation. Centers who hold on a routine basis case conferences to discuss in detail a patient's clinical condition, diagnostic findings, and recommendations for optimal treatment are beneficial to the patient's overall well-being and clinical outcome. This is a way to help ensure that the patient is being given individualized attention and care by utilizing maximum breast cancer knowledge, experience, and expertise by the breast center team.

Special Mammography Services

Appointments right away: If a woman is being referred by her family doctor or gynecologist for evaluation of a suspicious lump she wants to know right away if it is cancer. For that matter, if she finds the lump herself she doesn't want there to be any delay in getting answers about her situation. Mammography facilities should offer appointments for such patients immediately. Ideally the patient would be seen the same day or at the latest the following day. Often times radiologists are not readily available to read the films and talk with the patient about what the mammogram showed. You want to go to a

239

facility that has radiologists available to read the films while you are there and most importantly tell you what they show. Be sure to call and ask whether they offer this type of clinical service. It is one additional way to reduce your anxiety and speed the process along for you to get answers and proceed with treatment if it is determined to be cancer.

Percutaneous biopsy—mammotome, ABBI (advanced breast biopsy instrumentation), core biopsy, and fine needle biopsies: These are four types of biopsy procedures that can now to be done in mammography if the facility has the technology and medical expertise. This method of doing breast biopsies enables the patient to have a sample of tissue removed without having an open biopsy requiring an incision. Having the biopsy done this way required special equipment and devices that not all mammography facilities currently have. It also required special credentialing for the radiologist doing this type of procedure. Learning about these programs and services is an additional way to judge how up to date the facility it that you are considering going to for your care.

Inform the patient and referring physician of the findings right away: Once you have had a biopsy you want to know the results as soon as possible. Check to see what the "turn around time" is for pathology results. Many facilities can tell you or your doctor the results of a biopsy within 24 hours. The sooner you know what you are dealing with the sooner you can begin to makes plans about the best treatment options for you to pursue.

Clinical trials: Having the opportunity to have available to you as many treatment options as possible is important. Hospitals who participate in clinical trials can offer more innovative treatment options usually. In some cases these clinical trials are very new and the medical field is still learning about all of their benefits and value. If you are asked to participate in such a trial you are paving the way to the development of innovative research that will make an important impact on other women diagnosed in the future with breast cancer. You are also being closely monitored throughout your treatment process so that data can be collected about your experience with the chemotherapy agents you've been given. You might also be asked to participate in a study that already has proven to be very beneficial for treating breast cancer and now different dosages are being tested to determine the optimal dosage and frequency for you and other patients treated in the future. These new discoveries not only benefit you today but will make a big difference in how many lives we save in the future from breast cancer.

State of the art breast cancer surgery with minimal pain and nausea free: Most surgeons would say that doing a mastectomy or lumpectomy is not technically complicated surgery to perform. That doesn't mean however than any general surgeon does the procedure well. It is very important to have breast cancer surgery done by a surgeon who has chosen breast cancer surgery to be his or her surgical specialty and who does a large volume of breast surgeries on an annual basis. Historically, it was common for women to experience nausea and vomiting and postoperative pain following lumpectomy or mastectomy surgery, even those not having reconstruction done at the same time. There are breast centers who have solved this chronic problem and now are able to perform this type of surgery with minimal discomfort and without the GI side effects often times accompanying general anesthesia. It is important to ask questions related to this. The doctors who you are considering taking care of you should have quality of care data that describes their nausea/vomiting rate, pain management, length of time in the hospital on average for women having breast cancer surgery with and without reconstruction, complications that occur during or after surgery, and satisfaction data from prior patient's experience. All important information when choosing who you want to have take care of you. At Hopkins, for women who have breast cancer surgery without reconstruction, the majority of the patients feel so physically well after surgery that they choose to go home that same day. They are visited by a home health care nurse that evening and the next morning and are in constant contact with the nurse practitioner in the breast center for updates. What is nice about the option to go home is that it is the woman's choice. She is pain free and nausea free and able to concentrate on her emotional well-being which should be her primary focus postoperatively.

Radiation oncology: Patients who undergo lumpectomy surgery for treatment of their breast cancer almost always receive this form of adjuvant therapy afterwards. Most hospitals offer radiation oncology services. If the type of treatment that is advised for you to have includes radiation therapy you will want to ask questions about the radiation oncology physician's experience with treating breast cancer patients. Again, it is valuable to go to a facility that has extensive experience with treating this specific type of cancer. They should also have a physicist on staff who assists with this type of treatment to help ensure that the radiation is done in the precise location where the treatment is needed. As is the case with all your treatment, you as a patient should be given the opportunity to participate in the decision making about this type of treatment option. The physicians and nurses should be forthcoming with information about how this treatment is done, the risks and benefits of it, and how it will precisely be administered to you.

Plastic Surgery Offering the Latest Techniques

Free flap reconstructive surgery: Most hospitals and breast centers have plastic surgeons who can perform flap reconstruction by taking tissues from other parts of your body (usually tummy area) and creating from it a new breast. This in the past required the surgeon to maintain all of the vascular system (blood flow) attached during the procedure. There are new techniques now being used which enables the surgeon to transplant this tissue cutting the vessels free. By using intricate microvascular surgery the plastic surgeon is then able to reconnect the arteries and veins in their new location. The result for the patient is less pain after surgery. There are only a few facilities however who have a surgeon who has expertise with this type of procedure. If you are considering having this type of reconstruction done you may want to ask about this new method. Again, it is also important that the plastic surgeon you choose be someone who has done a large volume of flap and free flap reconstructive breast surgeries. Experience is a valuable asset when you want the very best cosmetic results that can be achieved.

Skin-sparing mastectomy: This is also a fairly new form of surgery which was developed at Hopkins and other major cancer centers. The affected breast is hollowed out, then the tissue from the abdominal area is used to fill the opening and created a new breast. There are few facilities that have the surgical expertise to perform this state of the art breast cancer surgery/reconstruction combination. Talk with your surgeon about it and discuss the pros and cons of taking this approach. Again the cosmetic appearance is amazing. When you are shown photographs of reconstructed breasts, you will be impressed with this surgical cosmetic effect. Often the patient doesn't look like she has had a mastectomy procedure done.

Medical oncology: Most, but not all, patients diagnosed with breast cancer need some form of chemotherapy as part of their treatment.

Again, most hospitals offer such clinical services. You want to make sure that the medical oncologist who is overseeing your treatment is specialized in the treatment of breast cancer. A medical oncologist may treat a wide variety of patients with various forms of cancer. You want to be cared for by someone who has chosen to specialize in breast cancer treatment. Someone who treats lots of women with this disease and has a track record for good outcomes. Ask the doctor about how many patients he or she treats in a given year for breast cancer and ask about the patients' experience with complications from treatment. You want to have a board certified medical oncologist who is readily accessible in the event you need to talk with him or her urgently while going through treatment. Ask questions about the doctor's procedure for addressing emergent calls as well as what type of monitoring will be done while you are undergoing this type of adjuvant therapy. Ask about the survival statistics for breast cancer patients treated at the facility you are considering too. All cancer patients' data is entered into a national database giving cancer specialists the ability to compare various treatment modalities and clinical outcomes. Hospitals that treat large volumes of cancer patients also study their own data and compare it to national statistics. You want to be in the hands of a team of professionals who have a history of good outcomes. Whenever possible seek care at a facility which can demonstrate that their survival rate is better than the national average. (For example at Hopkins, for women who are premenopausal and have positive lymph nodes, the survival rate is 10% higher than the national average.) You will have a higher sense of confidence and security being treated in a place which has these types of results.

Autologous bone marrow transplant (ABMT): This is a very specialized procedure which is done when very aggressive treatment is recommended. The patient has her healthy bone marrow harvested and stored away for safe keeping. She then receives high doses of chemotherapy which as a side effect destroys her remaining marrow. Afterwards her healthy bone marrow is returned to her. If a bone marrow transplant is advised for your type of breast cancer treatment you will want to select where you go carefully. Your insurance carrier may have a special arrangement with specific hospitals in your area or farther away since this type of treatment is not done at very many places. If given the option you want to be able to have all of your care at one facility where continuity of care can be provided smoothly. If you do need this type of treatment go to a facility that has experience with doing large volumes of bone marrow transplants specifically for the treatment of breast cancer. The more experienced the doctors and nurses are with this type of treatment the better your personal care and clinical outcomes will probably be. As a new state of the art approach for ABMT, a few, but very few, facilities are doing the procedure in the way that can reduce the amount of time the patient needs to spend hospitalized, which usually is several weeks. For example, Hopkins has a program called "IPOP" which stands for "inpatient/outpatient" bone marrow transplant. Breast cancer patients are kept in the acute hospital bed for as brief a time as is absolutely needed and receive a large majority of their treatment and intensive monitoring in an outpatient setting located at the hospital. This enables the patient to spend more time with family while receiving this life saving treatment to help eradicate her breast cancer.

Genetic counseling: This is a special program for women who have a family history of breast cancer or have other factors that make them higher risk for developing this disease. Counseling and genetic testing requires specialists who not only are experts in this field but also have excellent communication skills. The choice to have counseling and especially to decide to proceed with genetic testing is one to be taken seriously and with some caution. Though it can sound simple to be tested there are many things to consider before making such a choice. Physicians and nurses who have chosen to specialize in this field have expertise with helping women make these choices. Currently only a few facilities offer this type of program now. It is a growing field however. If this is an area of interest to you or your family you want to go to a facility that has many years of experience with genetic counseling and testing for breast cancer. Ask how long their program has existed and how many patients have been counseled and tested during that time. This will give you some idea as to their experience with this specialized type of service.

High risk assessment for breast cancer: Being evaluated for your risk of developing breast cancer or a family member getting this disease may be important for you to know. There are health care professionals who specialize in this type of screening and evaluation. Ask the breast center where you are contemplating going for your care if they offer this service, who performs the service, and how many patients they screen a year. The program should be conducted by a doctor or a nurse practitioner who specializes in breast health screening programs.

Pathology services: Patients don't always think about this particular service but it is a very important one. The pathologist who looks at your tissue specimen determines what type of breast cancer you have, how fast it is growing, whether it has spread to your lymph nodes, and provides other important pieces of clinical information to your breast surgeon, medical oncologist, and radiation oncologist. Accuracy and completeness is critical. It is difficult for a layperson to assess whether the pathology services being provide d at a hospital are of good quality or not. One source for this information is the JCAHO—Joint Commission for Accrediting Healthcare Organizations. They inspect hospitals on a tri-annual basis and write up reports on their findings. Included in their inspection are their findings for the pathology department. Though they don't actually look at slides and determine if they were accurately interpreted, they do look at the processes used by pathology to determine how effectively they work. They also review the credential files of the pathologists and other faculty at the facility. You can see the latest results of the hospital's inspection by going to the JCAHO website at http://www.jcaho.org or calling 630-792-5800 and requesting a copy of the report. This information became publicly accessible in 1997. There are some pathology departments who have made errors in reading the results of a breast tissue specimen. The worst case is when a specimen is read as benign tissue when in fact it contains cancer cells. You may wish to consider obtaining a second opinion about the pathology results by taking your pathology slides to a second facility that has extensive experience also in diagnosing and treating breast cancer. The pathologist should be considered one of the members of the breast center team and actively participate in the case conferences referenced earlier in this document. The information they provide serves as the road map for determining the treatment plan options best for your specific situation. Ask if the pathologist attends these conferences and what role he or she plays in the actual case discussion.

Patient satisfaction surveys: There are few breast centers who perform patient satisfaction surveys but all should. It is important to learn from patients how satisfied they were with their care and how can the center go about improving specific services and programs offered to make care even better than before. Conducting surveys is time and resource intensive. Centers who have chosen to survey their patients are sending an important message—that the health care professionals there care about their patients' opinions and want to hear from them. When asking a breast center whether they conduct surveys or not also ask what they do with the results they obtain. It is one thing to collect the data; it is another to do something constructive with it. Health care professionals need to take their patients' opinions seriously. All too often a patient may complain about a specific service or aspect of care she received and her words are not taken to heart. Seek out a place where the philosophy of the center is to use the results of their patient satisfaction surveys to determine what initiatives the center will work on to improve patient care. Go to a facility that considers the patient's opinions the most valuable—even more valuable than the health care professionals taking care of the patient. (A doctor may think it is acceptable for a patient to wait two weeks for an appointment when she has found a lump in her breast; the patient feels however that she should be able to get an appointment that same week. The patient is right!) Breast centers who truly have the patient's best interest in mind will demonstrate this philosophy by conducting surveys and acting on the results in real time.

Continuity of care: As more and more health care services are converted from an inpatient setting to an outpatient setting the need to ensure effective and efficient continuity of care heightens. Ask the facility how they go about keeping your primary care doctor or referring physician aware of your condition and treatment status. Check to see how they manage to keep track of how you are doing after you go home following surgery or chemotherapy treatments. Ask who is responsible for coordinating your care. You need to have confidence that you are being watched over even when you are not physically at the hospital. Some facilities have nurse practitioners who stay in touch with their patients via telephone once they are home. Some offer home health nursing care after surgical treatment is done. The team of professionals taking care of you also need to stay in close contact with one another—that's why they are a team. Ask them how they communicate with one another and keep each other informed about your progress and needs. You want to be cared for by a team who stay well connected with you and with one another, including your referring physician or doctor who functions as your family doctor. Feeling confident that you are receiving good continuity of care provides wonderful peace of mind to you and your family.

Urgent care needs services: When an urgent problem arises such as sickness that won't subside following a treatment you need to have ready access to a professional who can take care of this situation promptly. Ask what the breast center's procedures are for handling such emergencies. Also ask how often patients in the past have needed to utilize this special service. A breast center should have available for its patients a professional health care provider 24 hours a day, seven days a week to handle emergencies. In addition to this the patients should be well informed how to access this urgent care service and know they can confidently rely on it. You should not have to go to an Emergency Room to have such this urgent care needs attended. If their patient education program has been thorough and well done you and your family will know how to take care of most crises and head them off at the pass. (For example, taking an anti-nausea drug at a designated time to preventing vomiting later on.) There are unforeseen circumstances however that do arise on occasion which warrant prompt intervention by a doctor or nurse. Knowing and understanding how urgent care needs such as this are handled is important. Though you may never need to use it you want to know that such a program is in place and works well.

Long term follow up: Some doctors take care of your breast cancer and when treatment is done send you back to your referring physician. Their involvement with you ends when treatment ends. From a continuity of care perspective as well as peace of mind it is better to be cared for by professionals who will continue to see you for the rest of your life. Though we hope that your breast cancer does not reoccur there is a possibility that it might. Having the same health care team who treated you from the start continue to follow you at designated intervals to ensure that you remain well and healthy is a smart thing. Ask the center what their protocol is for following patients after their treatment is completed. You have been through a life threatening experience and need to continue to be seen, screened and evaluated by the people who are intimately familiar with your history and treatment that was done.

Psychological support for you and your family: Being diagnosed with breast cancer is devastating. Though some people don't openly express how they feel it is impossible to not be upset when told you have breast cancer. Those who love you are distressed too. Having ready access to professionals who can offer guidance, support, and help you and your family develop coping skills will make your breast cancer treatment go more smoothly for everyone. Ask the facility if they offer such services. You want to talk with professionals who have extensive experience with breast cancer patients and their families, who are familiar with the treatment you will be receiving and know

247

the doctors and nurses involved in your care. This provides for a better integrated approach to getting you well again physically and emotionally. A few facilities offer private counseling and psychotherapy. Most also have breast cancer support groups who generally meet monthly and are facilitated by a social worker or nurse. Some facilities also offer special support programs for family members including husbands and young children.

Survivor support: When confronted with a diagnosis of breast cancer your initial thought may be that you are alone in this battle. Feel assured you are not. There are 1.3 million women who are breast cancer survivors living in the United States today. Many breast centers arrange for a breast cancer survivor to talk with women who are newly diagnosed with this disease. The American Cancer Society offers as a free service a program called "Reach to Recovery." This program matches newly diagnosed women with women who are of the same or similar culture, ethnicity, and clinical condition (for example matching a 40 something year old with stage II breast cancer who is having a mastectomy and chemotherapy with a woman who is also in her forties and had the same treatment modality in the past and has completed her treatment at least a year ago.) This program is designed to help address the emotional needs you will be feeling. There is great benefit talking to someone who has been through what you are about to go through. Some breast centers have taken this program a step further and arrange for their own breast cancer survivor volunteers to also contact the patient. These survivor volunteers are very familiar with your situation because they have received their care from the same team of professionals you are receiving care from now. (Hopkins offers such a program. Though it is fairly new it has already proven to be very beneficial for our patients and their families.) Different facilities and doctors have sometimes different ways of doing certain types of treatments. Having a survivor who is familiar with the treatment program you are going to be receiving makes it easier to talk with and gain insight from her. This survivor volunteer becomes an extension of your breast cancer health care team. Ask the facility you are considering going to if they offer such a program and how it is organized. There are some facilities that discourage having newly diagnosed patients talk with women who have been previously diagnosed and treated. The belief in such situations is that the survivor may in some way negatively influence the patient in her decision making process. Health care professionals need to recognize the value of new patients talking with patients who have had similar treatment in the past and allow them time to exchange information. It is a patient's right to gain as much insight and understanding about her disease and its treatment as she can. This is one additional method it accomplish this goal.... and an additional way for you to evaluate the breast center you are considering.

Lymphedema prevention and management: A few patients, after having lymph nodes removed as part of their breast cancer surgery, develop lymphedema. This results in problems with swelling of their arm and hand on the side where their surgery was done. One way to prevent this from occurring is to be proactive in its management. Check to see if the breast center you are considering to going to offers a "lymphedema prevention and management program." Such centers will have a certified occupational therapist or physical therapist become certified and credentialed in lymphedema management. The therapist will see the patient prior to her surgery and teach her special exercises to do to help prevent the occurrence of lymphedema developing. She also will help in managing the problem should it occur anyway. A few breast centers also offer special support programs for lymphedema patients. Though lymphedema only occurs occasionally, knowing that the breast center offers programs designed to prevent it and manage it is a sign of the comprehensiveness of their services.

Rehabilitation medicine: Having breast cancer surgery, whether it be a mastectomy or lumpectomy with lymph node removal results in temporary difficulty with range of motion to your affected arm. It is smart to learn in advance of the surgery the best exercises to do to prevent range of motion problems from occurring. Some breast centers offer as part of their preoperative management and preparation a program specifically for this. It is usually conducted by the Rehabilitation and Physical Medicine Department which works in a coordinated manner with the breast center staff. Patients are trained in appropriate exercises to do by a physical therapist or occupational therapist. Patients who are experiencing problems with gaining their full range of motion back after their surgery are also seen by the same therapist. She works with the patient to restore her physical abilities to what they were before. Most patients do not need assistance after surgery if they have been trained well and follow the prescribed exercise program shown to them. It is good to know that such programs exist though should you be in need of these special services.

Continued education programs and seminars: When your treatment is over you will still want to stay on top of whatever is the latest treatment programs and research discoveries being made about breast cancer. Your continued good health may be dependent on it. For most women they thirst for information and want to learn as much as they can—it may make a difference for their own health or for someone in their family who they care about. Check to see what type of continued educational programs the facility offers related to breast cancer. Examples of seminars that might be offered include: hormone replacement therapy after breast cancer treatment; breast cancer gene research findings; the latest in breast reconstruction; coping with fear of reoccurrence of breast cancer. Though your treatment may be over the disease and its long term effects may continue. You will want to stay informed and should expect the center where you received your care to help in keeping you updated at routine intervals.

Other cancer screening programs for you and your family: Breast cancer, though it may be happening to you, effects your entire family. Usually a diagnosis of breast cancer is a surprise. This is the time to check out your health in general and that of your family's to make sure that there are no other surprises. Men at a minimum should be checked for colon cancer and prostate cancer. Women need to be also checked for colon cancer and uterine cancer. Take this opportunity to commit to yourself and your family to be properly screened for these types of cancer s and others that may apply due to family history or lifestyle. See what types of cancer screening programs are offered at the facility where you plan to receive your care. Your family will thank you and you will thank yourself for having had the screening done. The outcome for everyone will be a healthier future.

Image recovery: There are side effects, physical ones and psychological ones, that can take a toll on us as women when we are treated for breast cancer. For some of us we may lose a breast; for others we might lose our hair; many will lose both. These are symbols of femininity for many and are devastating to experience. Being prepared for these loses is a good way to adjust and cope. Some facilities offer on site or have an affiliation with an "Image Recovery" service. These places are sometimes referred to as mastectomy supply shops, wig shops, or called by some other name. Their purpose is to help restore (as in the case with a breast prosthesis) or temporarily replace (with a wig) that which is lost from your self image. If you anticipate needing a breast prosthesis be sure to be fitted by someone who is a certified fitter. This individual would have taken a special course to learn how to properly fit a woman for a breast prosthesis. An improper fit can result in poor body alignment, back pain, and lack of confidence in one's appearance. Check to see what the facility has to offer and go and visit it if possible. Many of them also offer special classes in make up and hair styling too as additional ways to improve our self image and help us to feel good a bout our appearance. Remember, you need to not just physically heal but also emotionally heal. Your treatments will go smoother if you can feel confident in the way you look during and after therapy.

Conclusion

I've tried to provide you some guidance and direction as to how to choose a breast center worthy of taking care of you—you are important.... your care is important.... it shouldn't be done just anywhere. After all, this is a life altering experience and depending on the accuracy of your diagnosis and effectiveness of your treatment a life saving experience. I want you to choose well. If you have questions or wish to discuss this one on one with me, you are welcome to reach me at the Johns Hopkins Breast Center. Remember, I am a breast cancer survivor. My mission is for there to be a lot more fellow survivors. Good luck to you and I wish you well as you embark on your road of transformation from victim to breast cancer survivor.

Chapter 30

Surgery for Breast Cancer

Chapter Contents

Section 30.1

Choosing between Breast-Sparing Surgery and Mastectomy

Excerpted from "Surgery Choices for Women with Early-Stage Breast Cancer," National Cancer Institute (www.cancer.gov), October 2004.

Introduction

As a woman with early-stage breast cancer (DCIS or Stage I, IIA, IIB, or IIIA breast cancer) you may be able to choose which type of breast surgery to have. Often, your choice is between breast-sparing surgery (surgery that takes out the cancer and leaves most of the breast) and a mastectomy (surgery that removes the whole breast). Research shows that women with early-stage breast cancer who have breast-sparing surgery along with radiation therapy live as long as those who have a mastectomy. Most women with breast cancer will lead long, healthy lives after treatment.

Treatment for breast cancer usually begins a few weeks after diagnosis. In these weeks, you should meet with a surgeon, learn the facts about your surgery choices, and think about what is important to you. Then choose which kind of surgery to have.

Most women want to make this choice. After all, the kind of surgery you have will affect how you look and feel. But it is often hard to decide what to do. The information in this section can help you make a choice you feel good about.

This information is for women who have early-stage breast cancer (DCIS or Stage I, IIA, IIB, or IIIA). If your cancer is Stage IIIB, IIIC, or IV this section does not have the information you need. To find information for you, visit the National Cancer Institute's website at http://www.cancer.gov.

Step 1: Talk with Your Surgeon

Talk to a surgeon about your breast cancer surgery choices. Find out what happens during surgery, types of problems that sometimes occur, and other kinds of treatment (if any) you will need after surgery.

Be sure to ask a lot of questions and learn as much as you can. You may also wish to talk with family members, friends, or others who have had breast cancer surgery.

After talking with a surgeon, you may want a second opinion. This means talking with another doctor who might tell you about other treatment options or simply give you information that can help you feel better about the choice you are making. Don't worry about hurting your surgeon's feelings. It is common practice to get a second opinion and some insurance companies require it. Plus, it is better to get a second opinion than worry that you made the wrong choice.

Step 2: Learn the Facts

Doctors talk about stages of cancer. This is a way of saying how big the tumor is and how far it has spread. If you are unsure of the stage of your cancer, ask your doctor or nurse.

Stage 0: This means that you either have DCIS or LCIS. DCIS (ductal carcinoma in situ) is very early breast cancer that is often too small to form a lump. Your doctor may refer to DCIS as noninvasive cancer. LCIS (lobular carcinoma in situ) is not cancer but may increase the chance that you will get breast cancer. Talk with your doctor about treatment options if you are diagnosed with LCIS.

Stage I: Your cancer is less than 1 inch across (2 centimeters), or about the size of a quarter. The cancer is only in the breast and has not spread to lymph nodes or other parts of your body.

Stage IIA: No cancer is found in your breast, but cancer is found in the lymph nodes under your arm. Or, your cancer is 1 inch (2 centimeters) or smaller and has spread to the lymph nodes under your arm. Or, your cancer is about 1–2 inches (2–5 centimeters) but has not spread to the lymph nodes under your arm.

Stage IIB: Your cancer is about 1–2 inches (2–5 centimeters) and has spread to the lymph nodes under your arm. Or, your cancer is larger than 2 inches (5 centimeters) and has not spread to the lymph nodes under your arm.

Stage IIIA: No cancer is found in the breast, but is found in lymph nodes under your arm, and the lymph nodes are attached to each other. Or, your cancer is 2 inches (5 centimeters) or smaller and has spread to lymph nodes under your arm, and the lymph nodes are attached to each other. Or, your cancer is larger than 2 inches (5 centimeters) and has spread to lymph nodes under your arm.

About Lymph Nodes

Lymph nodes are part of your body's immune system which helps fight infection and disease. Lymph nodes are small, round, and clustered (like a bunch of grapes) throughout your body.

Axillary lymph nodes are in the area under your arm. Breast cancer may spread to these lymph nodes even when the tumor in the breast is small. This is why most surgeons take out some of these lymph nodes.

Lymphedema is a swelling caused by a buildup of lymph fluid. You may have this type of swelling in your arm if your lymph nodes are taken out with surgery or damaged by radiation therapy. Here are some facts to know:

- Lymphedema can show up soon after surgery. The symptoms are often mild and last for a short time.

- Lymphedema can show up months or even years after cancer treatment is over. Often, lymphedema develops after an insect bite, minor injury, or burn on the arm where your lymph nodes were removed. Sometimes, this can be painful. One way to reduce the swelling is to work with a doctor who specializes in rehabilitation or a physical therapist.

- Sentinel lymph node biopsy is surgery to remove as few lymph nodes as possible from under the arm. The surgeon first injects a dye in the breast to see which lymph nodes the breast tumor drains into. Then, he or she removes these nodes to see if they have any cancer. If there is no cancer, the surgeon may leave the other lymph nodes in place. Talk with your surgeon if you want to learn more.

Step 3. Find Out about Your Breast Cancer Surgery Choices

Most women who have DCIS or Stage I, IIA, IIB, or IIIA breast cancer have three basic surgery choices. They are 1) breast-sparing surgery followed by radiation therapy, 2) mastectomy, or 3) mastectomy with breast reconstruction surgery.

Breast-sparing surgery: Breast-sparing surgery means that the surgeon removes only your cancer and some normal tissue around it. This kind of surgery keeps your breast intact—looking a lot like it did before surgery. Other words for breast-sparing surgery include "lumpectomy," "partial mastectomy," "breast-conserving surgery," or "segmental mastectomy."

After breast-sparing surgery, most women also get radiation therapy. This type of treatment is very important because it could keep cancer from coming back in the same breast. Some women also need chemotherapy and hormone therapy.

Mastectomy: In a mastectomy, the surgeon removes all of your breast and nipple. Sometimes, you will also need to have radiation therapy, chemotherapy, hormone therapy, or all three types of therapy. Here are some types of mastectomy:

- **Total (simple) mastectomy:** The surgeon removes all of your breast. Sometimes, the surgeon also takes out some of the lymph nodes under your arm.

- **Modified radical mastectomy:** The surgeon removes all of your breast, many of the lymph nodes under your arm, the lining over your chest muscles, and maybe a small chest muscle.

- **Double mastectomy:** The surgeon removes both your breasts at the same time, even if your cancer is in only one breast. This surgery is rare and mostly used when the surgeon feels you have a high risk for getting cancer in the breast that does not have cancer.

Breast reconstruction surgery: If you have a mastectomy, you can also choose to have breast reconstruction surgery. This surgery is done by a reconstructive plastic surgeon and gives you a new breast-like shape and nipple. Your surgeon can also add a tattoo that looks like the areola (the dark area around your nipple). Or you may not want any more surgery and prefer to wear a prosthesis (breast-like form) in your bra. To learn more about breast reconstruction, see Section 30.5 at the end of this chapter.

Step 4: Compare Your Choices

Below are some questions you may be thinking about.

Is this surgery right for me?

Breast-sparing surgery with radiation is a safe choice for most women who have early-stage breast cancer. This means that your cancer is DCIS or at Stage I, IIA, IIB, or IIIA. Mastectomy is a safe choice for women who have early-stage breast cancer (DCIS, Stage I, IIA, IIB, or IIIA). You may need a mastectomy if these conditions are present:

• You have small breasts and a large tumor

• You have cancer in more than one part of your breast

• The tumor is under the nipple

• You do not have access to radiation therapy

If you have a mastectomy, you might also want breast reconstruction surgery. You can choose to have reconstruction surgery at the same time as your mastectomy or wait and have it at a later date.

What will my breast look like after surgery?

Breast-sparing surgery: Your breast should look a lot like it did before surgery. But if your tumor is large, your breast may look different or smaller after breast-sparing surgery.

Mastectomy surgery: Your breast and nipple will be removed. You will have a flat chest on the side of your body where the breast was removed.

Mastectomy and breast reconstruction surgery: Although you will have a breast-like shape, your breast will not look the same as it did before surgery.

Will I have feeling in the area around my breast?

Breast-sparing surgery: Yes. You should still have feeling in your breast, nipple, and areola (the dark area around your nipple).

Mastectomy surgery: Maybe. After surgery, you will feel numb (have no feeling) in your chest wall and maybe also under your arm. This numb feeling should go away in one to two years, but it will never feel like it used to. Also, the skin where your breast was may feel tight.

Mastectomy and breast reconstruction surgery: No. The area around your breast will always be numb (have no feeling).

Will I have pain after the surgery?

You may have pain after breast-sparing surgery or mastectomy surgery, and you are likely to have pain after major surgery, such as mastectomy and reconstruction surgery. Talk with your surgeon or nurse if you have questions about pain and pain control.

What other problems can I expect?

Breast-sparing surgery: You may feel very tired after radiation therapy. You may get lymphedema—a problem in which your arm swells.

Mastectomy surgery: You may have pain in your neck or back. You may feel out of balance if you had large breasts and do not have reconstruction surgery. You may get lymphedema.

Mastectomy and breast reconstruction surgery: It may take you many weeks or even months to recover from breast reconstruction surgery. If you have an implant, you may get infections, pain, or hardness. Also, you may not like how your breast-like shape looks. You may need more surgery if your implant breaks or leaks. If you have tissue flap surgery, you may lose strength in the part of your body where the flap came from. You may get lymphedema.

Will I need more surgery?

Breast-sparing surgery: Maybe. You may need more surgery to remove lymph nodes from under your arm. Also, if the surgeon does not remove all your cancer the first time, you may need more surgery.

Mastectomy surgery: Maybe. You may need surgery to remove lymph nodes from under your arm. Also, if you have problems after your mastectomy, you may need to see your surgeon for treatment.

Mastectomy and breast reconstruction surgery: Yes. You will need surgery at least two more times to build a new breast-like shape. With implants, you may need more surgery months or years later. You may also need surgery to remove lymph nodes from under your arm.

What other types of treatment will I need?

Breast-sparing surgery: You will need radiation therapy, given almost every day for five to eight weeks. You also may need chemotherapy, hormone therapy, or both.

Mastectomy surgery: You also may need chemotherapy, hormone therapy, or radiation therapy. Some women get all three types of therapy.

Mastectomy and breast reconstruction surgery: You may need chemotherapy, hormone therapy, or radiation therapy. Some women get all three types of therapy.

Will insurance pay for my surgery?

Check with your insurance company to find out how much it pays for breast cancer surgery and other needed treatments. Check with your insurance company to find out if it pays for breast reconstruction surgery. You should also ask if your insurance will pay for problems that may result from breast reconstruction surgery.

Will the type of surgery I have affect how long I live?

Women with early-stage breast cancer who have breast-sparing surgery followed by radiation live just as long as women who have a mastectomy. Women with early-stage breast cancer who have a mastectomy live the same amount of time as women who have breast-sparing surgery followed by radiation therapy. Most women with breast cancer will lead long, healthy lives after treatment.

What are the chances that my cancer will come back after surgery?

Breast-sparing surgery: About 10% (one out of every 10) of women who have breast-sparing surgery along with radiation therapy get cancer in the same breast within 12 years. If this happens, you will need a mastectomy, but it will not affect how long you live.

Mastectomy surgery: About 5% (one out of every 20) of women who have a mastectomy will get cancer on the same side of their chest within 12 years.

Mastectomy and breast reconstruction surgery: About 5% (one out of every 20) of women who have a mastectomy will get cancer on the same side of their chest within 12 years. Breast reconstruction surgery does not affect the chances of your cancer coming back.

Step 5: Think about What Is Important to You

After you have talked with your surgeon and learned the facts, you may also want to talk with your spouse or partner, family, friends, or other women who have had breast cancer surgery. Then, think about what is important to you. Here are some questions to think about:

- Do I want to get a second opinion?

- How important is it to me how my breast looks after cancer surgery?

- How important is it to me how my breast feels after cancer surgery?

- If I have breast-sparing surgery, am I willing and able to also get radiation therapy?

- If I have a mastectomy, do I also want breast reconstruction surgery?

- If I have breast reconstruction surgery, do I want it at the same time as my mastectomy?

- What treatment does my insurance cover, and what do I have to pay for?

- Who would I like to talk with about my surgery choices?

- What else do I want to know, do, or learn before I make my choice about breast cancer surgery?

Step 6: Make Your Choice

Now that you have talked with your surgeon, learned the facts, and thought about what is important to you—it's time to make your breast cancer surgery choice.

Section 30.2

Hypnosis before Breast-Cancer Surgery Reduces Pain, Discomfort, and Cost

Clinical Trial Results, National Cancer Institute, September 12, 2007.

Women undergoing surgery for breast cancer who received a brief hypnosis session before entering the operating room required less anesthesia and pain medication during surgery and reported less pain, nausea, fatigue, and discomfort after surgery than women who did not receive hypnosis. The overall cost of surgery was also significantly less for women undergoing hypnosis.

—*Journal of the National Cancer Institute,* Sept. 5, 2007

Background

Surgery for breast cancer, either for diagnosis or treatment, can cause side effects, including pain, nausea, fatigue, and discomfort. While drugs including traditional pain medications can help provide relief, they can have side effects of their own and increase the overall cost of a surgical procedure.

Researchers have become interested in finding approaches other than drugs to help relieve the side effects of surgery. One technique under study is hypnosis, a type of guided relaxation in which participants become more open to suggestion.

The study described below tested whether a brief hypnosis session before breast cancer surgery could reduce the need for anesthesia and pain medication, reduce side effects experienced after surgery, or ease recovery.

The Study

Investigators from Mount Sinai Medical Center in New York City recruited 200 women scheduled to undergo either surgical breast biopsy for diagnosis or lumpectomy for treatment of breast cancer. The investigators randomly assigned participants to either the hypnosis group or a control group. Women scheduled for biopsy were randomized separately from women scheduled for lumpectomy, to evenly distribute the two types of surgery between the groups.

Women in the hypnosis group received a 15-minute hypnosis session within one hour prior to surgery. Psychologists trained in the use of hypnosis in the medical setting used a script including suggestions for relaxation, pleasant thoughts, and reduced experience of pain, nausea, and fatigue, as well as instructions on self-hypnosis for use after surgery. Women in the control group spent an equal amount of time with the psychologists within an hour of surgery to talk and receive emotional support.

All women received the drugs propofol and midazolam (anesthetics) and fentanyl and lidocaine (pain medications) during surgery. They also had access to additional pain medications after surgery, as needed.

Before leaving the hospital, the women reported their experiences of pain intensity, pain unpleasantness, fatigue, nausea, physical discomfort, and emotional upset. The investigators also collected information on the amount of anesthesia and pain medication used during and after surgery, the time spent in surgery, and the cost of the procedures, medications, and staff time.

Because the women knew their group assignment, the investigators took several precautions to reduce potential bias in the results.

- The same psychologists met with patients in both groups.

- The hypnosis and control sessions took place in a private room away from the anesthesiologists and surgeons, who did not know the group assignments.

- Data on anesthesia used was taken from computer records, not recorded by clinical staff.

- The psychologists did not collect the patient-reported data after surgery. Instead, research assistants who did not know the group assignments asked the women about their perceptions of pain and discomfort.

Results

Women in the hypnosis group required significantly less propofol and lidocaine, the doses of which were adjusted for individual patients as needed during surgery, than women in the control group. Use of fentanyl and midazolam did not differ significantly. Although use of pain medication after surgery did not differ between groups, women in the hypnosis group reported significantly less pain intensity, pain unpleasantness, nausea, fatigue, discomfort, and emotional upset than women in the control group.

Women in the hypnosis group also spent an average of about ten and a half fewer minutes in surgery than women in the control group. The researchers weren't able to say why this was so, only that the finding was statistically significant and resulted in cost savings. On average, the surgical procedures cost about $770 less per patient in the hypnosis group.

Limitations

One limitation of the study was that group assignment could not be hidden from participating women, since they actively participated in either the hypnosis or control sessions. When both participants and researchers in a study are unaware of the final group assignments, this is called a double-blind clinical trial, and is considered the best way to reduce potential bias in collecting results.

However, the researchers took precautions to make sure that the results were collected by staff that did not know which of the women had received hypnosis. The authors believed that their precautions "make it unlikely that either research or clinical staff were aware of study group assignment."

Also, in this study, the hypnosis was performed by specially trained psychologists, who may not be available at every hospital. More research is needed, explained the authors, to test whether other members of the clinical team could be taught to effectively give a similar hypnosis session.

The trial design did not allow for a definitive answer as to why the hypnosis group spent less time in surgery. "It is possible that the shorter procedure times in the hypnosis group were due to the patients being easier to prepare for surgery and to sedate or due to less time having been spent administering medications to patients," write the authors. "However, we did not investigate these mechanisms, and therefore, these possibilities are highly speculative."

Comments

"Overall, our results support the present hypnosis intervention as a brief, clinically effective means for controlling patients' pain, nausea, fatigue, discomfort, and emotional upset following breast cancer surgery beyond traditional pharmacotherapeutic approaches," stated the authors. "The present brief hypnosis intervention appears to be one of the rare clinical interventions that can simultaneously reduce both symptom burden and costs."

"If you can decrease the amount of pain using a technique such as hypnosis, and you can also at the same time reduce the cost involved in treating these patients, I think it's beneficial both ways," said Sonia Jakowlew, Ph.D., program director in the National Cancer Institute's (NCI) Cancer Cell Biology Branch. "It helps the patients and it helps the physicians as well."

Further studies are needed, explained the authors, to measure which specific parts of the hypnosis intervention are most effective, to see whether hypnosis had a long-term effect on the control of pain and discomfort, and to test hypnosis in patients with different types of cancer and from different demographic backgrounds. "Investigators should attempt to replicate [this study] and see if these are consistent findings," agreed Jeffrey White, M.D. director of NCI's Office of Cancer Complementary and Alternative Medicine.

Section 30.3

Practical Tips about What to Wear after Mastectomy Surgery

"What to Wear When You Have Breast Cancer" © 2008
CancerConsultants.com. Reprinted with permission.

From post-surgery camisoles to mastectomy-friendly workout wear, our expert has answers to questions you never even knew you had.

Q&A with Barbara Zarrell, RN, BSN, Woman's Personal Health Resource, Inc.

I will be undergoing a double mastectomy, and I haven't yet made up my mind about reconstruction. I've heard that there are now many prosthetic options available in breast forms and clothing. Can you describe what some of the most popular are?

There is a variety of options for breast prostheses. Generally, one can choose from breast forms made from regular-weight silicone or lightweight silicone or from various types of poly-fil forms. Some of the poly-fil forms are actually weighted to offer a nice mix between a superlight form and a silicone form.

After a double mastectomy, the issue of weight in a breast form is important. For the bra to stay in place and fit well, some weight is needed. In this case I might choose from one of the newer, lightweight silicone forms or the weighted poly-fils.

Are there specific clothing items or undergarments that I should consider purchasing to wear following my surgery to make my recovery easier or more comfortable?

An important garment to choose prior to breast surgery is a postmastectomy camisole. There are several on the market. This garment will provide support and comfort immediately after surgery and throughout your recovery. It has various pockets for the drain that your surgeon will place. The drain will remain in place for approximately seven to 10 days and can be uncomfortable and cumbersome. The pockets in these garments enable you to anchor the drain and have it hidden from your outer clothing. In addition, the camisoles are very soft, can be pulled up from your feet, come with two "puffs" that can be reconstructed by you to match the remaining breast, and are covered by insurance.

Along with a camisole, I highly recommend purchasing one or two leisure bras. These bras close in the front, can be used with the puffs from the camisole, and are a great addition right after surgery. One particular postmastectomy camisole has removable Velcro pockets that can also be anchored to your leisure bra. This offers a unique way to accommodate the drain.

I'm a very active person—I swim, run, and spend a lot of time outdoors. Are there breast forms that will accommodate my active lifestyle?

The wide variety of breast forms on the market today enables active women to continue their lifestyle. For swimming, we have swim forms that are silicone shells. These are light, reasonably priced, covered by insurance, and can be used in hot tubs, saltwater, and chlorine. Several of the lighter poly-fil forms or casual/leisure forms would work comfortably during exercise. Additionally, there is a wonderful new garment we call the bathing suit bra that can be worn under swimsuits and tank tops or used as a sports bra. It is constructed of a Lycra material similar to that of a bathing suit, and it enables women to feel confident and active as it keeps the forms in place.

I'm going to have a mastectomy, and I'm worried that no matter what kind of breast form I get, it won't look the same as my natural breast. How should I go about choosing a breast form to make sure I get the right fit and match?

After a mastectomy it is wise to wait four to six weeks before being fitted for a silicone form. It takes time for the swelling to decrease and for your chest area to feel comfortable so that you can wear a regular bra. The many silicone forms on the market today, ranging from very light to more weighted forms, and the skills of a certified fitter who can show you various types of forms will allow you to find one with which you're comfortable. By trying on various shapes and weights and using your eyes and a tape measure to compare, you will be able to choose the one that feels right. I always encourage my customers to think about comfort first. One must also allow for small imperfections. Remember, our natural breasts are not identical in size and shape.

I have been experiencing terrible night sweats as a result of my treatments. Do you have any ideas for sleepwear solutions that might keep me from waking up soaked?

Recently, several manufacturers have developed beautiful, comfortable sleepwear made from wicking fabric that pulls the excess moisture away from your skin. You can choose among nightgowns, nightshirts, and pajamas that have either long pants or shorts. There are also pillowcases and robes available that are made from the same type of fabric.

My hair has just started to really fall out fast, and I'm considering a wig. Are there different kinds of wigs I should consider? What other attractive options are available if I don't feel comfortable in a wig?

Hair loss as a result of chemotherapy and radiation can be one of the hardest side effects of treatment to handle. But the good news is that there are many options today for all types of women depending on your personal choice.

In the wig category, one can choose synthetic fibers, human-hair blends, or 100 percent human-hair wigs. The synthetic wigs are the easiest to care for. Many of these are made so well that one cannot tell they are synthetic. You will never have a "bad hair day" with a synthetic wig. The main drawback to these is that no heat can be applied. (That means not opening that oven door with your wig on and not using a hair dryer.) These wigs are prestyled and should not need any special treatment. The human-hair blends are 70 percent human hair and 30 percent synthetic, which allows the wig to act as a human-hair wig with the bonus that the synthetic fibers keep it perfectly styled. You may use a hair dryer with this type of wig. The 100 percent human-hair wigs are more costly and require a bit more care, although many women prefer them.

Not all women wish to purchase a wig. We have some wonderfully fashionable options. There are hats with hair, Velcro bangs, hoops of hair, and attractive scarves and turbans that can be layered for a chic, elegant look.

*All of these innovations in clothing and prosthetics seem
great, but I just don't have any extra money with all of the
medical bills left to pay. Are any of these items covered by
insurance or Medicare?*

Most commercial insurance companies cover wigs. Each policy is
different, and I encourage you to call and check with your insurance
company. All insurance companies, including Medicare, cover prosthetics and bras. Medicare covers one silicone prosthesis every two years,
one foam prosthesis every six months, and up to six bras per year.
Camisoles and bras with built-in forms are also covered.

*I was diagnosed with lymphedema after lymph nodes un-
der my arm were removed during my breast surgery. The
doctor has recommended a compression sleeve. Can you
tell me what they're all about?*

Women who have had breast surgery with lymph node removal are
more susceptible to arm swelling. If you notice a change, you should
be evaluated by a lymphedema specialist who has experience in lymphatic massage.

There are many types of sleeves, compressions, and products available. Your physician and lymphedema specialist can assist you in making the best choice. An excellent website for information is http://
www.lymphnet.org.

*I am undergoing radiation treatments, and my clothes are
uncomfortable because my skin is extremely sensitive. What
is the best type of clothing to wear? Also, I've heard that I
shouldn't use deodorant while receiving radiation—is this
true?*

The effects of radiation can be extremely irritating to skin. Radiation is also cumulative, which means that it continues to work after
treatments are completed. I recommend wearing a cotton or cotton-
blend camisole that will not irritate the area being treated. Several
of the immediate post-surgical camisoles would work. During this
period it is best to avoid tight-fitting garments and those with tight
elastic.

A non-metallic deodorant is recommended during radiation. One
good alternative is Alra deodorant, which has no aluminum or metallic salts to irritate the skin or interfere with medical treatments.

Section 30.4

Your Rights after a Mastectomy

"Your Rights after a Mastectomy... Women's Health and Cancer Rights
Act of 1998," U.S. Department of Labor (www.dol.gov), June 2006.

If you have had a mastectomy or expect to have one, you may be
entitled to special rights under the Women's Health and Cancer Rights
Act of 1998 (WHCRA). The following questions and answers clarify
your basic WHCRA rights. Under WHCRA, if your group health plan
covers mastectomies, the plan must provide certain reconstructive
surgery and other post-mastectomy benefits. Your health plan or is-
suer is required to provide you with a notice of your rights under
WHCRA when you enroll in the health plan, and then once each year.

I've been diagnosed with breast cancer and plan to have a mastectomy. How will WHCRA affect my benefits?

Under WHCRA, group health plans, insurance companies and health
maintenance organizations (HMOs) offering mastectomy coverage
also must provide coverage for certain services relating to the mastectomy in a manner determined in consultation with your attending physician and you. This required coverage includes all stages of
reconstruction of the breast on which the mastectomy was performed,
surgery and reconstruction of the other breast to produce a symmetrical appearance, prostheses and treatment of physical complications
of the mastectomy, including lymphedema.

Does WHCRA require all group health plans, insurance companies, and HMOs to provide reconstructive surgery benefits?

Generally, group health plans, as well as their insurance companies
and HMOs, that provide coverage for medical and surgical benefits
with respect to a mastectomy must comply with WHCRA. However,
if your coverage is provided by a "church plan" or "governmental plan",
check with your plan administrator. Certain plans that are church
plans or governmental plans may not be subject to this law.

May group health plans, insurance companies or HMOs impose deductibles or coinsurance requirements on the coverage specified in WHCRA?

Yes, but only if the deductibles and coinsurance are consistent with those established for other benefits under the plan or coverage.

I just changed jobs and am enrolled under my new employer's plan. I underwent a mastectomy and chemo-therapy treatment under my previous employer's plan. Now I want reconstructive surgery. Under WHCRA, is my new employer's plan required to cover my reconstructive surgery?

If your new employer's plan provides coverage for mastectomies and if you are receiving benefits under the plan that are related to your mastectomy, then your new employer's plan generally will be required to cover reconstructive surgery if you request it. In addition, your new employer's plan generally is required to cover other benefits specified under WHCRA. It does not matter that your mastectomy was not covered by your new employer's plan.

However, a group health plan may limit benefits relating to a health condition that was present before your enrollment date in your current employer's plan through a preexisting condition exclusion. A Federal law known as the Health Insurance Portability and Accountability Act of 1996 (HIPAA) limits the circumstances under which a preexisting condition exclusion may be applied. Specifically, HIPAA provides that a plan may impose a preexisting condition exclusion only if:

- The exclusion relates to a condition (whether physical or mental) for which medical advice, diagnosis, care or treatment was recommended or received within the six-month period ending on your enrollment date.

- The exclusion extends no more than 12 months (or 18 months in the case of a late enrollee in the new plan) after the enrollment date.

- The preexisting condition exclusion period is reduced by the days of prior creditable coverage (if any, which is defined in HIPAA as most health coverage).

- The plan also must provide you with written notification of the existence and terms of any preexisting condition exclusion under the plan and of your rights to demonstrate prior creditable coverage.

271

My employer's group health plan provides coverage through an insurance company. Following my mastectomy, my employer changed insurance companies. The new insurance company is refusing to cover my reconstructive surgery. Does WHCRA provide me with any protections?

Yes, as long as the new insurance company provides coverage for mastectomies, you are receiving benefits under the plan related to your mastectomy, and you elect to have reconstructive surgery. If these conditions apply, the new insurance company is required to provide coverage for breast reconstruction as well as the other benefits required under WHCRA. It does not matter that your mastectomy was not covered by the new insurance company.

I understand that my group health plan is required to provide me with a notice of my rights under WHCRA when I enroll in the plan. What information can I expect to find in this notice?

Plans must provide a notice to all employees when they enroll in the health plan describing the benefits that WHCRA requires the plan and its insurance companies or HMOs to cover. These benefits include coverage of all stages of reconstruction of the breast on which the mastectomy was performed, surgery and reconstruction of the other breast to produce a symmetrical appearance, prostheses, and treatment of physical complications of the mastectomy, including lymphedema.

The enrollment notice also must state that for the covered employee or their family member who is receiving mastectomy-related benefits, coverage will be provided in a manner determined in consultation with the attending physician and the patient.

Finally, the enrollment notice must describe any deductibles and coinsurance limitations that apply to the coverage specified under WHCRA. Deductibles and coinsurance limitations may be imposed only if they are consistent with those established for other benefits under the plan or coverage.

What can I expect to find in the annual WHCRA notice from my health plan?

Your annual notice should describe the four categories of coverage required under WHCRA and information on how to obtain a detailed description of the mastectomy-related benefits available under your plan. For example, an annual notice might look something like this:

"Do you know that your plan, as required by the Women's Health and Cancer Rights Act of 1998, provides benefits for mastectomy-related services including all stages of reconstruction and surgery to achieve symmetry between the breasts, prostheses, and complications resulting from a mastectomy, including lymphedema? Call your plan administrator [phone number here] for more information."

Your annual notice may be the same notice provided when you enrolled in the plan if it contains the information described above.

My state requires health insurance issuers to cover the benefits required by WHCRA and also requires health insurance issuers to cover minimum hospital stays in connection with a mastectomy (which is not required by WHCRA). If I have a mastectomy and breast reconstruction, am I also entitled to the minimum hospital stay?

If your employer's group health plan provides coverage through an insurance company or HMO, you are entitled to the minimum hospital stay required by the state law. Many state laws provide more protections than WHCRA. Those additional protections apply to coverage provided by an insurance company or HMO (known as "insured" coverage).

If your employer's plan does not provide coverage through an insurance company or HMO (in other words, your employer "self-insures" your coverage), then the state law does not apply. In that case, only the federal law, WHCRA, applies, and it does not require minimum hospital stays. To find out if your group health coverage is "insured" or "self-insured," check your health plan's Summary Plan Description or contact your plan administrator.

If your coverage is "insured" and you want to know if you have additional state law protections, check with your State insurance department.

My health coverage is through an individual policy, not through an employer. What rights, if any, do I have under WHCRA?

Health insurance companies and HMOs are generally required to provide WHCRA benefits to individual policies too. These requirements are generally within the jurisdiction of the state insurance department. Call your state insurance department or the Department of Health and Human Services toll free at 877-267-2323 extension 61565, for further information.

Section 30.5

Breast Reconstruction

This section begins with text excerpted from "Surgery Choices for Women with Early-Stage Breast Cancer," National Cancer Institute (www.cancer .gov), October 2004. "Questions about Breast Reconstruction" is excerpted from "Early Stage Breast Cancer: A Patient and Doctor Dialogue," Office on Women's Health, U.S. Department of Health and Human Services, March 2002. "Choices in Reconstructive Procedures" is excerpted from "Breast Implant Surgery and Related Issues," *FDA Breast Implant Consumer Handbook*, U.S. Food and Drug Administration (FDA), 2004. This section concludes with excerpts from "Breast Implant Questions and Answers," FDA, 2006.

Two Types of Breast Reconstruction Surgery

There are two types of breast reconstruction surgery:

Breast implants: In this kind of surgery, a reconstructive plastic surgeon puts an implant (filled with salt water or silicone gel) under your skin or chest muscle to build a new breast-like shape. While this shape looks like a breast, you will have little feeling in it because the nerves have been cut.

Breast implants do not last a lifetime. If you choose to have an implant, chances are you will need more surgery later on to remove or replace it. Implants can cause problems such as breast hardness, breast pain, and infection. The implant may also break, move, or shift. These problems can happen soon after surgery or years later.

Tissue flaps: In tissue flap surgery, a surgeon builds a new breast-like shape from muscle, fat, and skin taken from other parts of your body. This new breast-like shape should last the rest of your life. Women who are very thin or obese, smoke, or have other serious health problems often cannot have tissue flap surgery.

Tissue flap is major surgery. Healing often takes longer after this surgery than if you have breast implants. You may have other problems, as well. For example, you might lose strength in the part of your body where muscle was taken to build a new breast. Or you may get an infection or have trouble healing. Tissue flap surgery is best done by a reconstructive plastic surgeon who has done it many times before.

Questions about Breast Reconstruction

Can I have breast reconstruction at the same time as my mastectomy?

Most women can undergo at least part of the breast reconstruction procedure at the same time as their mastectomy. Breast reconstruction can be done later as well. For some kinds of reconstruction, more than one surgery is needed. Different breast reconstruction procedures have various complications that need to be discussed before a decision is made.

With reconstruction, can I change the size of my breasts? Can the plastic surgeon make the other breast match?

In many cases, a plastic surgeon can change the size of the breasts. Some plastic surgeons are more skilled than others at making the other breast match. Sometimes, it would be necessary to perform surgery on the healthy breast to help make them match. Usually, reconstruction with a woman's own tissue has a more natural appearance than implants, which tend to be higher and rounder than a natural breast. Women who are seriously considering reconstructive surgery should have a full consultation with the plastic surgeon before having a mastectomy and can bring a list of questions to ask.

Can I have reconstruction after radiation?

Breast reconstruction is possible after radiation but the surgery may be more difficult to perform, and this should be discussed with a plastic surgeon.

Choices in Reconstructive Procedures

The type of breast reconstruction procedures available to you depends on your medical situation, breast shape and size, general health, lifestyle, and goals. You can have your breast reconstructed with a breast implant, a tissue flap (your own tissues), or a combination of the two. If you have breast reconstruction, with or without breast implants, you will probably undergo several reoperations to improve symmetry and appearance.

For example, after your breast has healed from the original implant surgery, you may want to build a new nipple and darken the areola (skin around the nipple). This procedure can usually be performed on an outpatient basis. Ask your doctor to ex plain the various ways this can be done, such as using a skin graft from the opposite breast or by tattooing the area. Ask your doctor about the pros and cons of each implant technique. If you decide to have reconstruction for one breast, your doctor may suggest surgery on the other breast to achieve a similar appearance.

The following issues should be considered for women with breast cancer:

- The physical and cosmetic results with breast implants may be affected by chemotherapy, radiation therapy, or any other factor that significantly affects the healing process.

- Skin necrosis may occur because blood circulation to the remaining tissue has been changed by a mastectomy. Radiation treatment may also increase skin necrosis.

- It usually takes more than one operation to achieve the desired cosmetic outcome, especially if the reconstruction procedures include building a new nipple.

- Breast reconstruction is an optional procedure and is not needed to treat the cancer.

Breast Reconstruction with Breast Implants

The following information applies to reconstruction following mastectomy. However, similar considerations apply to reconstruction for breast trauma or congenital defects.

Your doctor will decide whether your health and medical condition makes you an appropriate candidate for breast reconstruction with breast implants. Women with larger breasts may require reconstruction with a combination of a tissue flap and an implant.

Your doctor may recommend a breast implant, reduction mammoplasty (breast reduction), or a mastopexy (breast lift) of your opposite, uninvolved breast to improve symmetry with your reconstructed breast. Reduction mammoplasty involves removal of breast tissue and skin. Mastopexy involves removing a strip of skin from under the breast or around the nipple and using it to lift and tighten the skin over the breast. If it is important to you not to alter the unaffected breast, you should discuss this with your doctor because it may affect the breast reconstruction procedures considered for your case.

The breast reconstruction process may begin at the time of your mastectomy (immediate reconstruction) or weeks to years afterwards (delayed reconstruction).

Immediate Reconstruction

- One-stage breast reconstruction may be done at the time of your mastectomy. After the general surgeon removes your breast tissue, the plastic surgeon will insert a breast implant under the skin where breast tissue was removed.

- Two-stage reconstruction is more typical. The first stage is a breast tissue expander placed at the time of your mastectomy to stretch your skin and create a pocket for a breast implant. Tissue expansion typically lasts four to six months. The tissue expander is then replaced several months later with a breast implant. This is considered immediate reconstruction because the tissue expander is placed at the time of mastectomy.

Delayed Reconstruction

Delayed reconstruction is a two-stage reconstruction starting with a breast tissue expander placed months or years later, which is then replaced several months later with a breast implant. This is considered delayed reconstruction because the tissue expander is placed after the mastectomy site has healed.

Immediate vs. Delayed Reconstruction

It is important to know that the one and two-stage references do not mean the number of surgeries involved. You should expect that any type of breast reconstruction will take several steps to complete. It could take months to years before your reconstruction is complete.

Two potential advantages to immediate reconstruction are that your breast reconstruction starts at the time of your mastectomy and that you may save money when you combine the mastectomy with the first stage of the reconstruction. However, with immediate reconstruction, there may be a higher risk of complications, such as rupture/deflation, as well as longer initial operation and healing times.

A potential advantage to delayed reconstruction is that you can delay your reconstruction decision and surgery until other treatments, such as radiation therapy and chemotherapy, are completed. Delayed reconstruction may be advisable if your surgeon anticipates healing problems with your mastectomy or if you just need more time to consider your options.

There are medical, financial, and emotional considerations to choosing immediate versus delayed reconstruction. You should discuss the pros and cons with the options available in your individual case with your surgeon, plastic surgeon, and oncologist.

Breast Reconstruction with Tissue Flaps

The breast can be reconstructed by surgically moving a section of skin, fat, muscle, and blood vessels from one area of your body to another. The tissue may be taken from such areas as your lower abdominal area, upper back, or buttocks. TRAM and latissimus dorsi are the most common types of tissue flaps:

- The TRAM (transverse rectus abdominus musculocutaneous) flap that uses tissue from the lower abdominal area.

- The latissimus dorsi flap that uses tissue from the upper back.

Flap surgery has the advantage of using your own tissue to construct a new breast. However, it is important for you to be aware that flap surgery, particularly TRAM flap surgery, is a major operation and more extensive than your mastectomy operation or breast implant surgery. It requires good general health and strong emotional motivation. If you are very overweight, smoke cigarettes, have had previous surgery at the flap site, or have any circulatory problems, you may not be a good candidate for a tissue flap procedure. Also, if you are very thin, you may not have enough tissue at the flap site to construct a breast mound.

Tissue flaps, in general, can be moved to the reconstruction site by one of two methods. The first method is when the flap is left attached to the muscle and blood vessels and tunneled under the skin to the reconstruction site. The second method is when the flap is completely removed and then transferred to the reconstruction site and reattached by microsurgery. More specifically, the TRAM flap can be done by either of these two methods while the latissimus dorsi flap procedure involves only the first method. In addition, for TRAM flap surgery, your surgeon may also need to build you a new belly button after the lower abdominal area is reshaped.

Flap surgery requires a hospital stay of several days and generally a longer recovery time than breast implant reconstruction. While you can resume normal daily activity after several weeks, some women report that it takes up to one year to resume a normal lifestyle.

Flap surgery also creates scars at the site where the flap was taken and possibly additional scars on the reconstructed breast. You may also have some temporary or permanent decreased muscle strength at the flap site.

As a special note regarding the TRAM flap procedure, if you are considering pregnancy after your reconstruction, you should discuss with your surgeon how this procedure may affect your abdominal muscle strength. In addition, although abdominal tissue feels like breast tissue to the touch, the nerves are cut during the surgery, so there may be little feeling or sensitivity in your breast. Also, you should know that a surgeon can take tissue from your abdomen only once. If you later need a mastectomy of your second breast and want to have a tissue flap procedure, then the tissue will have to come from another site, such as your back.

Breast Implant Questions and Answers

What are breast implants?

Breast implants are medical devices that are implanted either under breast tissue or under the chest muscle for breast augmentation or reconstruction. There are two major types: saline-filled and silicone gel-filled. Saline-filled breast implants are silicone shells that are either prefilled or filled with saline during surgery, and some of these allow for adjustments of the filler volume after surgery. Silicone gel-filled breast implants are silicone shells prefilled with silicone gel. Breast implants vary in profile, size, and shell surface (smooth or textured).

How are breast implants used?

Breast implants are used for the following purposes:

- Primary augmentation (to increase breast size for cosmetic reasons)

- Revision-augmentation (revision surgery to correct or improve the result of an original breast augmentation surgery)

- Primary reconstruction (to replace breast tissue that has been removed due to cancer or trauma or that has failed to develop properly due to a severe breast abnormality)

- Revision-reconstruction (revision surgery to correct or improve the result of an original breast reconstruction surgery).

What are the risks of breast implants?

Some of the risks of breast implants include the following:

- Reoperations (additional surgeries), with or without removal of the device

- Capsular contracture (hardening of the area around the implant)

- Breast pain

- Changes in nipple and breast sensation

- Rupture with deflation for saline-filled implants

- Rupture with or without symptoms for silicone gel-filled implants

- Migration of silicone gel for silicone gel-filled breast implants

What are some of the important factors I should consider when deciding whether or not to get breast implants?

- Breast implants do not last forever. If you decide to get breast implants, you will likely need additional surgeries on your breasts over your lifetime due to complications or unsatisfactory cosmetic outcomes.

- Many of the changes to your breasts following implantation cannot be undone. If you later choose to have your implants removed and not replaced, your breasts will not change back to the way they looked before your implant surgery. You may have permanent dimpling, puckering, wrinkling, or other cosmetic changes.

- When you have your implants replaced (revision), your risk of complications increases compared to your first (primary) surgery.

- Routine mammograms to screen for breast cancer will be more difficult with breast implants.

- Breast implants may affect your ability to breastfeed, either by reducing or eliminating milk production.

Factors to consider specifically about silicone gel-filled breast implants include the following:

- If your silicone gel-filled breast implant ruptures, you may have no symptoms. This is called a silent rupture because, most of the time, neither you nor your doctor will know that your implant has ruptured.

- The best way to determine whether or not your silicone gel-filled implant has ruptured is with an MRI examination. You should have your first MRI three years after your implant surgery and every two years thereafter.

- Over your lifetime, the cost of MRI screening may exceed the cost of your initial surgery. This cost may not be covered by medical insurance.

Chapter 31

Radiation Therapy

Chapter Contents

Section 31.1

Questions and Answers about Radiation Therapy

Excerpted from "Radiation Therapy and You: Support for People with Cancer," National Cancer Institute (www.cancer.gov), April 20, 2007.

What is radiation therapy?

Radiation therapy (also called radiotherapy) is a cancer treatment that uses high doses of radiation to kill cancer cells and stop them from spreading. At low doses, radiation is used as an x-ray to see inside your body and take pictures, such as x-rays of your teeth or broken bones. Radiation used in cancer treatment works in much the same way, except that it is given at higher doses.

How is radiation therapy given?

Radiation therapy can be external beam (when a machine outside your body aims radiation at cancer cells) or internal (when radiation is put inside your body, in or near the cancer cells). Sometimes people get both forms of radiation therapy.

Who gets radiation therapy?

Many people with cancer need radiation therapy. In fact, more than half (about 60 percent) of people with cancer get radiation therapy. Sometimes, radiation therapy is the only kind of cancer treatment people need.

What does radiation therapy do to cancer cells?

Given in high doses, radiation kills or slows the growth of cancer cells. Radiation therapy is used for these purposes:

- **Treat cancer:** Radiation can be used to cure, stop, or slow the growth of cancer.

- **Reduce symptoms:** When a cure is not possible, radiation may be used to shrink cancer tumors in order to reduce pressure.

Radiation therapy used in this way can treat problems such as pain, or it can prevent problems such as blindness or loss of bowel and bladder control.

How long does radiation therapy take to work?

Radiation therapy does not kill cancer cells right away. It takes days or weeks of treatment before cancer cells start to die. Then, cancer cells keep dying for weeks or months after radiation therapy ends.

What does radiation therapy do to healthy cells?

Radiation not only kills or slows the growth of cancer cells, it can also affect nearby healthy cells. The healthy cells almost always recover after treatment is over. But sometimes people may have side effects that do not get better or are severe. Doctors try to protect healthy cells during treatment by the following techniques:

- Using as low a dose of radiation as possible. The radiation dose is balanced between being high enough to kill cancer cells yet low enough to limit damage to healthy cells.

- Spreading out treatment over time. You may get radiation therapy once a day for several weeks or in smaller doses twice a day. Spreading out the radiation dose allows normal cells to recover while cancer cells die.

- Aiming radiation at a precise part of your body. New techniques, such as IMRT (intensity modulated radiation therapy) and 3-D conformal radiation therapy, allow your doctor to aim higher doses of radiation at your cancer while reducing the radiation to nearby healthy tissue.

- Using medicines. Some drugs can help protect certain parts of your body, such as the salivary glands that make saliva (spit).

Does radiation therapy hurt?

No, radiation therapy does not hurt while it is being given. But the side effects that people may get from radiation therapy can cause pain or discomfort.

Is radiation therapy used with other types of cancer treatment?

Yes, radiation therapy is often used with other cancer treatments. Here are some examples:

- **Radiation therapy and surgery:** Radiation may be given before, during, or after surgery. Doctors may use radiation to shrink the size of the cancer before surgery, or they may use radiation after surgery to kill any cancer cells that remain. Sometimes, radiation therapy is given during surgery so that it goes straight to the cancer without passing through the skin. This is called intraoperative radiation.

- **Radiation therapy and chemotherapy:** Radiation may be given before, during, or after chemotherapy. Before or during chemotherapy, radiation therapy can shrink the cancer so that chemotherapy works better. Sometimes, chemotherapy is given to help radiation therapy work better. After chemotherapy, radiation therapy can be used to kill any cancer cells that remain.

Who is on my radiation therapy team?

Many people help with your radiation treatment and care. This group of health care providers is often called the "radiation therapy team." They work together to provide care that is just right for you. Your radiation therapy team can include the following members:

- **Radiation oncologist:** This is a doctor who specializes in using radiation therapy to treat cancer. He or she prescribes how much radiation you will receive, plans how your treatment will be given, closely follows you during your course of treatment 10, and prescribes care you may need to help with side effects. He or she works closely with the other doctors, nurses, and health care providers on your team. After you are finished with radiation therapy, your radiation oncologist will see you for follow-up visits. During these visits, this doctor will check for late side effects and assess how well the radiation has worked.

- **Nurse practitioner:** This is a nurse with advanced training. He or she can take your medical history, do physical exams, order tests, manage side effects, and closely watch your response to treatment. After you are finished with radiation therapy, your nurse practitioner may see you for follow-up visits to check for late side effects and assess how well the radiation has worked.

- **Radiation nurse:** This person provides nursing care during radiation therapy, working with all the members of your radiation therapy team. He or she will talk with you about your radiation treatment and help you manage side effects.

- **Radiation therapist:** This person works with you during each radiation therapy session. He or she positions you for treatment and runs the machines to make sure you get the dose of radiation prescribed by your radiation oncologist.

- **Other health care providers:** Your team may also include a dietitian, physical therapist, social worker, and others.

- **You:** You are also part of the radiation therapy team. Your role is to arrive on time for all radiation therapy sessions; ask questions and talk about your concerns; let someone on your radiation therapy team know when you have side effects; tell your doctor or nurse if you are in pain; and follow the advice of your doctors and nurses about how to care for yourself at home, such as: taking care of your skin, drinking liquids, eating foods that they suggest, and keeping your weight the same.

Is radiation therapy expensive?

Yes, radiation therapy costs a lot of money. It uses complex machines and involves the services of many health care providers. The exact cost of your radiation therapy depends on the cost of health care where you live, what kind of radiation therapy you get, and how many treatments you need.

Talk with your health insurance company about what services it will pay for. Most insurance plans pay for radiation therapy for their members. To learn more, talk with the business office where you get treatment.

Should I follow a special diet while I am getting radiation therapy?

Your body uses a lot of energy to heal during radiation therapy. It is important that you eat enough calories and protein to keep your weight the same during this time. Ask your doctor or nurse if you need a special diet while you are getting radiation therapy. You might also find it helpful to speak with a dietitian.

You may want to read *Eating Hints,* a book from the National Cancer Institute. You can order a free copy online at https://cissecure.nci.nih.gov/ncipubs or by calling 800-4-CANCER.

Can I go to work during radiation therapy?

Some people are able to work full-time during radiation therapy. Others can only work part-time or not at all. How much you are able to work depends on how you feel. Ask your doctor or nurse what you may expect based on the treatment you are getting.

You are likely to feel well enough to work when you start radiation therapy. As time goes on, do not be surprised if you are more tired, have less energy, or feel weak. Once you have finished your treatment, it may take a few weeks or many months for you to feel better.

You may get to a point during your radiation therapy when you feel too sick to work. Talk with your employer to find out if you can go on medical leave. Make sure that your health insurance will pay for treatment when you are on medical leave.

What happens when radiation therapy is over?

Once you have finished radiation therapy, you will need follow-up care for the rest of your life. Follow-up care refers to checkups with your radiation oncologist or nurse practitioner after your course of radiation therapy is over. During these checkups, your doctor or nurse will see how well the radiation therapy worked, check for other signs of cancer, look for late side effects, and talk with you about your treatment and care. Your doctor or nurse will do the following:

- Examine you and review how you have been feeling. Your doctor or nurse practitioner can prescribe medicine or suggest other ways to treat any side effects you may have.

- Order lab and imaging tests. These may include blood tests, x-rays, or CT, MRI, or PET scans.

- Discuss treatment. Your doctor or nurse practitioner may suggest that you have more treatment, such as extra radiation treatments, chemotherapy, or both.

- Answer your questions and respond to your concerns. It may be helpful to write down your questions ahead of time and bring them with you.

After radiation therapy is over, what symptoms should I look for?

You have gone through a lot with cancer and radiation therapy. Now you may be even more aware of your body and how you feel each day. Pay attention to changes in your body and let your doctor or nurse know if you have any of these concerns:

- A pain that does not go away
- New lumps, bumps, swellings, rashes, bruises, or bleeding
- Appetite changes, nausea, vomiting, diarrhea, or constipation
- Weight loss that you cannot explain
- A fever, cough, or hoarseness that does not go away
- Any other symptoms that worry you

Section 31.2

Managing the Side Effects of Radiation Therapy

Excerpted from "Radiation Therapy and You: Support for People with Cancer," National Cancer Institute (www.cancer.gov), April 20, 2007.

Many people who get radiation therapy have skin changes and some fatigue. Other side effects depend on the part of your body being treated.

Skin changes may include dryness, itching, peeling, or blistering. These changes occur because radiation therapy damages healthy skin cells in the treatment area. You will need to take special care of your skin during radiation therapy.

Fatigue is often described as feeling worn out or exhausted. There are many ways to manage fatigue.

Depending on the part of your body being treated, you may also have any of the following:

- Diarrhea

- Hair loss in the treatment area
- Mouth problems
- Nausea and vomiting
- Sexual changes
- Swelling
- Trouble swallowing
- Urinary and bladder changes

Most of these side effects go away within two months after radiation therapy is finished.

Late side effects may first occur six or more months after radiation therapy is over. They vary by the part of your body that was treated and the dose of radiation you received. Late side effects may include infertility, joint problems, lymphedema, mouth problems, and secondary cancer. Everyone is different, so talk to your doctor or nurse about whether you might have late side effects and what signs to look for.

Breast Radiation Therapy Side Effects

Radiation therapy side effects depend on the part of your body being treated. Side effects most commonly associated with radiation therapy to the breast include fatigue, hair loss, skin changes, and tenderness and swelling.

Radiation Therapy Side Effects and Ways to Manage Them

Fatigue

What it is: Fatigue from radiation therapy can range from a mild to an extreme feeling of being tired. Many people describe fatigue as feeling weak, weary, worn out, heavy, or slow.

Why it occurs: Fatigue can happen for many reasons. These include the following:

- Anemia
- Anxiety
- Depression
- Infection

- Lack of activity
- Medicines

Fatigue can also come from the effort of going to radiation therapy each day or from stress. Most of the time, you will not know why you feel fatigue.

How long it lasts: When you first feel fatigue depends on a few factors, which include your age, health, level of activity, and how you felt before radiation therapy started.

Fatigue can last from six weeks to 12 months after your last radiation therapy session. Some people may always feel fatigue and, even after radiation therapy is over, will not have as much energy as they did before.

Ways to manage:

- Try to sleep at least eight hours each night. This may be more sleep than you needed before radiation therapy. One way to sleep better at night is to be active during the day. For example, you could go for walks, do yoga, or ride a bike. Another way to sleep better at night is to relax before going to bed. You might read a book, work on a jigsaw puzzle, listen to music, or do other calming hobbies.

- Plan time to rest. You may need to nap during the day. Many people say that it helps to rest for just 10 to 15 minutes. If you do nap, try to sleep for less than one hour at a time.

- Try not to do too much. With fatigue, you may not have enough energy to do all the things you want to do. Stay active, but choose the activities that are most important to you. For example, you might go to work but not do housework, or watch your children's sports events but not go out to dinner.

- Exercise. Most people feel better when they get some exercise each day. Go for a 15- to 30-minute walk or do stretches or yoga. Talk with your doctor or nurse about how much exercise you can do while having radiation therapy.

- Plan a work schedule that is right for you. Fatigue may affect the amount of energy you have for your job. You may feel well enough to work your full schedule, or you may need to work less— maybe just a few hours a day or a few days each week. You may want to talk with your boss about ways to work from home so you do not have to commute. And you may want to think about going on medical leave while you have radiation therapy.

- Plan a radiation therapy schedule that makes sense for you. You may want to schedule your radiation therapy around your work or family schedule. For example, you might want to have radiation therapy in the morning so you can go to work in the afternoon.

- Let others help you at home. Check with your insurance company to see whether it covers home care services. You can also ask family members and friends to help when you feel fatigue. Home care staff, family members, and friends can assist with household chores, running errands, or driving you to and from radiation therapy visits. They might also help by cooking meals for you to eat now or freeze for later.

- Learn from others who have cancer. People who have cancer can help each other by sharing ways to manage fatigue. One way to meet other people with cancer is by joining a support group—either in person or online. Talk with your doctor or nurse to learn more about support groups.

- Talk with your doctor or nurse. If you have trouble dealing with fatigue, your doctor may prescribe medicine (called psychostimulants) that can help decrease fatigue, give you a sense of well-being, and increase your appetite. Your doctor may also suggest treatments if you have anemia, depression, or are not able to sleep at night.

Hair Loss

What it is: Hair loss (also called alopecia) is when some or all of your hair falls out.

Why it occurs: Radiation therapy can cause hair loss because it damages cells that grow quickly, such as those in your hair roots.

Hair loss from radiation therapy only happens on the part of your body being treated. This is not the same as hair loss from chemotherapy, which happens all over your body. For instance, you may lose some or all of the hair on your head when you get radiation to your brain. But if you get radiation to your hip, you may lose pubic hair (between your legs) but not the hair on your head.

How long it lasts: You may start losing hair in your treatment area two to three weeks after your first radiation therapy session. It takes about a week for all the hair in your treatment area to fall out. Your hair may grow back three to six months after treatment is over. Sometimes, though, the dose of radiation is so high that your hair never grows back.

Once your hair starts to grow back, it may not look or feel the way it did before. Your hair may be thinner, or curly instead of straight. Or it may be darker or lighter in color than it was before.

Ways to manage hair loss on your head:

Before hair loss:

- Decide whether to cut your hair or shave your head. You may feel more in control of hair loss when you plan ahead. Use an electric razor to prevent nicking yourself if you decide to shave your head.

- If you plan to buy a wig, do so while you still have hair. The best time to select your wig is before radiation therapy begins or soon after it starts. This way, the wig will match the color and style of your own hair. Some people take their wig to their hair stylist. You will want to have your wig fitted once you have lost your hair. Make sure to choose a wig that feels comfortable and does not hurt your scalp.

- Check with your health insurance company to see whether it will pay for your wig. If it does not, you can deduct the cost of your wig as a medical expense on your income taxes. Some groups also sponsor free wig banks. Ask your doctor, nurse, or social worker if he or she can refer you to a free wig bank in your area.

- Be gentle when you wash your hair. Use a mild shampoo, such as a baby shampoo. Dry your hair by patting (not rubbing) it with a soft towel.

- Do not use curling irons, electric hair dryers, curlers, hair bands, clips, or hair sprays. These can hurt your scalp or cause early hair loss.

- Do not use products that are harsh on your hair. These include hair colors, perms, gels, mousse, oil, grease, or pomade.

After hair loss:

- Protect your scalp. Your scalp may feel tender after hair loss. Cover your head with a hat, turban, or scarf when you are outside.

Try not to be in places where the temperature is very cold or very hot. This means staying away from the direct sun, sun lamps, and very cold air.

- Stay warm. Your hair helps keep you warm, so you may feel colder once you lose it. You can stay warmer by wearing a hat, turban, scarf, or wig.

Skin Changes

What they are: Radiation therapy can cause skin changes in your treatment area. Here are some common skin changes:

- Redness: Your skin in the treatment area may look as if you have a mild to severe sunburn or tan. This can occur on any part of your body where you are getting radiation.

- Pruritus: The skin in your treatment area may itch so much that you always feel like scratching. This causes problems because scratching too much can lead to skin breakdown and infection.

- Dry and peeling skin: This is when the skin in your treatment area gets very dry—much drier than normal. In fact, your skin may be so dry that it peels like it does after a sunburn.

- Moist reaction: Radiation kills skin cells in your treatment area, causing your skin to peel off faster than it can grow back. When this happens, you can get sores or ulcers. The skin in your treatment area can also become wet, sore, or infected. This is more common where you have skin folds, such as your buttocks, behind your ears, under your breasts. It may also occur where your skin is very thin, such as your neck.

- Swollen skin: The skin in your treatment area may be swollen and puffy.

Why they occur: Radiation therapy causes skin cells to break down and die. When people get radiation almost every day, their skin cells do not have enough time to grow back between treatments. Skin changes can happen on any part of the body that gets radiation.

How long they last: Skin changes may start a few weeks after you begin radiation therapy. Many of these changes often go away a few weeks after treatment is over. But even after radiation therapy ends, you may still have skin changes. Your treated skin may always look darker and blotchy. It may feel very dry or thicker than before. And you may always burn quickly and be sensitive to the sun. You will always be at risk for skin cancer in the treatment area. Be sure to avoid tanning beds and protect yourself from the sun by wearing a hat, long sleeves, long pants, and sunscreen with an SPF of 30 or higher.

Ways to manage:

- Skin care. Take extra good care of your skin during radiation therapy. Be gentle and do not rub, scrub, or scratch in the treatment area. Also, use creams that your doctor prescribes.

- Take extra good care of your skin during radiation therapy. Be gentle and do not rub, scrub, or scratch.

- Do not put anything on your skin that is very hot or cold. This means not using heating pads, ice packs, or other hot or cold items on the treatment area. It also means washing with lukewarm water.

- Be gentle when you shower or take a bath. You can take a lukewarm shower every day. If you prefer to take a lukewarm bath, do so only every other day and soak for less than 30 minutes. Whether you take a shower or bath, make sure to use a mild soap that does not have fragrance or deodorant in it. Dry yourself with a soft towel by patting, not rubbing, your skin. Be careful not to wash off the ink markings that you need for radiation therapy.

- Use only those lotions and skin products that your doctor or nurse suggests. If you are using a prescribed cream for a skin problem or acne, you must tell your doctor or nurse before you begin radiation treatment. Check with your doctor or nurse before using any of the following skin products:

  - Bubble bath
  - Cornstarch
  - Cream
  - Deodorant
  - Hair removers
  - Makeup
  - Oil

- Ointment
- Perfume
- Powder
- Soap
- Sunscreen

If you use any skin products on days you have radiation therapy, use them at least four hours before your treatment session.

- Cool, humid places. Your skin may feel much better when you are in cool, humid places. You can make rooms more humid by putting a bowl of water on the radiator or using a humidifier. If you use a humidifier, be sure to follow the directions about cleaning it to prevent bacteria.

- Soft fabrics. Wear clothes and use bed sheets that are soft, such as those made from cotton.

- Do not wear clothes that are tight and do not breathe, such as girdles and pantyhose.

- Protect your skin from the sun every day. The sun can burn you even on cloudy days or when you are outside for just a few minutes. Do not go to the beach or sun bathe. Wear a broad-brimmed hat, long-sleeved shirt, and long pants when you are outside. Talk with your doctor or nurse about sunscreen lotions. He or she may suggest that you use a sunscreen with an SPF of 30 or higher. You will need to protect your skin from the sun even after radiation therapy is over, since you will have an increased risk of skin cancer for the rest of your life.

- Do not use tanning beds. Tanning beds expose you to the same harmful effects as the sun.

- Adhesive tape. Do not put bandages, BAND-AIDS®, or other types of sticky tape on your skin in the treatment area. Talk with your doctor or nurse about ways to bandage without tape.

- Shaving. Ask your doctor or nurse if you can shave the treated area. If you can shave, use an electric razor and do not use pre-shave lotion.

- Rectal area. If you have radiation therapy to the rectal area, you are likely to have skin problems. These problems are often worse after a bowel movement. Clean yourself with a baby wipe or squirt of water from a spray bottle. Also ask your nurse about sitz baths (a warm-water bath taken in a sitting position that covers only the hips and buttocks.)

- Talk with your doctor or nurse. Some skin changes can be very serious. Your treatment team will check for skin changes each time you have radiation therapy. Make sure to report any skin changes that you notice.

- Medicine. Medicines can help with some skin changes. They include lotions for dry or itchy skin, antibiotics to treat infection, and other drugs to reduce swelling or itching.

Late Radiation Therapy Side Effects

Late side effects are those that first occur at least six months after radiation therapy is over. Late side effects are rare, but they do happen. It is important to have follow-up care with a radiation oncologist or nurse practitioner for the rest of your life.

Whether you get late side effects will depend on the part of your body that was treated, the dose and length of your radiation therapy, and if you received chemotherapy before, during, or after radiation therapy. Your doctor or nurse will talk with you about late side effects and discuss ways to help prevent them, symptoms to look for, and how to treat them if they occur.

Secondary Cancer

What it is: Radiation therapy can cause a new cancer many years after you have finished treatment. This does not happen very often.

Ways to manage: You will need to have check-ups with your radiation oncologist or nurse practitioner for the rest of your life to check for cancer—the one you were treated for and any new cancer that may occur.

Questions to Ask Your Doctor or Nurse

Here are some questions you might want to ask your doctor or nurse. You may want to write down their answers so you can review them again later.

- What kind of radiation therapy will I get?
- How can radiation therapy help?

- How many weeks will my course of radiation therapy last?
- What kinds of side effects should I expect during my course of radiation therapy?
- Will these side effects go away after radiation therapy is over?
- What kind of late side effects should I expect after radiation therapy is over?
- What can I do to manage these side effects?
- What will you do to manage these side effects?
- How can I learn more about radiation therapy?

Section 31.3

Radiation Therapy for Breast Cancer Now Less Risky for the Heart

National Cancer Institute (www.cancer.gov), March 23, 2005.

The risk of death from heart disease caused by radiation therapy for breast cancer has declined steadily over the past 25 years, according to a new study.

About four out of every 10 women with breast cancer in the United States receive adjuvant (additional) radiation therapy after surgery. Studies have shown that giving radiation after lumpectomy reduces by two-thirds a woman's risk that her cancer will recur in the same breast. Survival rates for women treated with lumpectomy and radiation are the same as for women who have a mastectomy. Radiation may also be recommended after a mastectomy to reduce the risk of cancer recurrence.

Observational studies suggest that radiation therapy is underused in breast cancer patients, in part because of concerns about its adverse effects. In particular, several studies have shown that women treated with radiation have a higher risk of death from heart disease. These studies mostly involved patients treated in the 1960s and 1970s. Since that time, however, new techniques for giving radiation therapy have allowed doctors to minimize the radiation dose to the heart.

Radiation therapy to the left breast may deliver a higher dose of radiation to the heart than radiation therapy to the right breast. Previous studies have shown higher death rates from heart disease in women treated with radiation for cancer in the left breast than in those who received radiation to the right breast.

The current study was conducted to find out whether breast cancer patients' risk of death from heart disease caused by radiation therapy had changed over time.

The Study

Researchers analyzed information about more than 27,000 women who were diagnosed with breast cancer between 1973 and 1989 and were treated with radiation therapy in addition to surgery. The information was obtained from the National Cancer Institute (NCI's) Surveillance, Epidemiology, and End Results program.

The investigators grouped the women according to when their cancer was diagnosed and whether it was in the left or right breast. They then calculated death rates from heart disease both for the entire study population and for the subgroups.

The study's lead author is Sharon H. Giordano, M.D., MPH, of the University of Texas M.D. Anderson Cancer Center in Houston.

Results

In total, 8.7 percent of women with left-sided cancers died of heart disease within 15 years of their breast cancer diagnosis, compared with 7.5 percent of women with right-sided cancers. This difference was so small that it was not statistically significant—that is, it could have occurred by chance.

The overall death rate from heart disease among study participants declined steadily over the period of time covered by the study. The additional risk for women with left-sided cancers also fell steadily, dropping by six percent per year between 1979 and 1988. Among women diagnosed in 1988, death rates from heart disease were the same for women with left-sided and right-sided cancers.

Limitations

The researchers counted deaths from heart disease that occurred within 12 to 15 years of a breast cancer diagnosis. However, previous studies have shown that the risk of death from heart disease caused by radiation therapy persists for at least 20 years, points out Jack Cuzick, Ph.D., of Cancer Research UK in London, England, in an accompanying editorial. Longer follow-up is needed to show definitively whether or not radiation therapy still increases the risk of death from heart disease.

Also, the recent trend toward diagnosing more breast cancers early could have affected the study's findings, the authors note. Women whose cancer was detected before it had spread to the lymph nodes may have received less extensive radiation therapy and, for that reason, had a lower risk of heart disease.

Comment

"This is a well-done study which shows that the careful application of modern radiotherapy techniques reduces the risk of heart complications," says C. Norman Coleman, M.D., associate director of the radiation research program of the National Cancer Institute. "As with all studies of long-term outcome, additional follow-up data are important. These results mean that the decision to use or not use radiation as part of breast cancer therapy can be based on the clinical and biological features of the patient's disease and not on the fear of inducing a heart complication."

Chapter 32

Chemotherapy

Chapter Contents

Section 32.1

Questions and Answers about Chemotherapy

Excerpted from "Chemotherapy and You: Support for People with
Cancer," National Cancer Institute (www.cancer.gov); June 29, 2007.

What is chemotherapy?

Chemotherapy (also called chemo) is a type of cancer treatment
that uses drugs to destroy cancer cells.

How does chemotherapy work?

Chemotherapy works by stopping or slowing the growth of cancer
cells, which grow and divide quickly. But it can also harm healthy cells
that divide quickly, such as those that line your mouth and intestines
or cause your hair to grow. Damage to healthy cells may cause side effects. Often, side effects get better or go away after chemotherapy is over.

What does chemotherapy do?

Depending on your type of cancer and how advanced it is, chemotherapy can be use for the following:

- **Cure cancer:** When chemotherapy destroys cancer cells to the
  point that your doctor can no longer detect them in your body
  and they will not grow back.

- **Control cancer:** When chemotherapy keeps cancer from
  spreading, slows its growth, or destroys cancer cells that have
  spread to other parts of your body.

- **Ease cancer symptoms (also called palliative care):** When
  chemotherapy shrinks tumors that are causing pain or pressure.

How is chemotherapy used?

Sometimes, chemotherapy is used as the only cancer treatment.
But more often, you will get chemotherapy along with surgery, radiation

therapy, or biological therapy. Chemotherapy can be used for the following purposes:

- Make a tumor smaller before surgery or radiation therapy. This is called neoadjuvant chemotherapy.

- Destroy cancer cells that may remain after surgery or radiation therapy. This is called adjuvant chemotherapy.

- Help radiation therapy and biological therapy work better.

- Destroy cancer cells that have come back (recurrent cancer) or spread to other parts of your body (metastatic cancer).

How does my doctor decide which chemotherapy drugs to use?

This choice depends on these factors:

- The type of cancer you have. Some types of chemotherapy drugs are used for many types of cancer. Other drugs are used for just one or two types of cancer.

- Whether you have had chemotherapy before.

- Whether you have other health problems, such as diabetes or heart disease.

Where do I go for chemotherapy?

You may receive chemotherapy during a hospital stay, at home, or in a doctor's office, clinic, or outpatient unit in a hospital (which means you do not have to stay overnight). No matter where you go for chemotherapy, your doctor and nurse will watch for side effects and make any needed drug changes.

How often will I receive chemotherapy?

Treatment schedules for chemotherapy vary widely. How often and how long you get chemotherapy depends on your type of cancer and how advanced it is; the goals of treatment (whether chemotherapy is used to cure your cancer, control its growth, or ease the symptoms); the type of chemotherapy; and how your body reacts to chemotherapy.

You may receive chemotherapy in cycles. A cycle is a period of chemotherapy treatment followed by a period of rest. For instance, you might receive one week of chemotherapy followed by three weeks of rest. These four weeks make up one cycle. The rest period gives your body a chance to build new healthy cells.

Can I miss a dose of chemotherapy?

It is not good to skip a chemotherapy treatment. But sometimes your doctor or nurse may change your chemotherapy schedule. This can be due to side effects you are having. If this happens, your doctor or nurse will explain what to do and when to start treatment again.

How is chemotherapy given?

Chemotherapy may be given in many ways:

- **Injection:** The chemotherapy is given by a shot in a muscle in your arm, thigh, or hip or right under the skin in the fatty part of your arm, leg, or belly.

- **Intra-arterial (IA):** The chemotherapy goes directly into the artery that is feeding the cancer.

- **Intraperitoneal (IP):** The chemotherapy goes directly into the peritoneal cavity (the area that contains organs such as your intestines, stomach, liver, and ovaries).

- **Intravenous (IV):** The chemotherapy goes directly into a vein.

- **Topically:** The chemotherapy comes in a cream that you rub onto your skin.

- **Orally:** The chemotherapy comes in pills, capsules, or liquids that you swallow.

What are some things I should know about getting chemotherapy through an IV?

Chemotherapy is often given through a thin needle that is placed in a vein on your hand or lower arm. Your nurse will put the needle in at the start of each treatment and remove it when treatment is over. Let your doctor or nurse know right away if you feel pain or burning while you are getting IV chemotherapy.

IV chemotherapy is often given through catheters or ports, sometimes with the help of a pump.

- **Catheters:** A catheter is a soft, thin tube. A surgeon places one end of the catheter in a large vein, often in your chest area. The other end of the catheter stays outside your body. Most catheters stay in place until all your chemotherapy treatments are done. Catheters can also be used for drugs other than chemotherapy and to draw blood. Be sure to watch for signs of infection around your catheter.

- **Ports:** A port is a small, round disc made of plastic or metal that is placed under your skin. A catheter connects the port to a large vein, most often in your chest. Your nurse can insert a needle into your port to give you chemotherapy or draw blood. This needle can be left in place for chemotherapy treatments that are given for more than one day. Be sure to watch for signs of infection around your port.

- **Pumps:** Pumps are often attached to catheters or ports. They control how much and how fast chemotherapy goes into a catheter or port. Pumps can be internal or external. External pumps remain outside your body. Most people can carry these pumps with them. Internal pumps are placed under your skin during surgery.

How will I feel during chemotherapy?

Chemotherapy affects people in different ways. How you feel depends on how healthy you are before treatment, your type of cancer, how advanced it is, the kind of chemotherapy you are getting, and the dose. Doctors and nurses cannot know for certain how you will feel during chemotherapy.

Some people do not feel well right after chemotherapy. The most common side effect is fatigue, feeling exhausted and worn out. You can prepare for fatigue by asking someone to drive you to and from chemotherapy, planning time to rest on the day of and day after chemotherapy, and getting help with meals and childcare the day of and at least one day after chemotherapy.

Can I work during chemotherapy?

Many people can work during chemotherapy, as long as they match their schedule to how they feel. Whether or not you can work may depend on what kind of work you do. If your job allows, you may want to see if you can work part-time or work from home on days you do not feel well.

Many employers are required by law to change your work schedule to meet your needs during cancer treatment. Talk with your employer about ways to adjust your work during chemotherapy. You can learn more about these laws by talking with a social worker.

Can I take over-the-counter and prescription drugs while I get chemotherapy?

This depends on the type of chemotherapy you get and the other types of drugs you plan to take. Take only drugs that are approved by your doctor or nurse. Tell your doctor or nurse about all the over-the-counter and prescription drugs you take, including laxatives, allergy medicines, cold medicines, pain relievers, aspirin, and ibuprofen.

One way to let your doctor or nurse know about these drugs is by bringing in all your pill bottles. Your doctor or nurse needs to know the name of each drug, the reason you take it, how much you take, and how often you take it.

Can I take vitamins, minerals, dietary supplements, or herbs while I get chemotherapy?

Some of these products can change how chemotherapy works. For this reason, it is important to tell your doctor or nurse about all the vitamins, minerals, dietary supplements, and herbs that you take before you start chemotherapy. During chemotherapy, talk with your doctor before you take any of these products.

How will I know if my chemotherapy is working?

Your doctor will give you physical exams and medical tests (such as blood tests and x-rays). He or she will also ask you how you feel.

You cannot tell if chemotherapy is working based on its side effects. Some people think that severe side effects mean that chemotherapy is working well. Or that no side effects mean that chemotherapy is not working. The truth is that side effects have nothing to do with how well chemotherapy is fighting your cancer.

How much does chemotherapy cost?

It is hard to say how much chemotherapy will cost. It depends on the following:

- The types and doses of chemotherapy used
- How long and how often chemotherapy is given
- Whether you get chemotherapy at home, in a clinic or office, or during a hospital stay

- The part of the country where you live

Does my health insurance pay for chemotherapy?

Talk with your health insurance plan about what costs it will pay for. Questions to ask include the following:

- What will my insurance pay for?
- Do I or does the doctor's office need to call my insurance company before each treatment for it to be paid for?
- What do I have to pay for?
- Can I see any doctor I want or do I need to choose from a list of preferred providers?
- Do I need a written referral to see a specialist?
- Is there a co-pay (money I have to pay) each time I have an appointment?
- Is there a deductible (certain amount I need to pay) before my insurance pays?
- Where should I get my prescription drugs?
- Does my insurance pay for all my tests and treatments, whether I am an inpatient or outpatient?

How can I best work with my insurance plan?

- Read your insurance policy before treatment starts to find out what your plan will and will not pay for.
- Keep records of all your treatment costs and insurance claims.
- Send your insurance company all the paperwork it asks for. This may include receipts from doctors' visits, prescriptions, and lab work. Be sure to also keep copies for your own records.
- As needed, ask for help with the insurance paperwork. You can ask a friend, family member, social worker, or local group such as a senior center.
- If your insurance does not pay for something you think it should, find out why the plan refused to pay. Then talk with your doctor or nurse about what to do next. He or she may suggest ways to appeal the decision or other actions to take.

What are clinical trials and are they an option for me?

Cancer clinical trials (also called cancer treatment studies or research studies) test new treatments for people with cancer. These can be studies of new types of chemotherapy, other types of treatment, or new ways to combine treatments. The goal of all these clinical trials is to find better ways to help people with cancer.

Your doctor or nurse may suggest you take part in a clinical trial. You can also suggest the idea. Before you agree to be in a clinical trial, learn about its benefits, risks, and costs:

- **Benefits:** All clinical trials offer quality cancer care. Ask how this clinical trial could help you or others. For instance, you may be one of the first people to get a new treatment or drug.

- **Risks:** New treatments are not always better or even as good as standard treatments. And even if this new treatment is good, it may not work well for you.

- **Payment:** Your insurance company may or may not pay for treatment that is part of a clinical trial. Before you agree to be in a trial, check with your insurance company to make sure it will pay for this treatment.

Contact the National Cancer Institute's (NCI) Cancer Information Service (available online at www.cancer.gov) if you are interested in learning more about clinical trials.

Section 32.2

Managing the Side Effects of Chemotherapy

Excerpted from "Chemotherapy and You: Support for People with
Cancer," National Cancer Institute (www.cancer.gov); June 29, 2007.

Common Questions about Side Effects

What are side effects?

Side effects are problems caused by cancer treatment. Some common side effects from chemotherapy are fatigue, nausea, vomiting, decreased blood cell counts, hair loss, mouth sores, and pain.

What causes side effects?

Chemotherapy is designed to kill fast-growing cancer cells. But it can also affect healthy cells that grow quickly. These include cells that line your mouth and intestines, cells in your bone marrow that make blood cells, and cells that make your hair grow. Chemotherapy causes side effects when it harms these healthy cells.

Will I get side effects from chemotherapy?

You may have a lot of side effects, some, or none at all. This depends on the type and amount of chemotherapy you get and how your body reacts. Before you start chemotherapy, talk with your doctor or nurse about which side effects to expect.

How long do side effects last?

How long side effects last depends on your health and the kind of chemotherapy you get. Most side effects go away after chemotherapy is over. But sometimes it can take months or even years for them to go away.

Sometimes, chemotherapy causes long-term side effects that do not go away. These may include damage to your heart, lungs, nerves, kidneys, or reproductive organs. Some types of chemotherapy may cause a second cancer years later. Ask your doctor or nurse about your chance of having long-term side effects.

What can be done about side effects?

Doctors have many ways to prevent or treat chemotherapy side effects and help you heal after each treatment session. Talk with your doctor or nurse about which ones to expect and what to do about them. Make sure to let your doctor or nurse know about any changes you notice—they may be signs of a side effect.

Ways to Manage Chemotherapy Side Effects

Anemia

- Get plenty of rest. Try to sleep at least eight hours each night. You might also want to take one to two short naps (one hour or less) during the day.

- Limit your activities. This means doing only the activities that are most important to you. For example, you might go to work but not clean the house. Or you might order take-out food instead of cooking dinner.

- Accept help. When your family or friends offer to help, let them. They can help care for your children, pick up groceries, run errands, drive you to doctor's visits, or do other chores you feel too tired to do.

- Eat a well-balanced diet. Choose a diet that contains all the calories and protein your body needs. Calories will help keep your weight up, and extra protein can help repair tissues that have been harmed by cancer treatment. Talk to your doctor, nurse, or dietitian about the diet that is right for you.

- Stand up slowly. You may feel dizzy if you stand up too fast.

- When you get up from lying down, sit for a minute before you stand.

- Your doctor or nurse will check your blood cell count throughout your chemotherapy. You may need a blood transfusion if your red blood cell count falls too low. Your doctor may also prescribe a medicine to boost (speed up) the growth of red blood cells or suggest that you take iron or other vitamins.

Call your doctor or nurse if you experience the following:

- Your level of fatigue changes or you are not able to do your usual activities

- You feel dizzy or like you are going to faint

- You feel short of breath

- It feels like your heart is pounding or beating very fast

Appetite Changes

- Eat five to six small meals or snacks each day instead of three big meals. Choose foods and drinks that are high in calories and protein.

- Set a daily schedule for eating your meals and snacks. Eat when it is time to eat, rather than when you feel hungry. You may not feel hungry while you are on chemotherapy, but you still need to eat.

- Drink milkshakes, smoothies, juice, or soup if you do not feel like eating solid foods. Liquids like these can help provide the protein, vitamins, and calories your body needs.

- Use plastic forks and spoons. Some types of chemo give you a metal taste in your mouth. Eating with plastic can help decrease the metal taste. Cooking in glass pots and pans can also help.

- Increase your appetite by doing something active. For instance, you might have more of an appetite if you take a short walk before lunch. Also, be careful not to decrease your appetite by drinking too much liquid before or during meals.

- Change your routine. This may mean eating in a different place, such as the dining room rather than the kitchen. It can also mean eating with other people instead of eating alone. If you eat alone, you may want to listen to the radio or watch TV. You may also want to vary your diet by trying new foods and recipes.

- Talk with your doctor, nurse, or dietitian. He or she may want you to take extra vitamins or nutrition supplements (such as high protein drinks). If you cannot eat for a long time and are losing weight, you may need to take drugs that increase your appetite or receive nutrition through an IV or feeding tube.

Bleeding

Do

- Brush your teeth with a very soft toothbrush

- Soften the bristles of your toothbrush by running hot water over them before you brush

- Blow your nose gently

- Be careful when using scissors, knives, or other sharp objects

- Use an electric shaver instead of a razor

- Apply gentle but firm pressure to any cuts you get until the bleeding stops

- Wear shoes all the time, even inside the house or hospital

Do Not

- Use dental floss or toothpicks

- Play sports or do other activities during which you could get hurt

- Use tampons, enemas, suppositories, or rectal thermometers

- Wear clothes with tight collars, wrists, or waistbands

Check with your doctor or nurse before any of the following:

- Drinking beer, wine, or other types of alcohol

- Having sex

- Taking vitamins, herbs, minerals, dietary supplements, aspirin, or other over-the-counter medicines. Some of these products can change how chemotherapy works.

Let your doctor know if you are constipated. He or she may prescribe a stool softener to prevent straining and rectal bleeding when you go to the bathroom.

Your doctor or nurse will check your platelet count often. You may need medication, a platelet transfusion, or a delay in your chemotherapy treatment if your platelet count is too low.

Call your doctor or nurse if you have any of these symptoms:

- Bruises, especially if you did not bump into anything

- Small, red spots on your skin

- Red- or pink-colored urine

- Black or bloody bowel movements

- Bleeding from your gums or nose

- Heavy bleeding during your menstrual period or a prolonged period

- Vaginal bleeding not caused by your period

- Headaches or changes in your vision

- A warm or hot feeling in your arm or leg

- Feeling very sleepy or confused

Constipation

- Keep a record of your bowel movements. Show this record to your doctor or nurse and talk about what is normal for you. This makes it easier to figure out whether you have constipation.

- Drink at least eight cups of water or other fluids each day. Many people find that drinking warm or hot fluids, such as coffee and tea, helps with constipation. Fruit juices, such as prune juice, may also be helpful.

- Be active every day. You can be active by walking, riding a bike, or doing yoga. If you cannot walk, ask about exercises that you can do in a chair or bed. Talk with your doctor or nurse about ways you can be more active.

- Ask your doctor, nurse, or dietitian about foods that are high in fiber. Eating high-fiber foods and drinking lots of fluids can help soften your stools. Good sources of fiber include whole-grain breads and cereals, dried beans and peas, raw vegetables, fresh and dried fruit, nuts, seeds, and popcorn.

- Let your doctor or nurse know if you have not had a bowel movement in two days. Your doctor may suggest a fiber supplement, laxative, stool softener, or enema. Do not use these treatments without first checking with your doctor or nurse.

Diarrhea

- Eat five or six small meals and snacks each day instead of three large meals.

- Ask your doctor or nurse about foods that are high in salts such as sodium and potassium. Your body can lose these salts when you have diarrhea, and it is important to replace them. Foods that are high in sodium or potassium include bananas, oranges, peach and apricot nectar, and boiled or mashed potatoes.

- Drink eight to 12 cups of clear liquids each day. These include water, clear broth, ginger ale, or sports drinks such as Gatorade® or Propel®. Drink slowly, and choose drinks that are at room temperature. Let carbonated drinks lose their fizz before you drink them. Add extra water if drinks make you thirsty or nauseous (feeling like you are going to throw up).

- Eat low-fiber foods. Foods that are high in fiber can make diarrhea worse. Low-fiber foods include bananas, white rice, white toast, and plain or vanilla yogurt.

- Let your doctor or nurse know if your diarrhea lasts for more than 24 hours or if you have pain and cramping along with diarrhea. Your doctor may prescribe a medicine to control the diarrhea. You may also need IV fluids to replace the water and nutrients you lost. Do not take any medicine for diarrhea without first asking your doctor or nurse.

- Be gentle when you wipe yourself after a bowel movement. Instead of toilet paper, use a baby wipe or squirt of water from a spray bottle to clean yourself after bowel movements. Let your doctor or nurse know if your rectal area is sore or bleeds or if you have hemorrhoids.

- Ask your doctor if you should try a clear liquid diet. This can give your bowels time to rest. Most people stay on this type of diet for five days or less.

Stay away from the following:

- Drinks that are very hot or very cold

- Beer, wine, and other types of alcohol

- Milk or milk products, such as ice cream, milkshakes, sour cream, and cheese

- Spicy foods, such as hot sauce, salsa, chili, and curry dishes

- Greasy and fried foods, such as French fries and hamburgers

- Foods or drinks with caffeine, such as regular coffee, black tea, cola, and chocolate

- Foods or drinks that cause gas, such as cooked dried beans, cabbage, broccoli, and soy milk and other soy products

- Foods that are high in fiber, such as cooked dried beans, raw fruits and vegetables, nuts, and whole-wheat breads and cereals

Fatigue

- Relax. You might want to try meditation, prayer, yoga, guided imagery, visualization, or other ways to relax and decrease stress.

- Eat and drink well. Often, this means five to six small meals and snacks rather than three large meals. Keep foods around that are easy to fix, such as canned soups, frozen meals, yogurt, and cottage cheese. Drink plenty of fluids each day—about eight cups of water or juice.

- Plan time to rest. You may feel better when you rest or take a short nap during the day. Many people say that it helps to rest for just 10 to 15 minutes rather than nap for a long time. If you nap, try to sleep for less than one hour. Keeping naps short will help you sleep better at night.

- Be active. Research shows that exercise can ease fatigue and help you sleep better at night. Try going for a 15-minute walk, doing yoga, or riding an exercise bike. Plan to be active when you have the most energy. Talk with your doctor or nurse about ways you can be active while getting chemotherapy.

- Try not to do too much. With fatigue, you may not have enough energy to do all the things you want to do. Choose the activities you want to do and let someone else help with the others. Try quiet activities, such as reading, knitting, or learning a new language on tape.

- Sleep at least eight hours each night. This may be more sleep than you needed before chemotherapy. You are likely to sleep better at night when you are active during the day. You may also find it helpful to relax before going to bed. For instance, you might read a book, work on a jigsaw puzzle, listen to music, or do other quiet hobbies.

- Plan a work schedule that works for you. Fatigue may affect the amount of energy you have for your job. You may feel well enough to work your full schedule. Or you may need to work less— maybe just a few hours a day or a few days each week. If your job allows, you may want to talk with your boss about ways to work from home. Or you may want to go on medical leave (stop working for a while) while getting chemotherapy.

- Let others help. Ask family members and friends to help when you feel fatigue. Perhaps they can help with household chores or drive

315

you to and from doctor's visits. They might also help by shopping for food and cooking meals for you to eat now or freeze for later.

- Learn from others who have cancer. People who have cancer can help by sharing ways that they manage fatigue. One way to meet others is by joining a support group—either in person or online. Talk with your doctor or nurse to learn more.

- Keep a diary of how you feel each day. This will help you plan how to best use your time. Share your diary with your nurse. Let your doctor or nurse know if you notice changes in your energy level, whether you have lots of energy or are very tired.

- Talk with your doctor or nurse. Your doctor may prescribe medication that can help decrease fatigue, give you a sense of well-being, and increase your appetite. He or she may also suggest treatment if your fatigue is from anemia.

Hair Loss

Before Hair Loss

- Talk with your doctor or nurse. He or she will know if you are likely to have hair loss.

- Cut your hair short or shave your head. You might feel more in control of hair loss if you first cut your hair or shave your head. This often makes hair loss easier to manage. If you shave your head, use an electric shaver instead of a razor.

- If you plan to buy a wig, do so while you still have hair. The best time to choose your wig is before chemotherapy starts. This way, you can match the wig to the color and style of your hair. You might also take it to your hair dresser who can style the wig to look like your own hair. Make sure to choose a wig that feels comfortable and does not hurt your scalp.

- Ask if your insurance company will pay for a wig. If it will not, you can deduct the cost of your wig as a medical expense on your income tax. Some groups also have free "wig banks." Your doctor, nurse, or social worker will know if there is a wig bank near you.

- Be gentle when you wash your hair. Use a mild shampoo, such as a baby shampoo. Dry your hair by patting (not rubbing) it with a soft towel.

- Do not use items that can hurt your scalp. These include the following:
  - Straightening or curling irons
  - Brush rollers or curlers
  - Electric hair dryers
  - Hair bands and clips
  - Hairsprays
  - Hair dyes
  - Products to perm or relax your hair

After Hair Loss

- Protect your scalp. Your scalp may hurt during and after hair loss. Protect it by wearing a hat, turban, or scarf when you are outside. Try to avoid places that are very hot or very cold. This includes tanning beds and outside in the sun or cold air. And always apply sunscreen or sunblock to protect your scalp.

- Stay warm. You may feel colder once you lose your hair. Wear a hat, turban, scarf, or wig to help you stay warm.

- Sleep on a satin pillow case. Satin creates less friction than cotton when you sleep on it. Therefore, you may find satin pillow cases more comfortable.

- Talk about your feelings. Many people feel angry, depressed, or embarrassed about hair loss. If you are very worried or upset, you might want to talk about these feelings with a doctor, nurse, family member, close friend, or someone who has had hair loss caused by cancer treatment.

Infection

- Your doctor or nurse will check your white blood cell count throughout your treatment. If chemotherapy is likely to make your white blood cell count very low, you may get medicine to raise your white blood cell count and lower your risk of infection.

- Wash your hands often with soap and water. Be sure to wash your hands before cooking and eating, and after you use the bathroom, blow your nose, cough, sneeze, or touch animals. Carry hand sanitizer for times when you are not near soap and water.

- Use sanitizing wipes to clean surfaces and items that you touch. This includes public telephones, ATM machines, doorknobs, and other common items.

- Be gentle and thorough when you wipe yourself after a bowel movement. Instead of toilet paper, use a baby wipe or squirt of water from a spray bottle to clean yourself. Let your doctor or nurse know if your rectal area is sore or bleeds or if you have hemorrhoids.

- Stay away from people who are sick. This includes people with colds, flu, measles, or chicken pox. You also need to stay away from children who just had a "live virus" vaccine for chicken pox or polio. Call your doctor, nurse, or local health department if you have any questions.

- Stay away from crowds. Try not to be around a lot of people. For instance, plan to go shopping or to the movies when the stores and theaters are less crowded.

- Be careful not to cut or nick yourself. Do not cut or tear your nail cuticles. Use an electric shaver instead of a razor. And be extra careful when using scissors, needles, or knives.

- Watch for signs of infection around your catheter. Signs include drainage, redness, swelling, or soreness. Let your doctor or nurse know about any changes you notice near your catheter.

- Maintain good mouth care. Brush your teeth after meals and before you go to bed. Use a very soft toothbrush. You can make the bristles even softer by running hot water over them just before you brush. Use a mouth rinse that does not contain alcohol. Check with your doctor or nurse before going to the dentist.

- Take good care of your skin. Do not squeeze or scratch pimples. Use lotion to soften and heal dry, cracked skin. Dry yourself after a bath or shower by gently patting (not rubbing) your skin.

- Clean cuts right away. Use warm water, soap, and an antiseptic to clean your cuts. Do this every day until your cut has a scab over it.

- Be careful around animals. Do not clean your cat's litter box, pick up dog waste, or clean bird cages or fish tanks. Be sure to wash your hands after touching pets and other animals.

- Do not get a flu shot or other type of vaccine without first asking your doctor or nurse. Some vaccines contain a live virus, which you should not be exposed to.

- Keep hot foods hot and cold foods cold. Do not leave leftovers sitting out. Put them in the refrigerator as soon as you are done eating.

- Wash raw vegetables and fruits well before eating them.

- Do not eat raw or undercooked fish, seafood, meat, chicken, or eggs. These may have bacteria that can cause infection.

- Do not have food or drinks that are moldy, spoiled, or past the freshness date.

- Call your doctor right away (even on the weekend or in the middle of the night) if you think you have an infection. Be sure you know how to reach your doctor after office hours and on weekends. Call if you have a fever of 100.5°F or higher, or when you have chills or sweats. Do not take aspirin, acetaminophen (such as Tylenol®), ibuprofen products, or any other drugs that reduce fever without first talking with your doctor or nurse. Other signs of infection include:

  - Redness
  - Swelling
  - Rash
  - Chills
  - Cough
  - Earache
  - Headache
  - Stiff neck
  - Bloody or cloudy urine
  - Painful or frequent need to urinate
  - Sinus pain or pressure

Infertility

Talk with your doctor or nurse about these issues:

- Whether you want to have children. Before you start chemotherapy, let your doctor or nurse know if you might want to get pregnant in the future. He or she may talk with you about ways to preserve your eggs to use after treatment ends or refer you to a fertility specialist.

- Birth control. It is very important that you do not get pregnant while getting chemotherapy. These drugs can hurt the fetus, especially in the first three months of pregnancy. If you have not yet gone through menopause, talk with your doctor or nurse about birth control and ways to keep from getting pregnant.

- Pregnancy. If you still have menstrual periods, your doctor or nurse may ask you to have a pregnancy test before you start chemotherapy. If you are pregnant, your doctor or nurse will talk with you about other treatment options.

Mouth and Throat Changes

- Visit a dentist at least two weeks before starting chemotherapy. It is important to have your mouth as healthy as possible. This means getting all your dental work done before chemotherapy starts. If you cannot go to the dentist before chemotherapy starts, ask your doctor or nurse when it is safe to go. Be sure to tell your dentist that you have cancer and about your treatment plan.

- Check your mouth and tongue every day. This way, you can see or feel problems (such as mouth sores, white spots, or infections) as soon as they start. Inform your doctor or nurse about these problems right away.

- Keep your mouth moist. You can keep your mouth moist by sipping water throughout the day, sucking on ice chips or sugar-free hard candy, or chewing sugar-free gum. Ask your doctor or nurse about saliva substitutes if your mouth is always dry.

- Clean your mouth, teeth, gums, and tongue.

- Brush your teeth, gums, and tongue after each meal and at bedtime.

- Use an extra-soft toothbrush. You can make the bristles even softer by rinsing your toothbrush in hot water before you brush.

- If brushing is painful, try cleaning your teeth with cotton swabs or Toothettes®.

- Use a fluoride toothpaste or special fluoride gel that your dentist prescribes.

- Do not use mouthwash that has alcohol. Instead, rinse your mouth three to four times a day with a solution of 1/4 teaspoon baking soda and 1/8 teaspoon salt in one cup of warm water. Follow this with a plain water rinse.

- Gently floss your teeth every day. If your gums bleed or hurt, avoid those areas but floss your other teeth. Ask your doctor or nurse about flossing if your platelet count is low.

- If you wear dentures, make sure they fit well and keep them clean. Also, limit the length of time that you wear them.

- Be careful what you eat when your mouth is sore.

  - Choose foods that are moist, soft, and easy to chew or swallow. These include cooked cereals, mashed potatoes, and scrambled eggs.

  - Use a blender to puree cooked foods so that they are easier to eat. To help avoid infection, be sure to wash all blender parts before and after using them. If possible, it is best to wash them in a dishwasher.

  - Take small bites of food, chew slowly, and sip liquids while you eat.

  - Soften food with gravy, sauces, broth, yogurt, or other liquids.

  - Eat foods that are cool or at room temperature. You may find that warm and hot foods hurt your mouth or throat.

  - Suck on ice chips or popsicles. These can relieve mouth pain.

  - Ask your dietitian for ideas of foods that are easy to eat.

- Stay away from things that can hurt, scrape, or burn your mouth, such as the following:

  - Sharp or crunchy foods, such as crackers and potato or corn chips

  - Spicy foods, such as hot sauce, curry dishes, salsa, and chili

  - Citrus fruits or juices such as orange, lemon, and grapefruit

  - Food and drinks that have a lot of sugar, such as candy or soda

  - Beer, wine, and other types of alcohol

  - Toothpicks or other sharp objects

  - Tobacco products, including cigarettes, pipes, cigars, and chewing tobacco

Nausea and Vomiting

- Prevent nausea: One way to prevent vomiting is to prevent nausea. Try having bland, easy-to-digest foods and drinks that do not upset your stomach. These include plain crackers, toast, and gelatin.

- Plan when it's best for you to eat and drink. Some people feel better when they eat a light meal or snack before chemotherapy. Others feel better when they have chemotherapy on an empty stomach (nothing to eat or drink for two to three hours before treatment). After treatment, wait at least one hour before you eat or drink.

- Eat small meals and snacks. Instead of three large meals each day, you might feel better if you eat five or six small meals and snacks. Do not drink a lot before or during meals. Also, do not lie down right after you eat.

- Have foods and drinks that are warm or cool (not hot or cold). Give hot foods and drinks time to cool down, or make them colder by adding ice. You can warm up cold foods by taking them out of the refrigerator one hour before you eat or warming them slightly in a microwave. Drink cola or ginger ale that is warm and has lost its fizz.

- Stay away from foods and drinks with strong smells. These include coffee, fish, onions, garlic, and foods that are cooking.

- Try small bites of popsicles or fruit ices. You may also find sucking on ice chips helpful.

- Suck on sugar-free mints or tart candies. But do not use tart candies if you have mouth or throat sores.

- Relax before treatment. You may feel less nausea if you relax before each chemotherapy treatment. Meditate, do deep breathing exercises, or imagine scenes or experiences that make you feel peaceful. You can also do quiet hobbies such as reading, listening to music, or knitting.

- When you feel like vomiting, breathe deeply and slowly or get fresh air. You might also distract yourself by chatting with friends or family, listening to music, or watching a movie or TV.

- Talk with your doctor or nurse. Your doctor can give you drugs to help prevent nausea during and after chemotherapy. Be sure to take these drugs as ordered and let your doctor or nurse know if they do not work. You might also ask your doctor or nurse about acupuncture, which can help relieve nausea and vomiting caused by cancer treatment.

- Tell your doctor or nurse if you vomit for more than one day or right after you drink.

Nervous System Changes

- Let your doctor or nurse know right away if you notice any nervous system changes. It is important to treat these problems as soon as possible.

- Be careful when handling knives, scissors, and other sharp or dangerous objects.

- Avoid falling. Walk slowly, hold onto handrails when using the stairs, and put no-slip bath mats in your bathtub or shower. Make sure there are no area rugs or cords to trip over.

- Always wear sneakers, tennis shoes, or other footwear with rubber soles.

- Check the temperature of your bath water with a thermometer. This will keep you from getting burned by water that is too hot.

- Be extra careful to avoid burning or cutting yourself while cooking.

- Wear gloves when working in the garden, cooking, or washing dishes.

- Rest when you need to.

- Steady yourself when you walk by using a cane or other device.

- Talk to your doctor or nurse if you notice memory problems, feel confused, or are depressed.

- Ask your doctor for pain medicine if you need it.

Pain

- Talk about your pain with a doctor, nurse, or pharmacist. Be specific and describe:
  - Where you feel pain. Is it in one part of your body or all over?
  - What the pain feels like. Is it sharp, dull, or throbbing? Does it come and go, or is it steady?

- How strong the pain is. Describe it on a scale of 0 to 10.

- How long the pain lasts. Does it last for a few minutes, an hour, or longer?

- What makes the pain better or worse. For instance, does an ice pack help? Or does the pain get worse if you move a certain way?

- Which medicines you take for pain. Do they help? How long do they last? How much do you take? How often?

- Let your family and friends know about your pain. They need to know about your pain so they can help you. If you are very tired or in a lot of pain, they can call your doctor or nurse for you. Knowing about your pain can also help them understand why you may be acting differently.

- Practice pain control

  - Take your pain medicine on a regular schedule (by the clock) even when you are not in pain. This is very important when you have pain most of the time.

  - Do not skip doses of your pain medicine. Pain is harder to control and manage if you wait until you are in a lot of pain before taking medicine.

  - Try deep breathing, yoga, or other ways to relax. This can help reduce muscle tension, anxiety, and pain.

- Ask to meet with a pain or palliative care specialist. This can be an oncologist, anesthesiologist, neurologist, neurosurgeon, nurse, or pharmacist who will talk with you about ways to control your pain.

- Let your doctor, nurse, or pain specialist know if your pain changes. Your pain can change over the course of your treatment. When this happens, your pain medications may need to be changed.

Sexual Changes

- Talk with your doctor or nurse about:

  - Sex. Ask your doctor or nurse if it is okay for you to have sex during chemotherapy. Most women can have sex, but it is a good idea to ask.

- Birth control. It is very important that you not get pregnant while having chemotherapy. Chemotherapy may hurt the fetus, especially in the first three months of pregnancy. If you have not yet gone through menopause, talk with your doctor or nurse about birth control and ways to keep from getting pregnant.

- Medications. Talk with your doctor, nurse, or pharmacist about medications that help with sexual problems. These include products to relieve vaginal dryness or a vaginal cream or suppository to reduce the chance of infection.

- Wear cotton underwear (cotton underpants and pantyhose with cotton linings).

- Do not wear tight pants or shorts.

- Use a water-based vaginal lubricant (such as K-Y Jelly® or Astroglide®) when you have sex.

- If sex is still painful because of dryness, ask your doctor or nurse about medications to help restore moisture in your vagina.

- Cope with hot flashes by:
  - Dressing in layers, with an extra sweater or jacket that you can take off.
  - Being active. This includes walking, riding a bike, or other types of exercise.
  - Reducing stress. Try yoga, meditation, or other ways to relax.

Remember these tips:

- Be open and honest with your spouse or partner. Talk about your feelings and concerns.

- Explore new ways to show love. You and your spouse or partner may want to show your love for each other in new ways while you go through chemotherapy. For instance, if you are having sex less often, you may want to hug and cuddle more, bathe together, give each other massages, or try other activities that make you feel close to each other.

- Talk with a doctor, nurse, social worker, or counselor. If you and your spouse or partner are concerned about sexual problems, you may want to talk with someone who can help. This can be a psychiatrist, psychologist, social worker, marriage counselor, sex therapist, or clergy member.

Skin and Nail Changes

- Itching, dryness, redness, rashes, and peeling:
  - Apply cornstarch, as you would dusting powder.
  - Take quick showers or sponge baths instead of long, hot baths.
  - Pat (do not rub) yourself dry after bathing.
  - Wash with a mild, moisturizing soap.
  - Put on cream or lotion while your skin is still damp after washing. Tell your doctor or nurse if this does not help.
  - Do not use perfume, cologne, or aftershave lotion that has alcohol.
  - Take a colloidal oatmeal bath (special powder you add to bath water) when your whole body itches.
- Acne:
  - Keep your face clean and dry.
  - Ask your doctor or nurse if you can use medicated creams or soaps and which ones to use.
- Sensitivity to the sun:
  - Avoid direct sunlight. This means not being in the sun from 10 a.m. until 4 p.m. It is the time when the sun is strongest.
  - Use sunscreen lotion with an SPF (skin protection factor) of 15 or higher. Or use ointments that block the sun's rays, such as those with zinc oxide.
  - Keep your lips moist with a lip balm that has an SPF of 15 or higher.
  - Wear light-colored pants, long-sleeve cotton shirts, and hats with wide brims.
  - Do not use tanning beds.
- Nail problems:
  - Wear gloves when washing dishes, working in the garden, or cleaning the house.

- Use products to make your nails stronger. (Stop using these products if they hurt your nails or skin.)
- Let your doctor or nurse know if your cuticles are red and painful.
- Radiation recall:
  - Protect the area of your skin that received radiation therapy from the sun, and do not use tanning beds.
  - Place a cool, wet cloth where your skin hurts.
  - Wear clothes that are made of cotton or other soft fabrics. This includes your underwear (bras, underpants, and T-shirts).
  - Let your doctor or nurse know if you think you have radiation recall.

Urinary, Kidney, and Bladder Changes

- Your doctor or nurse will take urine and blood samples to check how well your bladder and kidneys are working.
- Drink plenty of fluids. Fluids will help flush the chemotherapy out of your bladder and kidneys. See the lists of clear liquids and liquid foods.
- Limit drinks that contain caffeine (such as black tea, coffee, and some cola products).
- Talk with your doctor or nurse if you have any of the problems listed above.

Other Side Effects

Flu-like symptoms: Some types of chemotherapy can make you feel like you have the flu. This is more likely to happen if you get chemotherapy along with biological therapy.

Flu-like symptoms may include the following:

- Muscle and joint aches
- Headache
- Fatigue
- Nausea
- Fever

- Chills
- Appetite loss

These symptoms may last from one to three days. An infection or the cancer itself can also cause them. Let your doctor or nurse know if you have any of these symptoms.

Fluid retention: Fluid retention is a buildup of fluid caused by chemotherapy, hormone changes caused by treatment, or your cancer. It can cause your face, hands, feet, or stomach to feel swollen and puffy. Sometimes fluid builds up around your lungs and heart, causing coughing, shortness of breath, or an irregular heart beat. Fluid can also build up in the lower part of your belly, which can cause bloating.

You and your doctor or nurse can help manage fluid retention by:

- weighing yourself at the same time each day, using the same scale. Let your doctor or nurse know if you gain weight quickly;
- avoiding table salt or salty foods;
- limiting the liquids you drink; or
- if you retain a lot of fluid, your doctor may prescribe medicine to get rid of the extra fluid.

Eye changes:

- Trouble wearing contact lenses: Some types of chemotherapy can bother your eyes and make wearing contact lenses painful. Ask your doctor or nurse if you can wear contact lenses while getting chemotherapy.
- Blurry vision: Some types of chemotherapy can clog your tear ducts, which can cause blurry vision.
- Watery eyes: Sometimes, chemotherapy can seep out in your tears, which can cause your eyes to water more than usual.

If your vision gets blurry or your eyes water more than usual, tell your doctor or nurse.

Section 32.3

Early Breast Cancer Patients Benefit from Shortened Chemotherapy

Clinical Trial Results, National Cancer Institute (www.cancer.gov),
January 19, 2005.

Women with one type of early breast cancer get the same benefit
from three months of one chemotherapy as they do from six months
of another drug combination, according to a large study presented at
the 2000 American Society for Clinical Oncology annual meeting.

The results mean that breast cancer patients who do not benefit
from the drug tamoxifen—which includes about half of all early
cases—can halve the duration of their drug therapy without dimin-
ishing the chances for long-term survival.

The study compared the chemotherapy combination AC (adriamycin
and cyclophosphamide) to the more widely used CMF (cyclophosphamide, methotrexate, and fluorouracil) in 2,000 women whose cancer had
not spread to their lymph nodes and who had tumors classified as estrogen receptor negative. Half received four cycles of AC over three
months; the other half received six cycles of CMF over six months.
Cancer-free survival after five years was 82 percent in both groups and
overall survival was 89 percent in both.

"There has been a swing toward using the AC regimen, and these
findings should accelerate that trend," said Bernard Fisher, M.D., the
lead researcher on the study conducted by the National Surgical Adjuvant Breast and Bowel Project in Pittsburgh.

Lori Goldstein, M.D., of Fox Chase Cancer Center in Philadelphia,
went a step further by saying, "This is one of the studies that will have
a direct and immediate impact on patients being treated today."

That impact includes three fewer months of side effects that can
include fatigue, nausea, and generally diminished quality of life.

Begun in 1991, the study originally sought to measure tamoxifen's
worth in women who had estrogen receptor negative breast tumors.
To that end, half of each of the two groups of women received tamoxifen
in addition to their AC or CMF regimens. In the intervening decade,

though, lab researchers discovered that tamoxifen acts directly on estrogen receptors to shut down tumor growth. It was no surprise, Fisher said, when tamoxifen offered no extra benefit to either group in the study.

He also took the opportunity to summarize progress against the disease. "I think we have made, in the last five or ten years, particularly in lymph node negative patients, greater strides than we have in all the years before. Early detection has made it possible for, not only for people to do better, but for therapeutic agents to work better."

Section 32.4

Chemotherapy with Anthracyclines for HER2-Positive Breast Cancer

"Anthracyclines Improve Survival for HER2-Positive, But Not HER2-Negative, Breast Cancer," Clinical Trial Results, National Cancer Institute (www.cancer.gov), January 30, 2008.

Combined data from eight randomized clinical trials shows that chemotherapy with an anthracycline drug such as doxorubicin or epirubicin extends survival for women with HER2-positive, but not HER2-negative, breast cancer. These results suggest that women with HER2-negative breast cancer may be spared these drugs, which carry a rare risk of potentially severe side effects including heart damage.

Background

Women with early-stage invasive breast cancer often receive chemotherapy in addition to surgery and radiation therapy. Several randomized clinical trials have shown that chemotherapy for breast cancer with a class of drugs called anthracyclines extends survival compared with non-anthracycline-based chemotherapy. However, the absolute increase in survival is not large and anthracycline chemotherapy can have severe side effects in some women, including heart damage and secondary leukemia.

Recent studies have suggested that women whose tumors produce too much of a protein called HER2 (called HER2-positive) may be the only ones who actually benefit from anthracycline chemotherapy. HER2-positive tumors are tumors that have HER2 gene amplification (too many copies of the HER2 gene) or protein over-expression (extra HER2 protein).

However, studies so far have not consistently shown a link between HER2 status (positive or negative) and the effectiveness of anthracycline chemotherapy. Many studies may have been too small to show a difference. In addition, studies have used different techniques to collect breast tissue samples and measure HER2 status, and used different chemotherapy regimens, making it difficult to compare results between them.

Knowing more certainly whether HER2 status influences the effectiveness of anthracycline chemotherapy would help physicians better personalize treatment for individual patients.

The Study

Investigators from the National Cancer Research Institute of Italy combined data (called a meta-analysis) from eight randomized clinical trials of chemotherapy for breast cancer. They found these eight trials by comprehensively searching databases of the medical literature and conference proceedings for published and unpublished clinical trials in English. All trials included in the meta-analysis had to meet three criteria:

- All patients included in the trial were randomly assigned to treatment

- The trial tested anthracycline-based chemotherapy against non-anthracycline-based chemotherapy after surgery for breast cancer

- The trial reported disease-free and overall survival rates based on HER2 status, or these rates could be calculated from the available data

The investigators then compared whether disease-free and overall survival differed for women receiving anthracycline-based chemotherapy depending on whether or not their tumors produced extra HER2.

Results

Out of 6,564 patients randomly assigned in one of the eight trials, 5,354 (82 percent) had their tumors tested for HER2 status. Of these,

331

1,536 (29 percent) had tumors that had extra HER2 protein or extra copies of the HER2 gene—that is, they were HER2 positive.

Six of the trials had data on disease-free survival. Seven trials had data on overall survival. When the meta-analysis was complete, the data showed that treatment with anthracycline-based chemotherapy significantly reduced the risk of relapse and reduced the risk of death from any cause compared with non-anthracycline-based chemotherapy.

However, when the results were broken into two groups by HER2 status, only women with HER2-positive tumors actually had a significantly reduced risk of relapse and death after anthracycline-based chemotherapy.

Limitations

The authors acknowledge several limitations to their study. They had to rely on results summarized by the other studies, and did not have access to the actual patient data. Therefore, they could not confirm the initial conclusions or perform additional statistical tests.

Also, the eight studies included in the meta-analysis did not all use the same methods for measuring HER2 status. However, this did not seem to influence the measured effectiveness of anthracycline-based chemotherapy when tested by the investigators.

Finally, there might have been unpublished clinical trials not found by the authors that failed to find a link between HER2 status and the success of anthracycline treatment. Not including these studies in the meta-analysis could cause a false-positive result (called publication bias). However, the authors did perform statistical tests designed to detect publication bias, and did not find any indication of such bias.

Comments

"Our results confirm that the added benefit of adjuvant chemotherapy with anthracyclines is confined to women who have breast tumors in which HER2 is over-expressed or amplified," concluded the authors. "The absence, in our study, of any effect of anthracyclines observed in patients with HER2-negative disease suggests that this group of patients could be spared unnecessary toxic effects related to the use of this class of agents."

JoAnne Zujewski, M.D., a breast cancer specialist with the National Cancer Institute's Division of Cancer Treatment and Diagnosis, agreed, saying "Women with estrogen-receptor-positive, HER2-negative breast cancer should ask their doctors about avoiding anthracycline-containing chemotherapy....The evidence is pretty consistent now that the benefit of anthracycline chemotherapy is seen in the HER2-positive cases but not in others."

Further clinical trials are needed, she explained, to determine what type of chemotherapy is best for women with so-called "triple-negative" breast cancer, which is HER2 negative, estrogen-receptor-negative, and progesterone-receptor negative. Some women with triple-negative disease may still derive a benefit from treatment with anthracyclines.

Section 32.5

Bevacizumab Combined with Chemotherapy for Patients with Advanced Breast Cancer

"Bevacizumab Combined With Chemotherapy Improves
Progression-Free Survival for Patients With Advanced Breast Cancer,"
National Cancer Institute (www.cancer.gov), June 16, 2005.

Preliminary results from a large, randomized clinical trial for patients with previously untreated recurrent or metastatic breast cancer—cancer that has spread from the breast to other parts of the body—show that those patients who received bevacizumab (Avastin™) in combination with standard chemotherapy had a longer time period before their cancer progressed than patients who received the same chemotherapy without bevacizumab.

The clinical trial was sponsored by the National Cancer Institute (NCI), part of the National Institutes of Health, and conducted by a network of researchers led by the Eastern Cooperative Oncology Group (ECOG). Genentech, Inc., South San Francisco, California, which manufactures bevacizumab, provided bevacizumab for the trial under the Cooperative Research and Development Agreement (CRADA) with NCI for the clinical development of bevacizumab.

The Data Monitoring Committee overseeing the trial (known as E2100) recommended that the results of a recent interim analysis be made public because the study had met its primary endpoint of increasing progression-free survival (the amount of time patients lived without the cancer getting worse).

Preliminary results suggest that patients in the study who received bevacizumab in combination with standard chemotherapy consisting of single-agent paclitaxel had a delay in worsening of their cancer by approximately five months, on average, compared to patients treated with paclitaxel chemotherapy alone. This difference is statistically significant. Detailed results about this trial were presented on May 16, 2005, at the American Society of Clinical Oncology meeting. The results include the facts that those on bevacizumab plus standard chemotherapy had progression-free survival of 10.97 months vs. 6.11 months on standard chemotherapy alone which is a 49 percent improvement in progression-free survival. There was a 28 percent response rate for those on bevacizumab plus standard chemotherapy vs. 14 percent for those on standard chemotherapy only.

"This study is the first to find a benefit of anti-angiogenic therapy in patients with breast cancer and represents a major advance in the treatment of patients with metastatic disease," said Study Chair Kathy D. Miller, M.D., of the Indiana University Medical Center in Indianapolis, Indiana. Anti-angiogenic drugs, also called angiogenesis inhibitors, are substances that may prevent angiogenesis, or the formation of blood vessels. In anticancer therapy, an angiogenesis inhibitor prevents the growth of blood vessels from surrounding tissue to a solid tumor.

"Recent clinical trials have shown that anti-angiogenic drugs have a favorable impact on colon and lung cancers," said NCI Director Andrew C. von Eschenbach, M.D. "This study demonstrates that when patients with recurrent or metastatic breast cancer received bevacizumab in addition to their chemotherapy, the period of time that they lived with their cancer under control was increased. This is an important step in our journey to ultimately eliminate the suffering and death due to cancer."

A total of 722 women with recurrent or metastatic breast cancer who had not previously received systemic chemotherapy for their recurrent or metastatic disease were enrolled in this study between December 2001 and May 2004. Patients were randomized to one of the two treatment arms. One patient group received standard treatment consisting of single-agent paclitaxel. The second group received the same regimen of paclitaxel with the addition of bevacizumab.

Patients whose tumors over-expressed HER2 were not included in the study unless they had previously received trastuzumab (Herceptin™) or were unable to receive trastuzumab. Also excluded were patients who had received preventive chemotherapy treatment with paclitaxel within the previous 12 months, as well as patients with a prior history of blood clots or who were on blood thinners. Serious bleeding and blood clots were rare in this study. Patients receiving the combination of paclitaxel and bevacizumab had slightly more neuropathy, or problem in peripheral nerve function (any part of the nervous system except the brain and spinal cord); abnormally high blood pressure; and proteinuria, a condition in which urine contains an abnormal amount of protein, than patients receiving paclitaxel alone. Other side effects were similar between the two treatment groups.

Bevacizumab, a humanized monoclonal antibody that already has been approved for metastatic colorectal cancer in combination with chemotherapy, is designed to bind to and inhibit vascular endothelial growth factor (VEGF). VEGF is a protein that plays a critical role in tumor angiogenesis.

"It is noteworthy that a previous company-sponsored trial in patients who received prior chemotherapy for advanced disease did not show a benefit with bevacizumab in combination with capecitabine, a different chemotherapy agent," said JoAnne Zujewski, M.D., who heads breast cancer trials for NCI's Cancer Therapy Evaluation Program. "It is fortunate that ECOG, assisted by multiple other NCI-sponsored Cooperative Groups, persisted with this trial in patients with newly diagnosed advanced breast cancer, as the agent is clearly active in this setting."

An estimated 211,240 women will be diagnosed with breast cancer in the United States in 2005. Breast cancer is the most commonly diagnosed cancer in women and the second leading cause of cancer-related death in women in this country. An estimated 40,110 deaths from female breast cancer will occur in 2005 in the United States, accounting for about 15 percent of all cancer-related deaths in women in the nation.

Section 32.6

Dose-Dense Chemotherapy for Patients with Metastatic Breast Cancer

"Dose-Dense Chemotherapy Helped Patients with Metastatic Breast Cancer," Clinical Trial Results, National Cancer Institute (www.cancer.gov), September 7, 2005.

Weekly administration of the drug paclitaxel (Taxol®) to patients with breast cancer that had spread to other parts of the body resulted in a higher response rate and a longer delay until patients' disease progressed, compared with conventional administration of the drug every three weeks. The same study found no benefit from adding the drug trastuzumab (Herceptin®) to paclitaxel for women with metastatic breast cancer whose tumors do not overproduce a protein called HER2.

Background

Conventional cancer chemotherapy is given at three-week intervals. In recent years, however, some researchers have begun to investigate "dose-dense" drug regimens where chemotherapy drugs are given more frequently, such as once a week or once every two weeks. The drug dose is either kept the same or is lowered slightly. The idea is that exposing cancer cells to the drugs more frequently may kill more cells and thus improve the effectiveness of chemotherapy.

Previous studies have suggested that giving the drug paclitaxel (Taxol) at weekly intervals might decrease side effects while improving outcomes for women with breast cancer that has spread (metastasized) to other parts of the body.

Studies have also shown that the drug trastuzumab (Herceptin), in combination with paclitaxel, improves response rates in patients with metastatic breast cancer whose tumors over-express (make too much of) a protein called HER2. About 25 percent of breast tumors are HER2-positive. These tumors tend to grow faster than other tumors.

Trastuzumab targets the cancer cells that over-express HER2 and slows or stops their growth.

The Study

The main goals of the study (called CALGB 9840) were to find out whether more patients would respond to treatment with weekly paclitaxel than to the standard paclitaxel regimen, and whether the addition of trastuzumab to paclitaxel would improve response rates in patients whose tumors did not over-express HER2.

A total of 585 patients were enrolled. When the trial began, patients were randomly assigned to receive either weekly paclitaxel or the standard paclitaxel regimen. While the trial was underway, trastuzumab became accepted as standard therapy for patients with HER2-positive tumors. From then on, all patients with HER2-positive tumors received trastuzumab in addition to paclitaxel. Other patients were randomly assigned to receive either paclitaxel alone or trastuzumab in addition to paclitaxel.

This study was conducted by the Cancer and Leukemia Group B (CALGB), one of several cooperative groups funded by the National Cancer Institute to conduct large cancer clinical trials. The principal investigator was Andrew Seidman, M.D., of Memorial Sloan-Kettering Cancer Center in New York.

Results

When the researchers calculated the study's results, they included an additional 158 patients who had been treated with the conventional three-weekly paclitaxel regimen in another CALGB study. This brought the total number of patients included in the calculation of results to 743.

Forty percent of patients treated with weekly paclitaxel responded to treatment, compared with 28 percent of those who received the standard regimen. Patients in the weekly paclitaxel group lived for nine months on average before their disease progressed. In patients receiving the standard paclitaxel regimen, by contrast, disease progressed after five months.

Among patients treated with weekly paclitaxel, there were more nervous-system side effects but fewer instances of low blood counts.

For patients with tumors that did not overproduce the HER2 protein, additional treatment with trastuzumab did not improve the response rate, a finding consistent with previous studies.

Comment

By design, the trial included in its final analysis 158 patients from another trial. These patients had received treatment similar to that given to patients who had been randomly assigned to the standard paclitaxel arm of the trial discussed here. However, some physicians at the American Society of Clinical Oncologist presentation questioned whether the inclusion of patients from another trial might not have biased the final result.

Chapter 33

Biological Therapies

What is biological therapy?

Biological therapy (sometimes called immunotherapy, biotherapy, or biological response modifier therapy) is a relatively new addition to the family of cancer treatments that also includes surgery, chemotherapy, and radiation therapy. Biological therapies use the body's immune system, either directly or indirectly, to fight cancer or to lessen the side effects that may be caused by some cancer treatments.

What is the immune system and what are its components?

The immune system is a complex network of cells and organs that work together to defend the body against attacks by "foreign" or "nonself" invaders. This network is one of the body's main defenses against infection and disease. The immune system works against diseases, including cancer, in a variety of ways. For example, the immune system may recognize the difference between healthy cells and cancer cells in the body and works to eliminate cancerous cells. However, the immune system does not always recognize cancer cells as "foreign." Also, cancer may develop when the immune system breaks down or does not function adequately. Biological therapies are designed to repair, stimulate, or enhance the immune system's responses.

Immune system cells include the following:

"Biological Therapies for Cancer: Questions and Answers," National Cancer Institute (www.cancer.gov), June 13, 2006.

- Lymphocytes are a type of white blood cell found in the blood and many other parts of the body. Types of lymphocytes include B cells, T cells, and natural killer cells.

  - B cells (B lymphocytes) mature into plasma cells that secrete proteins called antibodies (immunoglobulins). Antibodies recognize and attach to foreign substances known as antigens, fitting together much the way a key fits a lock. Each type of B cell makes one specific antibody, which recognizes one specific antigen.

  - T cells (T lymphocytes) work primarily by producing proteins called cytokines. Cytokines allow immune system cells to communicate with each other and include lymphokines, interferons, interleukins, and colony-stimulating factors. Some T cells, called cytotoxic T cells, release pore-forming proteins that directly attack infected, foreign, or cancerous cells. Other T cells, called helper T cells, regulate the immune response by releasing cytokines to signal other immune system defenders.

  - Natural killer cells (NK cells) produce powerful cytokines and pore-forming proteins that bind to and kill many foreign invaders, infected cells, and tumor cells. Unlike cytotoxic T cells, they are poised to attack quickly, upon their first encounter with their targets.

- Phagocytes are white blood cells that can swallow and digest microscopic organisms and particles in a process known as phagocytosis. There are several types of phagocytes, including monocytes, which circulate in the blood, and macrophages, which are located in tissues throughout the body.

What are biological response modifiers, and how can they be used to treat cancer?

Some antibodies, cytokines, and other immune system substances can be produced in the laboratory for use in cancer treatment. These substances are often called biological response modifiers (BRMs). They alter the interaction between the body's immune defenses and cancer cells to boost, direct, or restore the body's ability to fight the disease. BRMs include interferons, interleukins, colony-stimulating factors, monoclonal antibodies, vaccines, gene therapy, and nonspecific immunomodulating agents.

Researchers continue to discover new BRMs, to learn more about how they function, and to develop ways to use them in cancer therapy. Biological therapies may be used for these purposes:

- Stop, control, or suppress processes that permit cancer growth

- Make cancer cells more recognizable and, therefore, more susceptible to destruction by the immune system

- Boost the killing power of immune system cells, such as T cells, NK cells, and macrophages

- Alter the growth patterns of cancer cells to promote behavior like that of healthy cells

- Block or reverse the process that changes a normal cell or a precancerous cell into a cancerous cell

- Enhance the body's ability to repair or replace normal cells damaged or destroyed by other forms of cancer treatment, such as chemotherapy or radiation

- Prevent cancer cells from spreading to other parts of the body

Some BRMs are a standard part of treatment for certain types of cancer, while others are being studied in clinical trials (research studies). BRMs are being used alone or in combination with each other. They are also being used with other treatments, such as radiation therapy and chemotherapy.

What are interferons?

Interferons (IFNs) are types of cytokines that occur naturally in the body. They were the first cytokines produced in the laboratory for use as BRMs. There are three major types of interferons—interferon alpha, interferon beta, and interferon gamma; interferon alpha is the type most widely used in cancer treatment.

Researchers have found that interferons can improve the way a cancer patient's immune system acts against cancer cells. In addition, interferons may act directly on cancer cells by slowing their growth or promoting their development into cells with more normal behavior. Researchers believe that some interferons may also stimulate NK cells, T cells, and macrophages, boosting the immune system's anticancer function.

The U.S. Food and Drug Administration (FDA) has approved the use of interferon alpha for the treatment of certain types of cancer, including hairy cell leukemia, melanoma, chronic myeloid leukemia, and AIDS-related Kaposi sarcoma. Studies have shown that interferon alpha may also be effective in treating other cancers such as kidney cancer and non-Hodgkin lymphoma. Researchers are exploring combinations of interferon alpha and other BRMs or chemotherapy in clinical trials to treat a number of cancers.

What are interleukins?

Like interferons, interleukins (ILs) are cytokines that occur naturally in the body and can be made in the laboratory. Many interleukins have been identified; interleukin-2 (IL-2 or aldesleukin) has been the most widely studied in cancer treatment. IL-2 stimulates the growth and activity of many immune cells, such as lymphocytes, that can destroy cancer cells. The FDA has approved IL-2 for the treatment of metastatic kidney cancer and metastatic melanoma.

Researchers continue to study the benefits of interleukins to treat a number of other cancers, including leukemia, lymphoma, and brain, colorectal, ovarian, breast, and prostate cancers.

What are colony-stimulating factors?

Colony-stimulating factors (CSFs) (sometimes called hematopoietic growth factors) usually do not directly affect tumor cells; rather, they encourage bone marrow stem cells to divide and develop into white blood cells, platelets, and red blood cells. Bone marrow is critical to the body's immune system because it is the source of all blood cells.

Stimulation of the immune system by CSFs may benefit patients undergoing cancer treatment. Because anticancer drugs can damage the body's ability to make white blood cells, red blood cells, and platelets, patients receiving anticancer drugs have an increased risk of developing infections, becoming anemic, and bleeding more easily. By using CSFs to stimulate blood cell production, doctors can increase the doses of anticancer drugs without increasing the risk of infection or the need for transfusion with blood products. As a result, researchers have found CSFs particularly useful when combined with high-dose chemotherapy.

Some examples of CSFs and their use in cancer therapy are as follows:

- G-CSF (filgrastim) and GM-CSF (sargramostim) can increase the number of white blood cells, thereby reducing the risk of infection in patients receiving chemotherapy. G-CSF and GM-CSF can also stimulate the production of stem cells in preparation for stem cell or bone marrow transplants.

- Erythropoietin (epoetin) can increase the number of red blood cells and reduce the need for red blood cell transfusions in patients receiving chemotherapy.

- Interleukin-11 (oprelvekin) helps the body make platelets and can reduce the need for platelet transfusions in patients receiving chemotherapy.

Researchers are studying CSFs in clinical trials to treat a large variety of cancers, including lymphoma, leukemia, multiple myeloma, melanoma, and cancers of the brain, lung, esophagus, breast, uterus, ovary, prostate, kidney, colon, and rectum.

What are monoclonal antibodies?

Researchers are evaluating the effectiveness of certain antibodies made in the laboratory called monoclonal antibodies (MOABs or MoABs). These antibodies are produced by a single type of cell and are specific for a particular antigen. Researchers are examining ways to create MOABs specific to the antigens found on the surface of various cancer cells.

To create MOABs, scientists first inject human cancer cells into mice. In response, the mouse immune system makes antibodies against these cancer cells. The scientists then remove the mouse plasma cells that produce antibodies, and fuse them with laboratory-grown cells to create "hybrid" cells called hybridomas. Hybridomas can indefinitely produce large quantities of these pure antibodies, or MOABs.

MOABs may be used in cancer treatment in a number of ways:

- MOABs that react with specific types of cancer may enhance a patient's immune response to the cancer.

- MOABs can be programmed to act against cell growth factors, thus interfering with the growth of cancer cells.

- MOABs may be linked to anticancer drugs, radioisotopes (radioactive substances), other BRMs, or other toxins. When the antibodies latch onto cancer cells, they deliver these poisons directly to the tumor, helping to destroy it.

MOABs carrying radioisotopes may also prove useful in diagnosing certain cancers, such as colorectal, ovarian, and prostate.

Rituxan® (rituximab) and Herceptin® (trastuzumab) are examples of MOABs that have been approved by the FDA. Rituxan is used for the treatment of non-Hodgkin lymphoma. Herceptin is used to treat metastatic breast cancer in patients with tumors that produce excess amounts of a protein called HER2. In clinical trials, researchers are testing MOABs to treat lymphoma, leukemia, melanoma, and cancers of the brain, breast, lung, kidney, colon, rectum, ovary, prostate, and other areas.

What are cancer vaccines?

Cancer vaccines are another form of biological therapy currently under study. Vaccines for infectious diseases, such as measles, mumps, and tetanus, are injected into a person before the disease develops. These vaccines are effective because they expose the body's immune cells to weakened forms of antigens that are present on the surface of the infectious agent. This exposure causes the immune system to increase production of plasma cells that make antibodies specific to the infectious agent. The immune system also increases production of T cells that recognize the infectious agent. These activated immune cells remember the exposure, so that the next time the agent enters the body, the immune system is already prepared to respond and stop the infection.

Researchers are developing vaccines that may encourage the patient's immune system to recognize cancer cells. Cancer vaccines are designed to treat existing cancers (therapeutic vaccines) or to prevent the development of cancer (prophylactic vaccines). Therapeutic vaccines are injected in a person after cancer is diagnosed. These vaccines may stop the growth of existing tumors, prevent cancer from recurring, or eliminate cancer cells not killed by prior treatments. Cancer vaccines given when the tumor is small may be able to eradicate the cancer. On the other hand, prophylactic vaccines are given to healthy individuals before cancer develops. These vaccines are designed to stimulate the immune system to attack viruses that can cause cancer. By targeting these cancer-causing viruses, doctors hope to prevent the development of certain cancers.

Early cancer vaccine clinical trials involved mainly patients with melanoma. Therapeutic vaccines are also being studied in the treatment of many other types of cancer, including lymphoma, leukemia, and cancers of the brain, breast, lung, kidney, ovary, prostate, pancreas, colon, and rectum. Researchers are also studying prophylactic vaccines to prevent cancers of the cervix and liver. Moreover, scientists are investigating ways that cancer vaccines can be used in combination with other BRMs.

What is gene therapy?

Gene therapy is an experimental treatment that involves introducing genetic material into a person's cells to fight disease. Researchers are studying gene therapy methods that can improve a patient's immune response to cancer. For example, a gene may be inserted into an immune cell to enhance its ability to recognize and attack cancer cells. In another approach, scientists inject cancer cells with genes that cause the cancer cells to produce cytokines and stimulate the immune system. A number of clinical trials are currently studying gene therapy and its potential application to the biological treatment of cancer.

What are nonspecific immunomodulating agents?

Nonspecific immunomodulating agents are substances that stimulate or indirectly augment the immune system. Often, these agents target key immune system cells and cause secondary responses such as increased production of cytokines and immunoglobulins. Two nonspecific immunomodulating agents used in cancer treatment are bacillus Calmette-Guerin (BCG) and levamisole.

BCG, which has been widely used as a tuberculosis vaccine, is used in the treatment of superficial bladder cancer following surgery. BCG may work by stimulating an inflammatory, and possibly an immune, response. A solution of BCG is instilled in the bladder and stays there for about two hours before the patient is allowed to empty the bladder by urinating. This treatment is usually performed once a week for six weeks.

Levamisole is sometimes used along with fluorouracil (5-FU) chemotherapy in the treatment of stage III (Dukes' C) colon cancer following surgery. Levamisole may act to restore depressed immune function.

Do biological therapies have any side effects?

Like other forms of cancer treatment, biological therapies can cause a number of side effects, which can vary widely from agent to agent and patient to patient. Rashes or swelling may develop at the site where the BRMs are injected. Several BRMs, including interferons and interleukins, may cause flu-like symptoms including fever, chills, nausea, vomiting, and appetite loss. Fatigue is another common side effect of some BRMs. Blood pressure may also be affected. The side effects of IL-2 can often be severe, depending on the dosage given. Patients need to be closely monitored during treatment with high doses of IL-2. Side effects of CSFs may include bone pain, fatigue, fever, and appetite loss. The side effects of MOABs vary, and serious allergic reactions may occur. Cancer vaccines can cause muscle aches and fever.

Where can a person get more information about clinical trials?

Information about ongoing clinical trials involving these and other biological therapies is available from the Cancer Information Service or the clinical trials page of the NCI's website at http://www.cancer .gov/clinicaltrials on the internet.

Chapter 34

Complementary and Alternative Therapies

An "alternative" therapy is a treatment that is used in place of traditional medicine. A "complementary" therapy is a treatment that is used as a supplement to traditional medicine. Alternative and complementary medicines have become increasingly popular in recent years. According to the National Institutes of Health's National Center for Alternative and Complementary Medicine (NCCAM), Americans spent more than $27 billion on alternative or complementary therapies in 1997. This is more than all out-of-pocket hospital costs combined for 1997 (out-of-pocket costs are costs the patient may pay in addition to the costs covered by his or her health insurance or health plan).

While anecdotal evidence reveals that many alternative or complementary medicines may be beneficial to patients, extensive research is still needed to determine whether non-traditional medicines are truly effective. Therefore, most physicians recommend that patients who use non-traditional medicines use them only as supplements to traditional treatment options that have been scientifically proven to be effective. Currently, there is no scientific evidence that non-traditional therapies can cure breast cancer.

That is not to say that complementary medicines are not viable options for some patients. When used in conjunction with traditional medicines, some complementary therapies may be very beneficial to the physical or psychological well-being of a patient. There have been studies that show that non-traditional medicines can help alleviate

"Alternative/Complementary Medicine," reprinted with permission from www.imaginis.com. © 2008 Imaginis Corporation. All Rights Reserved.

the symptoms of cancer or ease the side effects of traditional thera-pies. For example, Chinese herbs have been shown to lessen the side effects of chemotherapy and acupuncture has been shown to reduce nausea (a possible side effect of chemotherapy and other drug thera-pies).

- **Alternative medicine:** A non-traditional therapy that is used in place of traditional medicine.

- **Complementary medicine:** A non-traditional therapy that is used as a supplement to traditional medicine.

However, it is important for patients to realize that not all alter-native or complementary medicines are safe. Patients who are con-sidering non-traditional medicines should thoroughly investigate the therapy and consult with their physicians or alternative medicine practitioners to make sure the therapy is safe and will not interact with other medicines they may be taking.

The National Cancer Institute recommends that patients ask the following questions when considering an alternative or complemen-tary therapy:

- What benefits can be expected from this therapy?
- What are the risks associated with this therapy?
- Do the known benefits outweigh the risks?
- What side effects can be expected?
- Will the therapy interfere with conventional treatment?
- Will the therapy be covered by health insurance?

Types of Alternative/Complementary Therapies

Mind-body/spiritual: These therapies often focus on the emo-tional and psychological aspects of a patient's health. Studies have shown that stress levels and emotional outlooks can impact a cancer patient's survival. In a recent study published in the *Journal of the National Cancer Institute*, researchers found that advanced breast cancer patients with high stress levels were less likely to live as long as patients who coped well with stress. Examples of mind-body or spiritual therapies include hypnosis, breathing techniques, dance, music, art therapy, poetry, prayer, and meditation. Many of these therapies originated in ancient Eastern cultures.

Oriental medicine: This category of medicine focuses on maintaining a balancing the body's energies: the "yin" and the "yang." It attempts to accomplish this balance by restoring the body's natural energy flow, called the qi (pronounced "chee").

Examples of oriental medicine include:

- Acupuncture: stimulating pressure points with needles.

- Acupressure: massage technique of pressure points.

- Moxibustion: heat therapy.

- Qi Gong: applying finger pressure to acupuncture points. Qi Gong involves using breathing techniques and medication to strengthen the qi (the body's natural immunity).

- Reiki ("Universal Life Energy"): involves channeling spiritual energy through the practitioner to help heal the body.

Ayurveda: This is India's traditional system of medicine. Ayurvedic means "science of life" and its system equally emphasizes the body, mind, and spirit to help restore harmony to the patient. Examples of Ayurvedic medicine include special diets, exercise, meditation, herbs, massage, exposure to sunlight, and controlled breathing.

Homeopathy: This Western therapy is based on the idea that a patient could be treated by using small doses of a medicine that produces the same symptoms as the patient's illness. Supporters of homeopathy believe that very diluted extracts from herbs, minerals, or animal substances can be potent remedies for illnesses and diseases.

Naturopathy: This therapy takes a natural approach to healing. Supporters of naturopathy see disease as an alteration of processes that can be healed naturally through diet, herbal remedies, exercise, homeopathy, massage, spinal and soft tissue manipulation, hydrotherapy (use of water to promote healing), counseling, light therapy, and other techniques. Some naturopaths practice Oriental medicine, including acupuncture.

Aromatherapy: This therapy was originally used in ancient Egypt and India and has become increasingly common in the United States since the early 1980s. Aromatherapy uses special scented oils to treat physical and emotional problems. The oils may be inhaled or applied topically to the skin, sometimes in the form of massage. Types of oils used during aromatherapy include eucalyptus, lavender, rosemary, and thyme. Aromatherapy is usually given by certified aromatherapists.

Biological therapies (vitamins, minerals, and herbs): This category of therapies involves the use of vitamins, minerals, or herbal supplements and is often used in conjunction with traditional therapies in cancer patients. An herb is a plant or an extract from the non-woody portion of a plant (the stems, leaves, flowers, etc.). Plant chemicals (called phytochemicals) are substances derived from plants that may have an effect on the body. In fact, many modern, traditional drugs were discovered from plants. For example, the breast cancer drug Taxol (generic name, paclitaxel) was first isolated from a Pacific yew tree in 1967.

Vitamins and minerals can help strengthen the body's immune system. The main antioxidant vitamins are vitamin A, vitamin C, and vitamin E. In addition, deficiencies of vitamin B1 (thiamin), vitamin B2 (riboflavin), vitamin B5 (pantothenic acid), and vitamin B12 can decrease white blood cell function. Some preliminary studies have shown that vitamins may help reduce risk of breast cancer or treat the disease. For example, clinical studies are investigating the effect of a drug called fenretinide, a derivative of vitamin A, on young women at high risk of breast cancer recurrence. However, further research is needed to definitely determine whether certain vitamins reduce breast cancer risk. Because high doses of some vitamins may be harmful for some breast cancer patients, patients should ask their physicians about taking vitamins and minerals while undergoing treatment.

Herbs and herbal supplements have also become more commonly used among breast cancer patients in recent years. Herbal remedies may consist of single or multiple herbal mixtures. Currently, there is little scientific research on the effectiveness of herbs on breast cancer. Still, some women find that taking herbal supplements is helpful during breast cancer treatment. However, women considering herbal diets should talk to their physicians since some herbs may interfere with other therapies or may be harmful if proper dosages are not followed.

Herbs and medicinal plants used for breast cancer include:

- astragalus root,
- burdock root,
- garlic,
- green tea, and
- licorice root.

Note, shark cartilage capsules became a popular alternative/complementary breast cancer therapy after the book, *Sharks Don't Get Cancer* by William Lance, was first published in 1993. However, researchers have since found that sharks do develop cancer, and now, a new study shows that shark cartilage does not have any effect on cancer.

This section outlined a few of the common schools of alternative and complementary medicine. There are many more therapies available. Although research on non-traditional medicine is limited at this time, many physicians are beginning to embrace some complementary medicines as useful supplements to traditional cancer treatment in selected cases. Women interested in learning more about alternative and complementary therapies should see the resources below and also speak with their physicians or alternative medicine practitioners.

Additional Resources and References

* To view a comprehensive listing of online resources for alternative and complementary therapies, please visit http://www .imaginis.com/breasthealth/links/alternative.asp

* The National Center for Complementary and Alternative Medicine (NCCAM), a division of the National Institutes of Health (NIH) supports and conducts basic and applied research on alternative and complementary therapies. The NCCAM website provides background information on alternative and complementary medicines, the latest research, and information on the organization at http://nccam.nih.gov

* Healingpeople.com provides information on a variety of alternative and complementary medicines and practices. The website also includes information on new research and articles written by medical doctors at http://www.healingpeople.com. A special section on cancer risk reduction is available at http://www .healingpeople.com/ht/topicResults.tmpl?ct=926&tt=cancer

* The National Cancer Institute provides information on alternative and complementary medicines at http://cancernet.nci.nih .gov/treatment/cam.shtml

* The NIH's Office of Dietary Supplements (ODS) supports and conducts research on dietary supplements. To learn more about the ODS, please visit http://odp.od.nih.gov/ods

* "An FDA Guide to Dietary Supplements" (1999) provides information on the dietary supplement industry, federally required

vitamin labeling, safety monitoring, claims of effects, quality of products, reporting harmful effects, and more. The document is available at http://vm.cfsan.fda.gov/~dms/fdsupp.html

- Healthfinder, a free website that directs users to reliable consumer health and human services information developed by the U.S. Department of Health and Human Services, provides resources on alternative and complementary medicines at http://www.healthfinder.gov/altmed

- *Prescription for Nutritional Healing: A Practical A–Z Reference to Drug-Free Remedies Using Vitamins, Minerals, Herbs, and Food Supplements* by James Balch, MD and Phyllis Balch, CNC is a comprehensive resource for information on vitamins, minerals, herbs, and other dietary supplements. To learn more about this book, visit http://www.imaginis.com/bookstore/breasthealth/diagnosis.asp#prescription

- *American Cancer Society's Guide to Complementary and Alternative Cancer Methods* published by the American Cancer Society provides information on herbs, vitamins, minerals, diets, manual healing, and alternative treatment methods. To learn more about this book, visit http://www.imaginis.com/bookstore/breasthealth/diagnosis.asp#ACSguide

- The medical study, "Trends in Alternative Medicine Use in the United States, 1990–1997," is published in the November 11, 1998 issue of the *Journal of the American Medical Association.* An abstract of the study is available at http://jama.ama-assn.org/issues/v280n18/abs/joc80870.html

Chapter 35

Nutrition in Cancer Care

Overview of Nutrition in Cancer Care

The diet is an important part of cancer treatment. Eating the right kinds of foods before, during, and after treatment can help the patient feel better and stay stronger. To ensure proper nutrition, a person has to eat and drink enough of the foods that contain key nutrients (vitamins, minerals, protein, carbohydrates, fat, and water). For many patients, however, some side effects of cancer and cancer treatments make it difficult to eat well. Symptoms that interfere with eating include anorexia, nausea, vomiting, diarrhea, constipation, mouth sores, trouble with swallowing, and pain. Appetite, taste, smell, and the ability to eat enough food or absorb the nutrients from food may be affected. Malnutrition (lack of key nutrients) can result, causing the patient to be weak, tired, and unable to resist infections or withstand cancer therapies. Eating too little protein and calories is the most common nutrition problem facing many cancer patients. Protein and calories are important for healing, fighting infection, and providing energy.

Anorexia (the loss of appetite or desire to eat) is a common symptom in people with cancer. Anorexia may occur early in the disease or later, when the tumor grows and spreads. Some patients may have anorexia when they are diagnosed with cancer. Almost all patients

Excerpted from PDQ® Cancer Information Summary. National Cancer Institute; Bethesda, MD. Nutrition in Cancer Care (PDQ®): Supportive Care - Patient. Updated 06/2007. Available at: http://cancer.gov. Accessed March 24, 2008.

who have widespread cancer will develop anorexia. Anorexia is the most common cause of malnutrition in cancer patients.

Cachexia is a wasting syndrome that causes weakness and a loss of weight, fat, and muscle. It commonly occurs in patients with tumors of the lung, pancreas, and upper gastrointestinal tract and less often in patients with breast cancer or lower gastrointestinal cancer. Anorexia and cachexia often occur together. Weight loss can be caused by eating fewer calories, using more calories, or a combination of the two. Cachexia can occur in people who are eating enough, but who cannot absorb the nutrients. Cachexia is not related to the tumor size, type, or extent. Cancer cachexia is not the same as starvation. A healthy person's body can adjust to starvation by slowing down its use of nutrients, but in cancer patients, the body does not make this adjustment.

Nutrition therapy can help cancer patients get the nutrients needed to maintain body weight and strength, prevent body tissue from breaking down, rebuild tissue, and fight infection. Eating guidelines for cancer patients can be very different from the usual suggestions for healthful eating. Nutrition recommendations for cancer patients are designed to help the patient cope with the effects of the cancer and its treatment. Some cancer treatments are more effective if the patient is well nourished and getting enough calories and protein in the diet. People who eat well during cancer treatment may even be able to handle higher doses of certain treatments. Being well-nourished has been linked to a better prognosis (chance of recovery).

Effect of Cancer on Nutrition

Tumors may produce chemicals that change the way the body uses certain nutrients. The body's use of protein, carbohydrates, and fat may be affected, especially by tumors of the stomach or intestines. A patient may appear to be eating enough, but the body may not be able to absorb all the nutrients from the food. Diets higher in protein and calories can help correct this and prevent the onset of cachexia. Drugs may also be helpful. It is important to monitor nutrition early, as cachexia is difficult to completely reverse.

Early treatment of cancer symptoms and side effects that affect eating and cause weight loss is important. Both nutrition therapy and drugs can help the patient maintain a healthy weight. The types of drugs commonly used to relieve these symptoms and side effects include the following:

- Medicines to prevent nausea and vomiting

- Medicines to prevent diarrhea
- Pancreatic enzymes
- Laxatives (to promote bowel movements)
- Medicines for mouth problems (to clean the mouth, stimulate saliva, prevent infections, relieve pain, and heal sores)
- Pain medications

Effect of Cancer Treatment on Nutrition

Effect of Surgery on Nutrition

The body needs extra energy and nutrients to heal wounds, fight infection, and recover from surgery. If the patient is malnourished before surgery, there may be complications during recovery, such as poor healing or infection. Patients with certain cancers, such as cancers of the head, neck, stomach, and intestines, may be malnourished at diagnosis. Nutrition care may therefore begin before surgery.

Nutrition-related side effects may occur as a result of surgery. More than half of cancer patients have cancer-related surgery. Surgery may include the removal of all or parts of certain organs, which may affect a patient's ability to eat and digest food. The following are nutrition problems related to specific surgeries:

- Surgery to the head and neck may cause chewing and swallowing problems. Mental stress due to the amount of tissue removed during surgery may affect appetite.

- Surgery involving cancer of organs in the digestive system may lessen the ability of the digestive system to work properly and may slow the digestion of food. Removal of part of the stomach may cause a feeling of fullness before enough food has been eaten. Stomach surgery may also cause dumping syndrome (emptying of the stomach into the intestines before food is digested). Some of the organs in the digestive system normally produce important hormones and chemicals that are necessary for digestion. If surgery affects these organs, the protein, fat, vitamins, and minerals in the diet may not be absorbed normally by the body. Levels of sugar, salt, and fluid in the body may become unbalanced.

Nutrition therapy can treat these problems and help cancer patients get the nutrients they need. Nutrition therapy may include the following:

- Nutritional supplement drinks

- Enteral nutrition (feeding liquid through a tube into the stomach or intestine)

- Parenteral nutrition (feeding through a catheter into the bloodstream)

- Medications to improve the appetite

It is common for patients to experience pain, tiredness, or loss of appetite after surgery. For a short time, some patients may not be able to eat their regular diet because of these symptoms. The following eating tips may help:

- Avoid carbonated drinks (such as sodas) and gas-producing foods (such as beans, peas, broccoli, cabbage, brussel sprouts, green peppers, radishes, and cucumbers).

- If regularity is a problem, increase fiber by small amounts and drink lots of water. Good sources of fiber include whole-grain cereals (such as oatmeal and bran), beans, vegetables, fruit, and whole grain breads.

- Choose high-protein and high-calorie foods to help wounds heal. Good choices include eggs, cheese, whole milk, ice cream, nuts, peanut butter, meat, poultry, and fish. Increase calories by frying foods and using gravies, mayonnaise, and salad dressings. Supplements high in calories and protein are available.

Effect of Chemotherapy on Nutrition

Chemotherapy is a cancer treatment that uses drugs to stop the growth of cancer cells, either by killing the cells or by stopping the cells from dividing. Because chemotherapy targets rapidly dividing cells, healthy cells that normally grow and divide rapidly may also be affected by the cancer treatments. These include cells in the mouth and digestive tract.

Side effects that interfere with eating and digestion may occur during chemotherapy. The following side effects are common:

- Anorexia

- Nausea

- Vomiting

- Diarrhea or constipation

- Inflammation and sores in the mouth
- Changes in the way food tastes
- Infections

The side effects of chemotherapy may make it difficult for a patient to obtain the nutrients needed to regain healthy blood counts between chemotherapy treatments. Nutrition therapy can treat these side effects and help chemotherapy patients get the nutrients they need to tolerate and recover from treatment, prevent weight loss, and maintain general health. Nutrition therapy may include the following:

- Supplements high in calories and protein
- Enteral nutrition (tube feedings)

Effect of Radiation Therapy on Nutrition

Radiation therapy is a cancer treatment that uses high energy x-rays or other types of radiation to kill cancer cells. There are two types of radiation therapy. External radiation therapy uses a machine outside the body to send radiation toward the cancer. Internal radiation therapy uses a radioactive substance sealed in needles, seeds, wires, or catheters that are placed directly into or near the cancer.

Healthy cells that are near the cancer may be affected by the radiation treatments, and side effects may occur. The side effects depend mostly on the radiation dose and the part of the body that is treated.

Radiation therapy to any part of the digestive system is likely to cause nutrition-related side effects. The following side effects may occur:

- Radiation therapy to the head and neck may cause anorexia, taste changes, dry mouth, inflammation of the mouth and gums, swallowing problems, jaw spasms, cavities, or infection.

- Radiation therapy to the chest may cause infection in the esophagus, swallowing problems, esophageal reflux (a backwards flow of the stomach contents into the esophagus), nausea, or vomiting.

- Radiation therapy to the abdomen or pelvis may cause diarrhea, nausea and vomiting, inflammation of the intestine or rectum, and fistula (holes) in the stomach or intestines. Long-term effects can include narrowing of the intestine, chronic inflamed intestines, poor absorption, or blockage in the stomach or intestine.

- Radiation therapy may also cause tiredness, which can lead to a decrease in appetite and a reduced desire to eat.

Nutrition therapy during radiation treatment can provide the patient with enough protein and calories to tolerate the treatment, prevent weight loss, and maintain general health. Nutrition therapy may include the following:

- Nutritional supplement drinks between meals
- Enteral nutrition (tube feedings)
- Other changes in the diet, such as eating small meals throughout the day and choosing certain kinds of foods

Effect of Immunotherapy on Nutrition

Immunotherapy is treatment that uses the patient's immune system to fight cancer. Substances made by the body or made in a laboratory are used to boost, direct, or restore the body's natural defenses against cancer. This type of cancer treatment is also called biologic therapy or biotherapy.

The following nutrition-related side effects are common during immunotherapy:

- Fever
- Nausea
- Vomiting
- Diarrhea
- Anorexia
- Tiredness

If the side effects of immunotherapy are not treated, weight loss and malnutrition may occur. These conditions can cause complications during recovery, such as poor healing or infection. Nutrition therapy can treat side effects from immunotherapy and help patients get the nutrients they need to tolerate treatment, prevent weight loss, and maintain general health.

Effect of Bone Marrow and Stem Cell Transplantation on Nutrition

Bone marrow and stem cell transplantation are methods of replacing blood-forming cells destroyed by cancer treatment with high doses of chemotherapy or radiation therapy. Stem cells (immature blood cells) are removed from the bone marrow of the patient or a donor and are frozen for storage. After the chemotherapy and radiation therapy are completed, the stored stem cells are thawed and given back to the patient through an infusion. Over a short time, these re-infused stem cells grow into (and restore) the body's blood cells.

Chemotherapy, radiation therapy, and medications used in the transplant process may cause side effects that prevent a patient from eating and digesting food as usual. These side effects include the following:

- Taste changes
- Dry mouth
- Thick saliva
- Mouth and throat sores
- Nausea and vomiting
- Diarrhea
- Constipation
- Lack of appetite
- Weight gain

Transplant patients also have a very high risk of infection. The high doses of chemotherapy and radiation therapy reduce the number of white blood cells, the cells that fight infection. Cancer patients should be especially careful to avoid infections and food-borne illnesses. Patients are advised to avoid eating certain foods that may carry harmful bacteria.

Patients undergoing the transplant process need adequate protein and calories to tolerate and recover from the treatment, prevent weight loss, fight infection, and maintain general health. Nutrition therapy is also designed to avoid possible infection from bacteria in food. Nutrition therapy during the transplant process may include the following:

- A diet of only cooked and processed foods, avoiding raw vegetables and fresh fruit
- Instruction on safe food handling
- Specific diet guidelines based on the type of transplant and the cancer site
- Parenteral nutrition (feeding through the bloodstream) during the first few weeks after the transplant is complete, to ensure the patient gets the calories, protein, vitamins, minerals and fluids needed for good health

Nutrition Therapy Overview

Early nutrition screening and assessment can identify problems that affect the success of anticancer therapy. Patients who are underweight or malnourished may not respond well to cancer treatments. Malnutrition may be caused by the cancer or made worse as the cancer progresses. Finding and treating nutrition problems early may help the patient gain or maintain weight, improve the patient's response to therapy, and reduce complications of treatment.

Because the ability to tolerate treatment is better for the well-nourished patient, screening and assessment are done before beginning anticancer therapy. Appropriate nutrition management is begun early, and nutritional status is checked often during treatment.

Screening is used to identify patients who may be at nutritional risk. Assessment determines the complete nutritional status of the patient and identifies if nutrition therapy is needed. The patient or caregiver may be asked for the following information:

- Weight changes over the past six months

- Changes in the amount and type of food eaten compared to what is usual for the patient

- Problems that have affected eating, such as nausea, vomiting, diarrhea, constipation, dry mouth, changes in taste and smell, mouth sores, pain, or loss of appetite

- Ability to walk and perform the activities of daily living

A physical exam is part of the assessment. The physical exam will check the body for general health and signs of disease, such as lumps or growths. The physician will look for loss of weight, fat, and muscle, and fluid buildup in the body.

A nutrition support team will monitor the patient's nutritional status during cancer treatment and recovery. The team may include the following specialists:

- Physician

- Nurse

- Registered dietitian

- Social worker

- Psychologist

Nutrition Suggestions for Symptom Relief

When side effects of cancer or cancer treatment interfere with normal eating, adjustments can be made to ensure the patient continues to get the necessary nutrition. Medications may be given to stimulate the appetite. Eating foods that are high in calories, protein, vitamins, and minerals is usually advised. Meal planning, however, should be individualized to meet the patient's nutritional needs and tastes in food.

Anorexia

Anorexia (lack of appetite) is one of the most common problems for cancer patients. The following suggestions may help cancer patients manage anorexia:

- Eat small high-protein and high-calorie meals every one to two hours instead of three larger meals

- Have help with preparing meals

- Add extra calories and protein to food (such as butter, skim milk powder, honey, or brown sugar)

- Take liquid supplements (special drinks containing nutrients), soups, milk, juices, shakes, and smoothies when eating solid food is a problem.

- Eat snacks that contain plenty of calories and protein

- Prepare and store small portions of favorite foods so they are ready to eat when hungry

- Eat breakfasts that contain one third of the calories and protein needed for the day

- Eat foods with odors that are appealing. Strong odors can be avoided by using boiling bags, cooking outdoors on the grill, using a kitchen fan when cooking, serving cold food instead of hot (since odors are in the rising steam), and taking off any food covers to release the odors before entering a patient's room. Small portable fans can be used to blow food odors away from patients. Cooking odors can be avoided by ordering take-out food.

- Try new foods. Be creative with desserts. Experiment with recipes, flavorings, spices, types, and consistencies of food. Food likes and dislikes may change from day to day.

The following high-calorie, high-protein foods are recommended:

- Cheese and crackers
- Muffins
- Puddings
- Nutritional supplements
- Milkshakes
- Yogurt
- Ice cream
- Powdered milk added to foods such as pudding, milkshakes, or any recipe using milk
- Finger foods (handy for snacking) such as deviled eggs, cream cheese or peanut butter on crackers or celery, or deviled ham on crackers

Taste Changes

Changes in how foods taste may be caused by radiation treatment, dental problems, or medicines. Cancer patients often complain of changes in their sense of taste when undergoing chemotherapy, in particular a bitter taste sensation. A sudden dislike for certain foods may occur. This may result in food avoidance, weight loss, and anorexia, which can greatly reduce the patients' quality of life. Some or all of the sense of taste may return, but it may be a year after treatment ends before the sense of taste is normal again. Drinking plenty of fluids, changing the types of foods eaten and adding spices or flavorings to food may help.

The following suggestions may help cancer patients manage changes in taste:

- Rinse mouth with water before eating
- Try citrus fruits (oranges, tangerines, lemons, grapefruit) unless mouth sores are present
- Eat small meals and healthy snacks several times a day
- Eat meals when hungry rather than at set mealtimes
- Use plastic utensils if foods taste metallic
- Try favorite foods
- Eat with family and friends

- Have others prepare the meal
- Try new foods when feeling best
- Substitute poultry, fish, eggs, and cheese for red meat
- Find nonmeat, high-protein recipes in a vegetarian or Chinese cookbook.
- Use sugar-free lemon drops, gum, or mints if there is a metallic or bitter taste in the mouth
- Add spices and sauces to foods
- Eat meat with something sweet, such as cranberry sauce, jelly, or applesauce

Taking zinc sulfate tablets during radiation therapy to the head and neck may speed the return of normal taste after treatment.

Dry Mouth

Dry mouth is often caused by radiation therapy to the head and neck. Some medicines may also cause dry mouth. Dry mouth may affect speech, taste, ability to swallow, and the use of dentures or braces. There is also an increased risk of cavities and gum disease because less saliva is produced to wash the teeth and gums.

The main treatment for dry mouth is drinking plenty of liquids, about ½ ounce per pound of body weight per day. Other suggestions to manage dry mouth include the following:

- Eat moist foods with extra sauces, gravies, butter, or margarine
- Suck on hard candy or chew gum
- Eat frozen desserts (such as frozen grapes and ice pops) or ice chips
- Clean teeth (including dentures) and rinse mouth at least four times per day (after each meal and before bedtime)
- Keep water handy at all times to moisten the mouth
- Avoid liquids and foods that contain a lot of sugar
- Avoid mouth rinses containing alcohol
- Drink fruit nectar instead of juice
- Use a straw to drink liquids

Mouth Sores and Infections

Mouth sores can result from chemotherapy and radiation therapy. These treatments target rapidly-growing cells because cancer cells grow rapidly. Normal cells inside the mouth may be damaged by these cancer treatments because they also grow rapidly. Mouth sores may become infected and bleed, making eating difficult. By choosing certain foods and taking good care of their mouths, patients can usually make eating easier. Suggestions to help manage mouth sores and infections include the following:

- Eat soft foods that are easy to chew and swallow, such as the following:
  - Soft fruits, including bananas, applesauce, and watermelon
  - Peach, pear, and apricot nectars
  - Cottage cheese
  - Mashed potatoes
  - Macaroni and cheese
  - Custards and puddings
  - Gelatin
  - Milkshakes
  - Scrambled eggs
  - Oatmeal or other cooked cereals
- Use the blender to process vegetables (such as potatoes, peas, and carrots) and meats until smooth.
- Avoid rough, coarse, or dry foods, including raw vegetables, granola, toast, and crackers.
- Avoid foods that are spicy or salty. Avoid foods that are acidic, such as vinegar, pickles, and olives.
- Avoid citrus fruits and juices, including orange, grapefruit, and tangerine.
- Cook foods until soft and tender.
- Cut foods into small pieces.
- Use a straw to drink liquids.
- Eat foods cold or at room temperature. Hot and warm foods can irritate a tender mouth.

- Clean teeth (including dentures) and rinse mouth at least four times per day (after each meal and before bedtime).

- Add gravy, broth, or sauces to food.

- Drink high-calorie, high-protein drinks in addition to meals.

- Numb the mouth with ice chips or flavored ice pops.

Using a mouth rinse that contains glutamine may reduce the number of mouth sores. Glutamine is a substance found in plant and animal proteins.

Nausea

Nausea caused by cancer treatment can affect the amount and kinds of food eaten. The following suggestions may help cancer patients manage nausea:

- Eat before cancer treatments.

- Avoid foods that are likely to cause nausea. For some patients, this includes spicy foods, greasy foods, and foods that have strong odors.

- Eat small meals several times a day.

- Slowly sip fluids throughout the day.

- Eat dry foods such as crackers, breadsticks, or toast throughout the day.

- Sit up or lie with the upper body raised for one hour after eating.

- Eat bland, soft, easy-to-digest foods rather than heavy meals.

- Avoid eating in a room that has cooking odors or that is overly warm. Keep the living space at a comfortable temperature and with plenty of fresh air.

- Rinse out the mouth before and after eating.

- Suck on hard candies such as peppermints or lemon drops if the mouth has a bad taste.

Diarrhea

Diarrhea may be caused by cancer treatments, surgery on the stomach or intestines, or by emotional stress. Long-term diarrhea may lead to dehydration (lack of water in the body) or low levels of salt and potassium, important minerals needed by the body.

The following suggestions may help cancer patients manage diarrhea:

- Eat broth, soups, sports drinks, bananas, and canned fruits to help replace salt and potassium lost by diarrhea.

- Avoid greasy foods, hot or cold liquids, and caffeine.

- Avoid high-fiber foods—especially dried beans and cruciferous vegetables (such as broccoli, cauliflower, and cabbage).

- Drink plenty of fluids through the day. Room temperature liquids may cause fewer problems than hot or cold liquids.

- Limit milk to two cups or eliminate milk and milk products until the source of the problem is found.

- Limit gas-forming foods and beverages such as peas, lentils, cruciferous vegetables, chewing gum, and soda.

- Limit sugar-free candies or gum made with sorbitol (sugar alcohol).

- Drink at least one cup of liquid after each loose bowel movement.

Taking oral glutamine may help keep the intestines healthy when taking the anticancer drug fluorouracil.

Low White Blood Cell Count

Cancer patients may have a low white blood cell count for a variety of reasons, some of which include radiation therapy, chemotherapy, or the cancer itself. Patients who have a low white blood cell count are at an increased risk of infection. The following suggestions may help cancer patients prevent infections when white blood cell counts are low:

- Check dates on food and do not buy or use the food if it is out of date.

- Do not buy or use food in cans that are swollen, dented, or damaged.

- Thaw foods in the refrigerator or microwave. Never thaw foods at room temperature. Cook foods immediately after thawing.

- Refrigerate all leftovers within two hours of cooking and eat them within 24 hours.

- Keep hot foods hot and cold foods cold.

- Avoid old, moldy, or damaged fruits and vegetables.

- Avoid unpackaged tofu sold in open bins or containers.

- Cook all meat, poultry, and fish thoroughly. Avoid raw eggs or raw fish.

- Buy foods packed as single servings to avoid leftovers.

- Avoid salad bars and buffets when eating out.

- Avoid large groups of people and people who have infections.

- Wash hands often to prevent the spread of bacteria.

Hot Flashes

Hot flashes occur in most women with breast cancer and men with prostate cancer. When caused by natural or treatment-related menopause, hot flashes can be relieved with estrogen replacement. Many women, however, (including women with breast cancer), are not able to take estrogen replacement. Eating soy foods, which contain an estrogen-like substance, is sometimes suggested to relieve hot flashes in patients who cannot take estrogen replacement, but no benefit has been proven.

Fluid Intake

The body needs plenty of water to replace the fluids lost every day. Long-term diarrhea, nausea and vomiting, and pain may prevent the patient from drinking and eating enough to get the water needed by the body. One of the first signs of dehydration (lack of water in the body) is extreme tiredness. The following suggestions may help cancer patients prevent dehydration:

- Drink eight to 12 cups of liquids a day. This can be water, juice, milk, or foods that contain a large amount of liquid such as puddings, ice cream, ice pops, flavored ices, and gelatins.

- Take a water bottle whenever leaving home. It is important to drink even if not thirsty, as thirst is not a good sign of fluid needs.

- Limit drinks that contain caffeine, such as sodas, coffee, and tea (both hot and cold).

- Drink most liquids after and between meals.

- Use medicines that help relieve nausea and vomiting.

Constipation

Constipation is defined as fewer than three bowel movements per week. It is a very common problem for cancer patients and may result from lack of water or fiber in the diet; lack of physical activity; anticancer therapies such as chemotherapy; and medications.

Prevention of constipation is a part of cancer care. The following suggestions may help cancer patients prevent constipation:

- Eat more fiber-containing foods on a regular basis. The recommended fiber intake is 25 to 35 grams per day. Increase fiber gradually and drink plenty of fluids at the same time to keep the fiber moving through the intestines.

- Drink eight to ten cups of fluid each day. Water, prune juice, warm juices, lemonade, and teas without caffeine can be very helpful.

- Take walks and exercise regularly. Proper footwear is important.

If constipation does occur, the following suggestions for diet, exercise, and medication may help correct it:

- Continue to eat high-fiber foods and drink plenty of fluids. Try adding wheat bran to the diet; begin with two heaping tablespoons each day for three days, then increase by one tablespoon each day until constipation is relieved. Do not exceed six tablespoons per day.

- Maintain physical activity.

- Include over-the-counter constipation treatments, if necessary. This refers to bulk-forming products (such as Citrucel, Metamucil, Fiberall, FiberCon, and Fiber-Lax); stimulants (such as Dulcolax tablets or suppositories and Senokot); stool softeners (such as Colace, Surfak, and Dialose); and osmotics (such as milk of magnesia). Cottonseed and aerosol enemas can also help relieve the problem. Lubricants such as mineral oil are not recommended because they may prevent the body's use of important nutrients.

Drug-Nutrient Interactions

Cancer patients may be treated with a number of drugs throughout their care. Some foods or nutritional supplements do not mix safely with certain drugs. The combination of these foods and drugs may reduce or change the effectiveness of anticancer therapy or cause life-threatening side effects. Table 35.1 provides information on some of the drug-nutrient interactions that may occur with certain anticancer drugs:

The combination of some herbs with certain foods and drugs may reduce or change the effectiveness of anticancer therapy or cause life-threatening side effects. Table 35.2 (found on page 370) provides information about herbs commonly taken by cancer patients. The information provided covers known interactions only; additional side effects are possible for these herbs. A pharmacist or updated herbal supplement references may provide more information.

Table 35.1. Anticancer Drug-Food Interactions

Trade Name	Generic Name	Food Interactions
Targretin	bexarotene	Grapefruit juice may increase a drug's effects.
Folex; Rheumatrex	methotrexate	Alcohol may cause liver damage.
Mithracin	plicamycin	Supplements of calcium and vitamin D may decrease the drug's effect.
Matulane	procarbazine	Alcohol may cause a reaction that includes flushing of the skin, breathing difficulty, nausea, and low blood pressure. Caffeine may raise blood pressure.
Temodar	temozolomide	Food may slow or decrease the drug's effect.

Table 35.2. Common Herbs Used by Cancer Patients and Possible Food/Drug Interactions

Herbal	Possible Food/Drug Interactions
Black cohosh	May lower blood fat or blood pressure when taken with certain drugs. May increase the effect of tamoxifen.
Chamomile	May increase bleeding when used with blood-thinners. May increase the effect of certain tranquilizers.
Dong quai	May increase effects of warfarin (a blood-thinner).
Echinacea	May interfere with therapy that uses the immune system to fight cancer.
Garlic	May increase bleeding when used with aspirin, dipyridamole, and warfarin. May increase the effects of drugs that treat high blood sugar.
Ginkgo biloba	May increase bleeding when used with aspirin, dipyridamole, and warfarin. May raise blood pressure when used with certain diuretics (drugs that cause the body to lose water through the kidneys).
Ginseng	May prevent the blood from clotting normally. May decrease blood sugar if taken with insulin. May interfere with drugs used to treat a mental disorder. May cause high blood pressure with long-term use of caffeine.
Kava kava	May increase the effect of certain tranquilizers. May cause liver damage.
St. John's wort	May cause life-threatening side effects when used with drugs that raise the level of serotonin in the brain, such as many antidepressants. May reduce the effect of certain drugs used for cancer, AIDS, organ transplants, heart disease, and birth control.
Ma huang (ephedra)	May cause high blood pressure, increased heart rate, or death if used with beta-blockers (drugs used for high blood pressure and heart conditions), monoamine oxidase inhibitors (antidepressants), caffeine, and St. John's wort.
Yohimbe	Reduces the effect of St. John's wort and drugs for depression, high blood pressure, and high blood sugar.

Part Five

Recurrent and
Metastatic Cancer:
Special Considerations

Chapter 36

If Cancer Returns

Adjusting to the News

Maybe in the back of your mind, you feared that your cancer might return. Now you might be thinking, "How can this be happening to me again? Haven't I been through enough?"

You may be feeling shocked, angry, sad, or scared. Many people have these feelings. But you have something now that you didn't have before—experience. You've lived through cancer once. You know a lot about what to expect and hope for.

Also remember that treatments may have improved since you had your first cancer. New drugs or methods may help with your treatment or in managing side effects. In fact, cancer is now often thought of as a chronic disease, one which people manage for many years.

Why and Where Cancer Returns

When cancer comes back, doctors call it a recurrence (or recurrent cancer). Some things you should know are the following:

- A recurrent cancer starts with cancer cells that the first treatment didn't fully remove or destroy. Some may have been too small to be seen in follow-up. This doesn't mean that the treatment you received was wrong. And it doesn't mean that you did anything wrong, either. It just means that a small number of

Excerpted from "When Cancer Returns," National Cancer Institute (www.cancer.gov), August 23, 2005.

cancer cells survived the treatment. These cells grew over time into tumors or cancer that your doctor can now detect.

- When cancer comes back, it doesn't always show up in the same part of the body. For example, if you had colon cancer, it may come back in your liver. But the cancer is still called colon cancer. When the original cancer spreads to a new place, it is called a metastasis.

- It is possible to develop a completely new cancer that has nothing to do with your original cancer. But this doesn't happen very often. Recurrences are more common.

Where Cancer Can Return

Doctors define recurrent cancers by where they develop. There are different types of recurrence:

- **Local recurrence:** This means that the cancer is in the same place as the original cancer or is very close to it.

- **Regional recurrence:** This is when tumors grow in lymph nodes or tissues near the place of the original cancer.

- **Distant recurrence:** In these cases, the cancer has spread (metastasized) to organs or tissues far from the place of the original cancer.

Local cancer may be easier to treat than regional or distant cancer. But this can be different for each patient. Talk with your doctor about your options.

Taking Control: Your Care and Treatment

Cancer that returns can affect all parts of your life. You may feel weak and no longer in control. But you don't have to feel that way. You can take part in your care and in making decisions. You can also talk with your health care team and loved ones as you decide about your care. This may help you feel a sense of control and well-being.

Talking with Your Health Care Team

Many people have a treatment team of health providers who work together to help them. This team may include doctors, nurses, oncology social workers, dietitians, or other specialists. Some people don't like to ask about treatment choices or side effects. They think that doctors don't like being questioned. But this is not true. Most doctors want their patients to be involved in their own care. They want patients to discuss concerns with them.

Here are a few topics you may want to discuss with your health care team:

- **Pain or other symptoms:** Be honest and open about how you feel. Tell your doctors if you have pain and where. Tell them what you expect in the way of pain relief.

- **Communication:** Some people want to know details about their care. Others prefer to know as little as possible. Some people with cancer want their family members to make most of their decisions. What would you prefer? Decide what you want to know, how much you want to know, and when you've heard enough. Choose what is most comfortable for you. Then tell your doctor and family members. Ask that they follow through with your wishes.

- **Family wishes:** Some family members may have trouble dealing with cancer. They don't want to know how far the disease has advanced. Find out from your family members how much they want to know. And be sure to tell your doctors and nurses. Do this as soon as possible. It will help avoid conflicts or distress among your loved ones.

Here are some additional tips for talking with your health care team:

- Speak openly about your needs, questions, and concerns. Don't be embarrassed to ask your doctor to repeat or explain something.

- Keep a file or notebook of all the papers and test results that your doctor has given you. Take this file to your visits. Also keep records or a diary of all your visits. List the drugs and tests you have taken. Then you can refer to your records when you need to. Many patients say this is helpful, especially when you meet with a new doctor for the first time.

- Write down your questions before you see your doctors so you will remember them.

- Ask a family member or friend to go to the doctor's office with you. They can help you ask questions to get a clear sense of what to expect. This can be an emotional time. You may have trouble focusing on what the doctor says. It may be easier for someone else to take notes. Then you can review them later.

- Ask your doctor if it's okay to tape-record your talks.

- Tell your doctor if you want to get dressed before talking about your results. Wearing a gown or robe is distracting for some patients. They find it harder to focus on what the doctor is saying.

Treatment Choices

There are many treatment choices for recurrent cancer. Your treatment will depend partly on the type of cancer and the treatment you had before. It will also depend on where the cancer has recurred:

- A local recurrence may be best treated by surgery or radiation therapy. This means that the doctor removes the tumor or destroys it with radiation.

- A distant recurrence may need chemotherapy, biological therapy, or radiation therapy.

It's important to ask your doctor questions about all your treatment choices. You may want to get a second opinion as well. You may also want to ask whether a clinical trial is an option for you.

Second Opinions

Some patients worry that doctors will be offended if they ask for a second opinion. Usually the opposite is true. Most doctors welcome a second opinion. And many health insurance companies will pay for them.

If you get a second opinion, the doctor may agree with your first doctor's treatment plan. Or the second doctor may suggest another approach. Either way, you have more information and perhaps a greater sense of control. You can feel more confident about the decisions you make, knowing that you've looked at your options.

Clinical Trials

Treatment clinical trials are research studies that try to find better ways to treat cancer. Every day, cancer researchers learn more about treatment options from clinical trials.

Each study has rules about who can take part. These rules include the person's age and type of cancer. They also cover earlier treatments and where the cancer has returned.

Clinical trials have both benefits and risks. Your doctor should tell you about them before you make any decisions about taking part.

There are different phases of clinical trials. They include the following:

- Phase I trials test what dose of a treatment is safe and how it should be given.

- Phase II trials discover how cancer responds to a new drug or treatment.

- Phase III trials compare an accepted cancer treatment (standard treatment) with a new treatment that researchers hope is better.

Taking part in a clinical trial could help you and others who get cancer in the future. But insurance and managed care plans do not always cover the costs. What they cover varies by plan and by study. If you want to learn more about clinical trials, talk with your health care team.

Questions to Ask Your Doctor or Nurse about Treatment Choices

Decide on the most important things you need to ask your doctor or nurse. Here are some ideas:

- What are my treatment choices?

- Which do you suggest for me?

- How is this treatment the same as or different from my last treatment?

- How successful is the treatment you recommend? Why is it best for me?

- Will I still be able to do things I enjoy with the treatment? Without the treatment?

- How long will I be on this treatment?

- Will I have side effects? If so, how long will they last?

- How can I manage the side effects?

- Will I have to stay in the hospital?

- Is a clinical trial available to me?

- Will I have to pay any costs in a clinical trial?

- If the treatment doesn't work, then what will I do?

Making Your Wishes Known

When cancer returns, the treatment goals may change, or they may be the same as they were for your first cancer. But for many people, it's the second cancer diagnosis that finally prompts them to make their wishes known. Although it can be tough to think about, and maybe even tougher to talk about, having recurrent cancer may prompt you to make certain decisions about what you want done for you if you are unable to speak for yourself.

Everyone should make a will and talk about end-of-life choices with loved ones. This is one of the most important things you can do. Also, think about giving someone you trust some rights to make medical decisions for you. You give these rights through legal documents called advance directives. These papers tell your loved ones and doctors what to do if you can't tell them yourself. They let you decide ahead of time how you want to be treated. These papers may include a living will and a durable power of attorney for health care.

Setting up an advance directive is not the same as giving up. Making such decisions at this time keeps you in control. You are making your wishes known for all to follow. This can help you worry less about the future and live each day to the fullest.

It's hard to talk about these issues. But it often comforts family members to know what you want. And it saves them from having to bring up the subject themselves. You may also gain peace of mind. You are making these hard choices for yourself instead of leaving them to your loved ones.

Make copies of your advance directives. Give them to your family members, your health care team, and your hospital medical records department. That way, everyone will know your decisions.

Legal Papers

Advance Directives

- A living will lets people know what kind of medical care you want if you are unable to speak for yourself.

- A durable power of attorney for health care names a person to make medical decisions for you if you can't make them yourself. This person is called a health care proxy.

Other Legal Papers

- A will tells how you want to divide your money and property among your heirs. (Heirs are usually the family members who survive you. You may also name other people as heirs in your will.)

- A trust appoints a person you choose to manage your money for you.

- Power of attorney appoints a person to make financial decisions for you when you can't make them yourself.

Note: You do not always need a lawyer present to fill out these papers. But you may need a notary public. Each state has its own laws about advance directives. Check with your lawyer or social worker about the laws in your state.

Chapter 37

Metastatic Cancer

Questions and Answers about Metastatic Cancer

What is cancer?

Cancer is a group of many related diseases. All cancers begin in cells, the building blocks that make up tissues. Cancer that arises from organs and solid tissues is called a solid tumor. Cancer that begins in blood cells is called leukemia, multiple myeloma, or lymphoma.

Normally, cells grow and divide to form new cells as the body needs them. When cells grow old and die, new cells take their place. Sometimes this orderly process goes wrong. New cells form when the body does not need them, and old cells do not die when they should.

The extra cells form a mass of tissue, called a growth or tumor. Tumors can be either benign (not cancerous) or malignant (cancerous). Benign tumors do not spread to other parts of the body, and they are rarely a threat to life. Malignant tumors can spread (metastasize) and may be life threatening.

What is primary cancer?

Cancer can begin in any organ or tissue of the body. The original tumor is called the primary cancer or primary tumor. It is usually named for the part of the body or the type of cell in which it begins.

This chapter includes text from "Metastatic Cancer: Questions and Answers," National Cancer Institute (NCI), September 1, 2004; and "Two Studies Identify Drivers of Metastases," *NCI Cancer Bulletin*, January 22, 2008.

What is metastasis, and how does it happen?

Metastasis means the spread of cancer. Cancer cells can break away from a primary tumor and enter the bloodstream or lymphatic system (the system that produces, stores, and carries the cells that fight infections). That is how cancer cells spread to other parts of the body.

When cancer cells spread and form a new tumor in a different organ, the new tumor is a metastatic tumor. The cells in the metastatic tumor come from the original tumor. This means, for example, that if breast cancer spreads to the lungs, the metastatic tumor in the lung is made up of cancerous breast cells (not lung cells). In this case, the disease in the lungs is metastatic breast cancer (not lung cancer). Under a microscope, metastatic breast cancer cells generally look the same as the cancer cells in the breast.

Where does cancer spread?

Cancer cells can spread to almost any part of the body. Cancer cells frequently spread to lymph nodes (rounded masses of lymphatic tissue) near the primary tumor (regional lymph nodes). This is called lymph node involvement or regional disease. Cancer that spreads to other organs or to lymph nodes far from the primary tumor is called metastatic disease. Doctors sometimes also call this distant disease.

The most common sites of metastasis from solid tumors are the lungs, bones, liver, and brain. Some cancers tend to spread to certain parts of the body. For example, lung cancer often metastasizes to the brain or bones, and colon cancer frequently spreads to the liver. Prostate cancer tends to spread to the bones. Breast cancer commonly spreads to the bones, lungs, liver, or brain. However, each of these cancers can spread to other parts of the body as well.

Because blood cells travel throughout the body, leukemia, multiple myeloma, and lymphoma cells are usually not localized when the cancer is diagnosed. Tumor cells may be found in the blood, several lymph nodes, or other parts of the body such as the liver or bones. This type of spread is not referred to as metastasis.

Are there symptoms of metastatic cancer?

Some people with metastatic cancer do not have symptoms. Their metastases are found by x-rays and other tests performed for other reasons.

When symptoms of metastatic cancer occur, the type and frequency of the symptoms will depend on the size and location of the metastasis.

For example, cancer that spreads to the bones is likely to cause pain and can lead to bone fractures. Cancer that spreads to the brain can cause a variety of symptoms, including headaches, seizures, and unsteadiness. Shortness of breath may be a sign of lung involvement. Abdominal swelling or jaundice (yellowing of the skin) can indicate that cancer has spread to the liver.

Sometimes a person's primary cancer is discovered only after the metastatic tumor causes symptoms. For example, a man whose prostate cancer has spread to the bones in his pelvis may have lower back pain (caused by the cancer in his bones) before he experiences any symptoms from the primary tumor in his prostate.

How does a doctor know whether a cancer is a primary or a metastatic tumor?

To determine whether a tumor is primary or metastatic, a pathologist examines a sample of the tumor under a microscope. In general, cancer cells look like abnormal versions of cells in the tissue where the cancer began. Using specialized diagnostic tests, a pathologist is often able to tell where the cancer cells came from. Markers or antigens found in or on the cancer cells can indicate the primary site of the cancer.

Metastatic cancers may be found before or at the same time as the primary tumor, or months or years later. When a new tumor is found in a patient who has been treated for cancer in the past, it is more often a metastasis than another primary tumor.

Is it possible to have a metastatic tumor without having a primary cancer?

No. A metastatic tumor always starts from cancer cells in another part of the body. In most cases, when a metastatic tumor is found first, the primary tumor can be found. The search for the primary tumor may involve lab tests, x-rays, and other procedures. However, in a small number of cases, a metastatic tumor is diagnosed but the primary tumor cannot be found, in spite of extensive tests. The pathologist knows the tumor is metastatic because the cells are not like those in the organ or tissue in which the tumor is found. Doctors refer to the primary tumor as unknown or occult (hidden), and the patient is said to have cancer of unknown primary origin (CUP). Because diagnostic techniques are constantly improving, the number of cases of CUP is going down.

What treatments are used for metastatic cancer?

When cancer has metastasized, it may be treated with chemo-therapy, radiation therapy, biological therapy, hormone therapy, sur-gery, cryosurgery, or a combination of these. The choice of treatment generally depends on the type of primary cancer, the size and loca-tion of the metastasis, the patient's age and general health, and the types of treatments the patient has had in the past. In patients with CUP, it is possible to treat the disease even though the primary tu-mor has not been located. The goal of treatment may be to control the cancer, or to relieve symptoms or side effects of treatment.

Are new treatments for metastatic cancer being developed?

Yes, many new cancer treatments are under study. To develop new treatments, the National Cancer Institute (NCI) sponsors clinical tri-als (research studies) with cancer patients in many hospitals, univer-sities, medical schools, and cancer centers around the country. Clinical trials are a critical step in the improvement of treatment. Before any new treatment can be recommended for general use, doctors conduct studies to find out whether the treatment is both safe for patients and effective against the disease. The results of such studies have led to progress not only in the treatment of cancer, but in the detection, di-agnosis, and prevention of the disease as well. Patients interested in taking part in a clinical trial should talk with their doctor.

Two Studies Identify Drivers of Metastases

A study published in *Nature* (January 10, 2008) has pinpointed several microRNAs (miRNAs)—tiny RNA strands that regulate gene expression—that help suppress breast cancer metastases.

Researchers from Memorial Sloan-Kettering Cancer Center exam-ined miRNAs in breast cancer cell lines that were highly metastatic to bone and lung compared with control breast cancer cell lines. They chose to focus further studies on the six miRNAs whose expression was most decreased in the metastatic cells.

Restoring the function of three of these miRNAs—called miR-335, miR-206, and miR-126—by gene therapy significantly reduced the formation of bone metastases in mice implanted with the breast can-cer cell lines. Rare cells that did metastasize had decreased expres-sion of the three miRNAs.

To measure the expression of these miRNAs in human tumors, the investigators used archived tissue samples from 11 women with metastatic breast cancer and nine women whose cancer did not metastasize. They found that patients whose primary tumors had low expression of the three miRNAs "had a shorter median time to metastatic relapse."

In particular, low levels of miR-335 or miR-126 "were associated with very poor overall metastasis-free survival compared to the group whose tumors expressed a high level of these miRNAs." Further studies identified genes regulated by miR-335 that are directly associated with relapse.

A second study published in *Science* (January 11, 2008) identified a specific contribution of cells in the tumor microenvironment involved in the angiogenic switch—the generation of a tumor blood supply—and the associated progression of lung micrometastases to deadly macrometastases.

Researchers from Cold Spring Harbor Laboratory found that micrometastases that recruit a type of cell called a bone marrow-derived endothelial progenitor cell (EPC) to their immature blood vessels undergo development of a blood supply, in both xenograft and spontaneous mouse models of cancer.

The researchers also identified a protein called Id1 that is needed to draw the EPCs to the tumor site. When this protein was suppressed in a mouse model, the number of EPCs in the bloodstream was significantly reduced, and tumor blood vessel growth was suppressed. "These findings ...suggest that the efficacy of antiangiogenic inhibitors used in clinical trials...may be a consequence of directly targeting [bone marrow]-derived EPCs, as well as the nascent tumor vasculature," conclude the authors.

Chapter 38

Making Choices about Care for Advanced Cancer

People have different goals for care when dealing with advanced cancer. And your goals for care may be changing. Perhaps you had been hoping for a remission. Yet now you need to think more about controlling the spread or growth of the cancer. Your decisions about treatment will be very personal. You will want to seek the help of your loved ones and health care providers. But only you can decide what to do. Your desire to avoid future regrets should be measured against the positives and negatives of treatment.

Questions you may want to ask:

- What's the best we can hope for by trying another treatment? What is the goal?

- Is this treatment plan meant to help side effects, slow the spread of cancer, or both?

- Is there a chance that a new treatment will be found while we try the old one?

- What's the most likely result of trying this treatment?

- What are the possible side effects and other downsides of the treatment? How likely are they?

- Are the possible rewards bigger than the possible drawbacks?

Excerpted from "Coping with Advanced Cancer," National Cancer Institute (www.cancer.gov), September 2005.

It is important to ask your health care team what to expect in the future. It's also important to be clear with them about how much information you want to receive from them.

Comfort Care

You have a right to comfort care both during and after treatment. This kind of care is often called palliative care. It includes treating or preventing cancer symptoms and the side effects caused by treatment. Comfort care can also mean getting help with emotional and spiritual problems during and after cancer treatment. Sometimes patients don't want to tell the doctor about their symptoms. They only want to focus on the cancer. Yet you can improve your quality of life with comfort care.

People once thought of palliative care as a way to comfort those dying of cancer. Doctors now offer this care to all cancer patients, beginning when the cancer is diagnosed. You should receive palliative care through treatment, survival, and advanced disease. Your oncologist may be able to help you. But a palliative care specialist may be the best person to treat some problems. Ask your doctor or nurse if there is a specialist you can go to.

Your Choices

You have a number of options for your care. These depend on the type of cancer you have and the goals you have for your care. Your health care team should tell you about any procedures and treatments available, as well as the benefits and risks of those treatments. Options include the following:

- Clinical trials
- Palliative radiation, chemotherapy, or surgery
- Hospice care
- Home care

Many patients choose more than one option. Ask all the questions you need to.

Try to base your decision on your own feelings about life and death, and the pros and cons of cancer treatment. If you choose not to receive any more active cancer treatment, it does not necessarily mean a quick decline and death. It also does not mean you will stop being given palliative care. Your health care team can offer information and advice on options. You also may want to talk about these options with family members and others who are close to you.

Clinical Trials

Treatment clinical trials are research studies that try to find better ways to treat cancer. Every day, cancer researchers learn more about treatment options from clinical trials. The different types of clinical trials are as follows:

- Phase 1 trials test how to give a drug, how often it should be given, and what dose is safe. Usually, only a small number of patients take part.

- Phase 2 trials discover how cancer responds to a new drug treatment. More patients take part.

- Phase 3 trials compare an accepted cancer treatment (standard treatment) with a new treatment that researchers hope is better. More treatment centers and patients take part.

If you decide to try a clinical trial, the trial you choose will depend on the type of cancer you have. It will also depend on the treatments you have already received. Each study has rules about who can take part. These rules may include the patient's age, health, and type of cancer. Clinical trials have both benefits and risks. Your doctor and the study doctors should tell you about these before you make any decisions.

Taking part in a clinical trial could help you and help others who get cancer in the future. But insurance and managed care plans do not always cover costs. What they cover varies by plan and by study. Talk with your health care team to learn more about coverage for clinical trials for your type of cancer.

Palliative Radiation, Chemotherapy, or Surgery

Some palliative chemotherapy and palliative radiation may help relieve pain and other symptoms. In this way, they may improve your quality of life even if they don't stop your cancer. These treatments may be given to remove or shrink a tumor. Or they may be given to slow down a tumor's spread. Palliative surgery is sometimes used to relieve pain or other problems.

Hospice

Hospice care is an option if you feel you are no longer benefiting from cancer treatments. Choosing hospice care doesn't mean that you've given up. It just means the treatment goals are different at this point. It does not mean giving up hope, but rather changing what you hope for. But be sure to check with the hospice you use to learn what treatments and services are covered. Check with your insurance company also.

The goal of hospice is to help patients live each day to the fullest by making them comfortable and lessen their symptoms. Hospice doctors, nurses, spiritual leaders, social workers, and volunteers are specially trained. They are dedicated to supporting their patients' and families' emotional, social, and spiritual needs as well as dealing with patients' medical symptoms.

People usually qualify for hospice services when their doctor signs a statement that says that patients with their type and stage of disease, on average, aren't likely to survive beyond six months. Many people don't realize that they can use hospice services for a number of months, not just a few weeks. In fact, many say they wish they had gotten hospice care much sooner than they did. They were surprised by the expert care and understanding that they got. Often, control of symptoms not only improves quality of life but also helps people live longer. You will be reviewed periodically to see if hospice care is still right for you. Services may include the following:

- Doctor services (You may still keep your own doctors, too.)
- Nursing care
- Medical supplies and equipment
- Drugs to manage cancer-related symptoms and pain
- Short-term in-patient care
- Homemaker and home health aide services
- Respite (relief) services for caregivers. This means someone else helps with care for awhile, so the caregiver can take a break.
- Counseling
- Social work services
- Spiritual care
- Bereavement (grief) counseling and support
- Volunteer services

You can get hospice services at home, in special facilities, in hospitals, and in nursing homes. They have specialists to help guide care. They also have nurses on call 24 hours a day in case you need advice. And they have many volunteers who help families care for their loved one. Some hospices will give palliative chemotherapy at home as well. Hospice care doesn't seek to treat cancer, but it does treat reversible problems with brief hospital stays if needed. An example might be pneumonia or a bladder infection. Medicare, Medicaid, and most private insurers cover hospice services. For those without coverage and in financial need, many hospices provide care for free. To learn more about hospice care, call the National Hospice and Palliative Care Organization at 800-658-8898. Or visit their website at http://www.nhpco.org. The website can also help you find a hospice in your community.

Hospice and home care professionals can help you and your family work through some tough emotional issues. A social worker can offer emotional support, help in planning hospice or home care, and ease the move between types of care. Many people prefer the comfort of their own home, familiar surroundings, and having friends and family members nearby. Getting health care at home gives family members, friends, and neighbors the chance to spend time with you and help with your care.

Home Care

Home care services are for people who are at home rather than in a hospital. Home care services may include the following:

- Monitoring care
- Managing symptoms
- Providing medical equipment
- Physical and other therapies

You may have to pay for home care services yourself. Check with your insurance company. Medicare, Medicaid, and private insurance will sometimes cover home care services when ordered by your doctor. But some rules apply. So talk to your social worker and other members of your health care team to find out more.

Part Six

Breast Cancer Research

Chapter 39

Breast Cancer Advances

Cancer Advances In Focus

Thirty-Five Years Ago

- Approximately 75% of women diagnosed with breast cancer survived their disease at least five years.

- Mastectomy was the only accepted surgical option for breast cancer treatment.

- Only one randomized trial of mammography for breast cancer screening had been conducted.

- Clinical investigation of combination chemotherapy, using multiple drugs with different mechanisms of action, and of hormonal therapy as post-surgical (adjuvant) treatment for breast cancer was in its earliest stages.

- Hormonal treatment of inoperable or advanced breast cancer with tamoxifen, a selective estrogen receptor modulator (SERM), was being investigated but had not yet been approved by the U.S. Food and Drug Administration (FDA).

- Genes associated with an increased risk of breast cancer had not yet been identified.

Excerpted from two documents produced by the National Cancer Institute (www.cancer.gov): "Cancer Advances in Focus," 2006, and "A Snapshot of Breast Cancer," December 2007.

Today

- Nearly 90% of women diagnosed with breast cancer will survive their disease at least five years.

- Breast-conserving surgery (lumpectomy) followed by local radiation therapy has replaced mastectomy as the preferred surgical approach for treating women with early stage breast cancer.

- Routine mammographic screening is an accepted standard for the early detection of breast cancer. The results of eight randomized trials and of the National Cancer Institute–American Cancer Society (NCI-ACS) Breast Cancer Detection Demonstration Projects established that mammographic screening can reduce mortality from breast cancer.

- Combination chemotherapy has become standard in the adjuvant treatment of women with early stage breast cancer. The goal of this systemic therapy is to eradicate cancer cells that may have spread beyond the breast. Neoadjuvant chemotherapy, or chemotherapy given before surgery to reduce the size of the tumor and to increase the chance of breast-conserving surgery, is being studied in clinical trials.

- Hormonal therapy with SERMs, such as tamoxifen, and aromatase inhibitors is now standard in the treatment of women with estrogen receptor-positive breast cancer, both as adjuvant therapy and in the treatment of advanced disease. Estrogen receptor-positive breast cancer cells can be stimulated to grow by the hormone estrogen. SERMs interfere with this growth stimulation by preventing estrogen from binding to its receptor. In contrast, aromatase inhibitors block estrogen production by the body. FDA-approved aromatase inhibitors include anastrozole, exemestane, and letrozole.

- Tamoxifen and another SERM, raloxifene, have been shown in clinical trials to prevent the development of invasive breast cancer in women at high risk of this disease. Tamoxifen has already been approved by the FDA as a breast cancer prevention drug.

- The monoclonal antibody trastuzumab is being used to treat breast cancers that overproduce a protein called human epidermal growth factor receptor 2 or HER2. This protein is overproduced in about 20% of breast cancers. These HER2-overproducing cancers tend to be more aggressive and are more likely to recur.

Trastuzumab targets the HER2 protein, and this antibody, in conjunction with adjuvant chemotherapy, can lower the risk of HER2-overproducing breast cancer recurrence by 50% compared to chemotherapy alone.

- The study of large groups of related individuals (kindreds) has led to the identification of several breast cancer susceptibility genes, including BRCA1, BRCA2, TP53, and PTEN/MMAC1. Mutations in BRCA1 and BRCA2 account for approximately 80–90% of all hereditary breast cancers, and women who carry mutations in these genes have a lifetime risk of breast cancer that is roughly 10 times greater than that of the general population.

Tomorrow

We will exploit our rapidly increasing knowledge of genetics, molecular biology, and immunology to develop even more effective and less toxic treatments for breast cancer. We will expand our ability to target and disrupt the effects of molecular changes that cause breast cells to become cancerous. In addition, we will use this knowledge to personalize breast cancer therapy. For example:

- Gene expression analysis has led to the identification of five subtypes of breast cancer that have distinct biological features, clinical outcomes, and responses to chemotherapy. This knowledge should allow the development of treatment strategies based on an individual's tumor characteristics.

- A patient's response to chemotherapy is influenced not only by the tumor's genetic characteristics but also by inherited variation in genes that affect a person's ability to absorb, metabolize, and eliminate drugs. This knowledge should allow prediction of tumor response to and the likelihood of severe adverse effects from individual chemotherapy drugs or classes of drugs. It should also aid in the design of more effective and less toxic chemotherapeutic agents.

Examples of NCI Research Initiatives Relevant to Breast Cancer

- Eleven breast cancer-specific Specialized Programs of Research Excellence (SPOREs) are moving results from the laboratory to the clinical setting (http://spores.nci.nih.gov/current/breast/breast.html).

- The Breast and Prostate Cancer and Hormone-Related Gene Variants Cohort Consortium Study is pooling data and biospecimens from six large prospective cohorts to examine the role of interactions between genes and the environment in the development of breast and prostate cancer (http://epi.grants.cancer.gov/BPC3).

- Cancer Genetic Markers of Susceptibility (CGEMS) is identifying genetic alterations that make people susceptible to prostate and breast cancer. Scientists are using DNA from five large studies of prostate cancer and five large studies of breast cancer to scan the genome for common genetic differences between patients who have these cancers and those who do not have cancer (http://cgems.cancer.gov/index.asp).

- The national I-SPY trial is identifying biomarkers that can predict response to therapy in women with Stage III breast cancer. The investigators are using contrast-enhanced magnetic resonance imaging (MRI) to evaluate locally advanced breast cancers. They are correlating the MRI results with molecular markers to identify the best surrogate marker for early response (http://tr.nci.nih.gov/iSpy).

- The Trial Assigning IndividuaLized Options for Treatment (Rx), or TAILORx, is determining whether genes associated with risk of recurrence in women with early-stage breast cancer can be used to identify the most appropriate and effective treatments for these women (http://www.cancer.gov/newscenter/pressreleases/TAILORxRelease).

- NCI's Strategic Partnering to Evaluate Cancer Signatures (SPECS) program is exploring the use of comprehensive molecular analyses to improve treatment outcomes. One SPECS project is refining and validating molecular signatures to identify five subtypes of breast cancer (http://cancerdiagnosis.nci.nih.gov/specs/index.htm).

- The Breast Cancer Home Page directs visitors to up-to-date information on breast cancer treatment, prevention, genetics, causes, screening, testing, and other topics (http://www.cancer.gov/breast).

Selected Advances in Breast Cancer Research

- The Study of Tamoxifen and Raloxifene (STAR) trial showed that Evista® (raloxifene) is as effective as tamoxifen in reducing breast cancer risk in high-risk premenopausal women and has fewer dangerous side effects (http://www.nci.nih.gov/ncicancerbulletin/NCI_Cancer_Bulletin_041806/page2).

- Adding magnetic resonance imaging to a standard mammography and clinical breast exam finds more cancers in women who already have breast cancer in the opposite breast (http://www.cancer.gov/ncicancerbulletin/NCI_Cancer_Bulletin_040307/page2).

- Breast cancer incidence declined sharply in 2003 after increasing for more than 20 years because of a drop in the use of hormone replacement therapy (http://www.cancer.gov/ncicancerbulletin/NCI_Cancer_Bulletin_050107/page2).

- Radiation therapy after breast-conserving surgery and five years of tamoxifen therapy reduces the risk of breast cancer recurrence in older women (http://www.cancer.gov/ncicancerbulletin/NCI_Cancer_Bulletin_013007/page4).

Chapter 40

Studying Breast Cancer Risks and Prevention

Chapter Contents

Section 40.1

Breast Cancer Prevention Trial: Final Results

"Final Results from the NSABP Breast Cancer Prevention
Trial Reported," National Cancer Institute (www.cancer.gov),
November 15, 2005.

Researchers from the National Surgical Adjuvant Breast and Bowel Project (NSABP) who conducted the landmark Breast Cancer Prevention Trial (BCPT), report a seven-year and final update of the trial results in the November 16, 2005, *Journal of the National Cancer Institute*. In this final report, reductions in breast cancer incidence among participants taking tamoxifen were found to be very similar compared to those reported in 1998 when initial findings from the BCPT were released. The conclusion is supported by the observation that the incidence rate of breast cancer was relatively constant through seven years of follow-up among women who received tamoxifen and by the fact that the rate remained stable for at least two years beyond the time that women stopped taking the drug. The risks of stroke, deep-vein thrombosis, and cataracts—possible side-effects of tamoxifen treatment—were also similar to those reported previously.

"The BCPT should be viewed not only as the first study that demonstrated that breast cancer can be prevented, but also as a beginning from which a new paradigm for breast cancer prevention can evolve," said Bernard Fisher, M.D., first author of the initial and final reports, and principal investigator for the trial. "Cohorts of women at increased risk for breast cancer, who could derive a net benefit from receiving tamoxifen, have been clearly defined."

The BCPT was designed to see whether the drug tamoxifen could prevent breast cancer in women who were at an increased risk of developing the disease. Women in the study were randomly assigned to receive tamoxifen or a placebo, and neither participants nor their physicians were aware of the treatment assignment, a process called double-blinding. Since 1998, BCPT participants have been followed by the NSABP, the Pittsburgh-based research network that conducted the trial with support from the National Cancer Institute (NCI), part of the National Institutes of Health.

When the initial results of the BCPT were first announced, researchers found a 49 percent reduction in invasive breast cancer (cancer that has spread and is growing into surrounding, healthy tissues) incidence among participants at increased risk for the disease who took tamoxifen (Nolvadex®, AstraZeneca Pharmaceuticals, Wilmington, Delaware), a drug that had been used for over twenty years to treat breast cancer. The initial study results also showed a 45 percent reduction in non-invasive breast cancer incidence.

By 2005, after seven years of follow-up, investigators found that healthy women assigned to take tamoxifen developed 145 cases of invasive breast cancer compared to 250 cases in the women assigned to take placebo. This final analysis confirms that tamoxifen reduces the risk of invasive breast cancer in both pre- and postmenopausal women at increased risk for the disease. Additionally, risk of pulmonary embolism was 11 percent lower than initially reported and risk of endometrial cancer was about 29 percent higher, but neither of these differences was statistically significant.

"The NCI is very pleased with the ultimate results of the BCPT, in part because there is proof of a benefit from tamoxifen beyond the time a woman is taking the pills," said Leslie Ford, M.D., associate director for NCI's Division of Cancer Prevention and co-author of the study. "We hope that other breast cancer prevention clinical trials, such as STAR, the Study of Tamoxifen and Raloxifene, help us identify drugs that maximize the benefits and minimize the side effects for women interested in reducing their risk of developing breast cancer."

Launched in April 1992, the BCPT also looked at whether taking tamoxifen decreased the number of heart attacks and reduced the number of certain common types of bone fractures in these women. There was almost no difference in the number of heart attacks between the tamoxifen and placebo group, but women in the tamoxifen group had fewer bone fractures of the hip, wrist, and spine (80 cases in the tamoxifen group vs. 116 cases in the placebo group) as reported in 2005.

Only women at increased risk of developing breast cancer participated in the study. Because the risk of breast cancer increases with age, women 60 years of age and older qualified to participate based on age alone. At age 60, about 17 of every 1,000 women are expected to develop breast cancer within five years. Women between the ages of 35 and 59, who demonstrated an increased risk of breast cancer equivalent to or greater than that of an average 60-year-old woman, were also eligible.

Section 40.2

Weight Gain Increases Risk of Breast Cancer after Menopause

National Cancer Institute, *NCI Cancer Bulletin*, Vol. 3, No. 29, July 18, 2006.

Gaining weight after age 18, specifically after menopause, increases a woman's risk of breast cancer after menopause, whereas losing weight after menopause can reduce the risk, researchers at Harvard Medical School have found. They say that many cases of breast cancer could be avoided by women losing weight after menopause.

The researchers suggest that women should be advised to avoid weight gain during adulthood to decrease their postmenopausal breast cancer risk. Hormones are directly related to breast cancer risk, and associations found in the study may be explained in part by the effect of gaining weight on hormones, the researchers report in the July 12, 2006, issue of the *Journal of the American Medical Association.*

Dr. A. Heather Eliassen and her colleagues tracked participants in the Nurses' Health Study. To assess weight change since age 18, they followed 87,000 women for up to 26 years. They followed 49,500 women for up to 24 years to assess weight change since menopause.

Among the women, 4,400 had invasive breast cancer. After adjusting for multiple breast cancer risk factors, the researchers found that women who gained 55 lbs. or more after age 18 had almost 1½ times the risk of cancer compared with those who maintained their weight. A gain of 22 lbs. after menopause was associated with an increased risk of 18 percent. Losing 22 lbs. after menopause decreased the risk by 57 percent.

"Although these data suggest that it is never too late to lose weight to decrease risk, given the difficulty in losing weight, the emphasis must also remain on weight maintenance throughout adult life," they conclude.

Section 40.3

Evista Approved for Reducing Breast Cancer Risk

Consumer Update, U.S. Food and Drug Administration (FDA),
September 17, 2007.

The U.S. Food and Drug Administration (FDA) has approved Evista (raloxifene hydrochloride) for reducing the risk of invasive breast cancer in postmenopausal women with osteoporosis and in postmenopausal women at high risk for invasive breast cancer. Invasive breast cancer develops when abnormal cells spread into the surrounding breast tissue.

Evista, which is manufactured by Eli Lilly and Company, Indianapolis, Ind., is only the second drug approved to reduce the risk of breast cancer. The drug was already approved for preventing and treating osteoporosis in postmenopausal women.

Effectiveness

Evista is commonly referred to as a selective estrogen receptor modulator (SERM). In reducing the risk of invasive breast cancer, SERMs may act by blocking estrogen receptors in the breast.

Three clinical trials in 15,234 postmenopausal women comparing Evista to placebo (no drug) demonstrated that Evista reduces the risk of invasive breast cancer by 44 to 71 percent. A fourth clinical trial in 19,747 postmenopausal women at high risk for developing breast cancer compared Evista to tamoxifen. In this trial, the risk of developing invasive breast cancer was similar for the two treatments.

Evista does not completely prevent breast cancer. Breast examinations and mammograms should be done before starting Evista and regularly thereafter.

Evaluating Benefits and Risks

Because Evista can cause serious side effects, the benefits and risks of taking the drug should be carefully evaluated for each woman.

Women should talk with their health care providers about whether the drug is right for them.

Evista can cause serious side effects, including blood clots in the legs and lungs and death due to stroke. Women with current or prior blood clots in the legs, lungs, or eyes should not take Evista.

Other potential side effects include hot flashes, leg cramps, swelling of the legs and feet, flu-like symptoms, joint pain, and sweating.

Evista should not be taken by premenopausal women and women who are or may become pregnant, because it may cause harm to the unborn baby.

Evista should not be taken with cholestyramine (a drug used to lower cholesterol levels) or estrogens.

Chapter 41

Improvements in Monitoring Breast Cancer

Chapter Contents

Section 41.1

Breast Cancer Specific Molecular Prognostic Test

"FDA Clears Breast Cancer Specific Molecular Prognostic Test,"
FDA News, U. S. Food and Drug Administration (FDA), February 6, 2007.

In February 2007, the U.S. Food and Drug Administration (FDA) cleared for marketing a test that determines the likelihood of breast cancer returning within five to 10 years after a woman's initial cancer. It is the first cleared molecular test that profiles genetic activity.

The MammaPrint test uses the latest in molecular technology to predict whether existing cancer will metastasize (spread to other parts of a patient's body). The test relies on microarray analysis, a powerful tool for simultaneously studying the patterns of behavior of large numbers of genes in biological specimens.

The recurrence of cancer is partly dependent on the activation and suppression of certain genes located in the tumor. Prognostic tests like the MammaPrint can measure the activity of these genes, and thus help physicians understand their patients' odds of the cancer spreading.

MammaPrint was developed by Agendia, a laboratory located in Amsterdam, Netherlands, where the product has been on the market since 2005.

"Clearance of the MammaPrint test marks a step forward in the initiative to bring molecular-based medicine into current practice," said Andrew C. von Eschenbach, M.D., Commissioner of Food and Drugs. "MammaPrint results will provide patients and physicians with more information about the prospects for the outcome of the disease. This information will support treatment decisions.

Agendia compared the genetic profiles of a large number of women suffering from breast cancer and identified a set of 70 genes whose activity confers information about the likelihood of tumor recurrence. The MammaPrint test measures the level of activity of each of these genes in a sample of a woman's surgically removed breast cancer tumor, then uses a specific formula, known as an algorithm, to produce a score that determines whether the patient is deemed low risk or high risk for spread of the cancer to another site. The result may help a doctor in planning appropriate follow-up for a patient when used with other clinical information and laboratory tests.

The MammaPrint is the first cleared in vitro diagnostic multivariate index assay (IVDMIA) device. Several months ago, FDA issued a draft guidance document concerning the need for these complex molecular tests to meet pre-market review and post-market device requirements even when the tests are developed and used by a single laboratory. Although FDA regulates diagnostic tests sold to laboratories, hospitals and physicians, it uses discretion when regulating tests developed and performed by single laboratories.

"There have been rapid advances in microarrays and other pioneering diagnostics, and a corresponding increase in the use and impact of these complex tests. This has prompted FDA to take a closer look at the potential risks as well as the benefits associated with such tests when they are developed and used in laboratories," remarked Steven Gutman, M.D., Director, Office of In Vitro Diagnostic Device Evaluation. "This test clearance takes into account the development of these innovative technologies and ensures public health by carefully evaluating their performance."

Prior to clearance, FDA requested evidence that the MammaPrint had been properly validated for its intended use. Agendia submitted data from a study using tumor samples and clinical data from 302 patients at five European centers. These studies confirmed that the test was useful in predicting time to distant metastasis in women who are under age 61 and in the two earliest stages of the disease (Stage I and Stage II) and who have tumor size equal to or less than five centimeters and no evidence that the cancer has spread to nearby lymph nodes (lymph node–negative). FDA plans to publish a special controls guidance document within the next 60 days describing types of data that should support claims for genetic profiling for breast cancer prognosis.

According to the American Cancer Society, an estimated 178,480 new cases of invasive breast cancer will be diagnosed among women in the United States this year and over 40,000 women are expected to die from the disease.

Section 41.2

Predicting Risk of Breast Cancer Recurrence and Who Will Benefit from Chemotherapy

"Molecular Test Can Predict both the Risk of Breast Cancer Recurrence and Who Will Benefit from Chemotherapy," National Cancer Institute (www.cancer.gov), December, 10, 2004.

A new test can predict both the risk of breast cancer recurrence and may identify women who will benefit most from chemotherapy, according to research supported by the National Cancer Institute (NCI), part of the National Institutes of Health, and performed in collaboration with the National Surgical Adjuvant Breast and Bowel Project (NSABP) and Genomic Health Inc. These results suggest that almost half of over 50,000 U.S. women diagnosed with estrogen-dependent, lymph node–negative breast cancer* every year are at low risk for recurrence and may not need to go through the discomfort and side effects of chemotherapy.

The test is based on levels of expression (increased or decreased) of a panel of cancer-related genes. This panel is used to predict whether estrogen-dependent breast cancer will come back, according to a study published online in the *New England Journal of Medicine* on Friday, December 10, 2004.** Scientists on this study also will present new results on that day at San Antonio Breast Cancer Symposium indicating that the same test can predict which women benefit most from chemotherapy. Women with low risk of breast cancer recurrence—about half of the women in the recent study—do not appear to derive much benefit from chemotherapy.

The researchers used tissue samples and medical records from women enrolled in clinical trials of the cancer drug tamoxifen, which blocks the effect of estrogen on breast cancer cells. These women had a kind of breast cancer defined as estrogen receptor-positive, lymph node–negative. Each year, over 50,000 women are diagnosed with this kind of breast cancer, which needs estrogen to grow but has not spread to the lymph nodes. Currently, many women with this type of breast cancer in the United States do receive chemotherapy in addition to hormonal therapy.

410

Using samples from 447 patients and a collection of 250 genes in three independent preliminary studies, 16 cancer-related genes were found that worked best. The scientists created a formula that generates a "recurrence score" based on the expression patterns of these genes in a tumor sample. Ranging from one to 100, the recurrence score is a measure of the risk that a given cancer will recur.***

Prior to this research, analysis of the expression of genes was performed on tumor specimens that were frozen rather than on tissue prepared for routine pathologic evaluation (fixed and embedded). The expression analysis depended on measurement of RNA (the molecule necessary for the translation of a gene into a protein), and RNA is altered when tissues are fixed and embedded. Frozen tissues are generally not readily available in routine practice. Researchers at Genomic Health Inc. developed a method for performing these analyses on tissues embedded in paraffin wax. Their method allows them to use the altered RNA that is found in fixed tissue.

The results published in the *New England Journal of Medicine* validate the ability of the recurrence score to predict risk of recurrence. Using biopsy tissue and medical records from another NSABP tamoxifen trial, researchers divided 668 women into low, intermediate, and high risk of recurrence groups. Fifty-one percent were in the low risk group (with a score of less than 18); 22 percent were at intermediate risk (recurrence score 18 or higher but less than 31); 27 percent were at high risk (a score of 31 or higher).

These risk group divisions correlated well with the actual rates of recurrence of breast cancer after 10 years. There was a significant difference in recurrence rates between women in the low and high risk groups. In the low risk group, there was a 6.8 percent rate of recurrence at 10 years; in the intermediate and high risk categories these rates were 14.3 and 30.5 percent, respectively. Up to a recurrence score of 50, rates of recurrence increased continuously as the recurrence score increased. These trends held across age groups and tumor size.

"These results were generated perhaps a decade earlier than would have been possible if the researchers had not had access to biopsy tissue from the NSABP trials," notes Sheila E. Taube, Ph.D., associate director of NCI's Cancer Diagnosis Program.

The same 21-gene test has also been used to predict how beneficial chemotherapy will be for women with estrogen receptor-positive, lymph node–negative breast cancer for women on tamoxifen in NSABP trials. These results were presented at the San Antonio Breast Cancer Symposium on December 10, 2004.

411

"NCI staff worked with the company, NSABP and experts from other NCI Cooperative Groups to develop an overall strategy to validate the test; this plan was fruitful and may lead to providing an important tool for physicians and women to use in considering breast cancer treatment decisions," said Taube.

In the treatment study, women with high recurrence scores, who are representative of about 25 percent of patients with this kind of breast cancer, had a large benefit from chemotherapy in terms of 10 year recurrence-free rates. Women with low recurrence scores, who represent about 50 percent of these patients, derived minimal benefits from chemotherapy. The group under study was not large enough to determine whether chemotherapy is detrimental to the low risk group.

"The test has the potential to change medical practice by sparing thousands of women each year from the harmful short- and long-term side effects associated with chemotherapy," said JoAnne Zujewski, M.D., senior investigator in NCI's Cancer Therapy Evaluation Program.

Notes

*Tumor size can affect the estimate of the number of women diagnosed with this type of cancer. This estimate is based on tumors larger than one centimeter and smaller than five centimeters.

**Print version: Paik S, Shak S, Wolmark N, et al. A Multigene Assay to Predict Recurrence of Tamoxifen-Treated, Node-Negative Breast Cancer. *New England Journal of Medicine*, 351(27). December 30, 2004.

***This technology is called the Oncotype DXTM.

Section 41.3

Detecting the Spread of Breast Cancer

"Test Detects the Spread of Breast Cancer," Consumer Update,
U.S. Food and Drug Administration (FDA), July 16, 2007.

The first molecular-based laboratory test for detecting whether breast cancer has spread (metastasized) to nearby lymph nodes was approved by FDA on July 16, 2007. The GeneSearch BLN Assay, manufactured by Veridex, a Johnson & Johnson Company, of Warren, New Jersey, detects molecules that are abundant in breast tissue but scarce in a normal lymph node.

The Importance of Lymph Nodes

Lymph nodes are part of the system that helps protect the body against infection. The first lymph node that filters fluid from the breast is called the "sentinel node," because that is where breast cancer cells are likely to spread first.

The presence or absence of breast cancer cells in underarm lymph nodes is a powerful predictor of whether the cancer has spread and is used to help decide the appropriate treatment for a woman with metastatic breast cancer.

"The GeneSearch BLN Assay offers a new approach to sentinel node testing," says Daniel Schultz, M.D., Director of FDA's Center for Devices and Radiological Health. "Results of this rapid test are available while patients are on the operating table, providing a way for some women to avoid a second operation."

During a lumpectomy or mastectomy to remove a breast tumor, surgeons commonly remove the sentinel node for examination under a microscope. Sometimes the sentinel node is examined immediately, and if tumor cells are found, additional lymph nodes are removed.

A more extensive microscopic examination, requiring one to two days for results, is almost always performed. If tumor cells are only found with the later microscopic examination, the woman may require a second surgery to remove the remaining lymph nodes.

413

Test Effectiveness

In a clinical trial, the GeneSearch BLN Assay showed strong agreement with results from extensive microscopic examination of the lymph nodes of 416 women. The test accurately predicted nearly 88% of the time that breast cancer had spread in women with metastasis. Women without metastasis were identified accurately 94% of the time.

Chapter 42

Treatment Implications of Breast Cancer Genomes

As normal cells turn cancerous and develop into tumors, their genomes accumulate tell-tale changes. Some changes involve gene amplification, meaning they accumulate multiple copies and cause genes to overexpress the proteins they code for. Other changes involve gene deletion, which leads to reduced gene expression. Many of these changes may affect genes that normally regulate cell survival and cell proliferation, processes that, uncontrolled, are hallmarks of cancer.

These genomic aberrations are complex but not random. By studying their patterns, researchers are uncovering clues to the many genes involved in breast cancer, how different kinds of breast cancer may progress, and which treatments may be most effective—including targets for promising new drugs.

Scientists at Berkeley Lab and the University of California at San Francisco, with colleagues at other institutions, have now linked genomic aberrations in breast cancers to likely clinical outcomes, identified new genes involved in breast cancer, and specified new targets for therapy. In closely related research, they have demonstrated that many of the revealing aberrant patterns found in tumor genomes are well modeled by breast cancer cell lines.

"Our goal is to understand how these abnormalities occur and how the genes associated with them function in breast cancer, so we can

"Decoding Breast Cancer Genomes," by Paul Preuss, *Science@Berkeley Lab*, January 2007. Reprinted with permission from Lawrence Berkeley National Laboratory (www.lbl.gov).

identify molecular differences among clinically similar tumors and design effective therapeutic agents against them," says Joe W. Gray, who is director of Berkeley Lab's Life Sciences Division, Associate Laboratory Director for Life and Environmental sciences, and co-leader of the Breast Oncology Program at the UCSF Comprehensive Cancer Center. The new breast cancer genome results were developed in Gray's laboratory.

How Genome Aberrations Reflect Cancer Pathophysiology

The University of California at San Francisco (UCSF) Comprehensive Cancer Center's Koei Chin, a member of the Gray lab who is a guest in Berkeley Lab's Life Sciences Division, has conducted research in concert with a score of colleagues from groups at UCSF, Berkeley Lab, the California Pacific Medical Center, and Affymetrix, Inc. Led by Chin, these researchers have shown that analyzing a tumor's genome copy numbers and gene expression can help predict how well a patient's tumor will respond to current aggressive treatments; the same factors can identify specific genes that can be attacked to improve therapy in patients whose tumors do not respond well to current treatment methods.

"Both high-level amplification of some genes—meaning multiple copies of them—and loss of other genes contribute to how breast cancers develop and progress," says Chin. "In some types of breast cancer that don't respond well to current treatments, our research pinpoints genes overexpressed by high amplification in specific regions of the tumor genome, which are potential targets for new or different drug therapies."

Chin says that although analysis of gene expression is a powerful method of subtyping breast cancers these days—assays can look at the expression of up to 20,000 genes on a single microassay chip—the power of these gene-based assays to predict treatment outcomes is still not as great as one might hope. "By concentrating on combined analysis of genome copy number and expression, we have been able to identify a small number of genes that improve our ability to better predict clinical outcomes for some cancer subtypes."

Chin and his colleagues applied microarray techniques to measure changes in genome copy number and gene expression in tumor genomes. By mapping genome copy number abnormalities in tumors from 145 patients, and gene expression in 130 tumors, they were able to identify regions of amplification and deletion that were associated

416

with good and bad clinical outcome. These results may eventually be developed into clinical assays that will allow patients and their physicians to make informed decisions about treatment options.

Surgery and radiation have long been the standard treatments for breast cancer; depending on the stage, chemotherapy may be aggressively applied in addition. Anticancer drugs are a significant burden for post-surgery patients, however. Ideally, only the most appropriate therapeutic agents would be selected to treat individual tumors, based on their molecular signatures.

Chin and his colleagues found that as the number of genome abnormalities in a breast cancer tumor increases, so does the likelihood of poor treatment outcome. In some tumor subtypes, high-level gene amplification was strongly associated with reduced survival. While patterns of gene amplification and expression correlate well with the known tumor subtypes, the new and more detailed analysis of changes in gene amplification and expression produce more accurate predictions of likely clinical outcomes, by focusing on specific sites and specific genes.

In four high-level amplification regions on chromosomes 8, 11, 17, and 20 (namely the regions designated 8p11-12, 11q13-14, 17q11-12, and 20q13), the researchers found 66 genes whose expression had been deregulated. These 66 genes appear to play important functional roles in breast cancer. Although patients with the types of tumors in which there is amplification of these sites generally do not fare well under present therapies, at least nine of the newly identified genes in these regions offer excellent "druggable" targets for new breast cancer therapies.

A Cell-Line System

Research led by Richard Neve of the Life Sciences Division, in collaboration with colleagues from Berkeley Lab, UCSF, the University of California at Berkeley, the Wayne State University School of Medicine, the University of Texas Southwestern Medical Center, the Georgetown University School of Medicine, and the University of Michigan Medical School, has established that genome analyses based on a library of 51 breast cancer cell lines maintained in vitro are substantially similar to analyses based on tumor tissues. Thus, information gained from cell-line experiments can greatly complement the analysis of a primary tumor and improve clinical decisions.

"By using data from a growing library of cell lines, we can better understand how specific genomic or gene expression abnormalities influence cancer behavior," says Neve. "This can lead to a better treatment plan and a better understanding of possible outcomes, resulting in a better choice of therapeutic drugs."

Because the cell lines retain most of the recurrent patterns of genomic changes present in primary tumors, says Neve, "The genomic characteristics of the cell lines reflect those of the tumors—not perfectly, but quite well, so we can use these to investigate how these characteristics influence the cancer biology."

Oncogenes associated with the development of cancer are among those amplified in the genomes of cancerous cells, while tumor suppressors are among those deleted or suppressed, Neve says. "We come out with a long list of potential oncogenes and tumor suppressors—a list that identifies many genes not previously thought to be associated with breast cancer." Not only does this information suggest novel drug targets, it can improve patient selection for clinical trials of a range of new drugs. "We can pull out a gene profile and find the patients most likely to respond, which could save money and could also get much better results for those patients."

Neve says, "Research using cell lines has suffered from poorly maintained and annotated stocks. We have developed a well characterized reference stock of cell lines, and we've found that the best way to track and identify a particular cell line is to look at its DNA fingerprint. We have also amassed a large body of biological information for these cell lines. The more people who share this data, the better, so we are putting all our information on the web."

Focusing on gene amplification and gene expression in both primary tumors and in a wide range of existing cell lines opens a new path for studying how breast cancers develop, for predicting the outcomes of breast cancer treatments, for suggesting promising new targets of drug therapy, and for honing clinical trials for more meaningful results.

Koei Chin and his colleagues were supported in this work by the National Institutes of Health, the Department of Energy's Office of Science, and the Avon Foundation. Research by Neve and his colleagues was supported by the Department of Energy (DOE)'s Office of Science and the National Institutes of Health.

Additional Information

- "Genomic and transcriptional aberrations linked to breast cancer pathologies," by Koei Chin, Sandy DeVries, Jane Fridyland, Paul Spellman, Ritu Roydasgupta, Wen-Lin Kuo, Anna Lapuk, Richard Neve, Zuwei Qian, Tom Ryder, Fanqing Chen, Heidi Feiler,

Taku Tokuyasu, Chris Kingsley, Shanaz Dairkee, Zhenhang Meng, Karen Chew, Daniel Pinkel, Ajay Jain, Britt Marie Ljung, Laura Esserman, Donna Albertson, Frederic Waldman, and Joe W. Gray, appears in the December, 2006 issue of *Cancer Cell* and is available online to subscribers.

- "A breast cancer cell line 'system' for functional cancer genomics," by Richard M. Neve, Koei Chin, Jane Fridyland, Jennifer Yeh, Frederick L. Baehner, Tea Fevr, Laura Clark, Nora Bayani, Jean-Philippe Coppe, Frances Tong, Terry Speed, Paul T. Spellman, Sandy DeVries, Anna Lapuk, Wen-Lin Kuo, Jackie L. Stillwell, Daniel Pinkel, Donna G. Albertson, Frederick M. Waldman, Frank McCormick, Robert B. Dickson, Michael D. Johnson, Marc Lippman, Stephen Ethier, Adi Gazdar, and Joe W. Gray, appears in the December, 2006 issue of *Cancer Cell* and is available online to subscribers.

Chapter 43

Trial Assigning IndividuaLized Options for Treatment (TAILORx)

What is the purpose of the trial?

TAILORx—the Trial Assigning IndividuaLized Options for Treatment (Rx)—is designed to determine whether adjuvant hormonal therapy alone is as effective as adjuvant hormonal therapy in combination with chemotherapy for certain women with early-stage breast cancer. Trial results will help individualize treatment for each breast cancer patient in order to achieve improved clinical outcomes.

Who is eligible to enroll in TAILORx?

Women with estrogen receptor or progesterone receptor positive, lymph node negative (cancer that has not spread to the lymph nodes), HER2/neu negative breast cancer are eligible to enroll in TAILORx. The tumor size must be 1.1 to 5.0 cm (or 0.5 mm to 1.0 cm, with unfavorable histologic features). Participants must meet standard clinical criteria and be medically suitable candidates for adjuvant chemotherapy.

What does the trial involve?

All patients who agree to participate in the trial will have a molecular test performed on a sample of the tumor that has already been removed. This test does not require an additional biopsy or

"TAILORx (Trial Assigning IndividuaLized Options for Treatment): Questions and Answers," National Cancer Institute (www.cancer.gov), May 23, 2006.

other procedures. The specimen will be sent to a laboratory for the test to be done. It takes about seven to 10 days from the time a specimen is received at the laboratory for a doctor to get the result of the test. These results will be used to guide therapy.

What are the primary objectives of the trial?

The primary objectives of TAILORx are twofold:

- To determine whether adjuvant hormonal therapy with chemotherapy is better than adjuvant hormonal therapy alone in women whose tumors fall in a range where the benefit from chemotherapy is uncertain as indicated by a molecular test. The primary study endpoint is disease-free survival. Another primary endpoint is overall survival.

- To create a tissue and specimen bank for patients enrolled in this trial, including formalin-fixed, paraffin-embedded tumor specimens, tissue microarrays, plasma, and DNA obtained from peripheral blood. This resource will be critical for evaluating emerging clinical cancer tests.

What is the molecular test used in this trial?

The molecular test is called Oncotype DXTM. It is a test that analyzes the expression pattern of certain genes in breast tumors. The test can more precisely estimate a woman's risk of cancer recurrence than standard characteristics that doctors normally use to assess recurrence risk (for example, tumor size, tumor grade, and other characteristics of the tumor). The Oncotype DXTM test that is being used in this trial has been commercially available since 2004. Genomic Health, Inc. (Redwood City, California), the company that developed the test, performs the assay in its own laboratory. It has been performed on tumor specimens from over 10,000 breast cancer patients thus far.

How will the Oncotype DXTM test be used to guide therapy?

The test result is expressed as a "Recurrence Score." The higher the score, the greater the chance of having a recurrence of breast cancer if a woman is treated with hormonal therapy alone. The treatment that patients will receive in this trial will depend upon the results of the Recurrence Score.

- If the Recurrence Score is 10 or less, it is estimated that approximately 95 percent of patients or more may live long term without a distant disease recurrence with hormonal therapy alone. These patients will only receive hormonal therapy. About 25 percent of patients are estimated to have a Recurrence Score in this range.

- If the Recurrence Score is 26 or higher, the risk of recurrence is about 30 percent with hormonal therapy alone, and may be reduced to about 10 percent with the addition of chemotherapy. These patients will receive chemotherapy and hormonal therapy. About 30 percent of patients are estimated to have a Recurrence Score in this range.

- If the Recurrence Score is 11 to 25, the risk of recurrence is about seven percent to 16 percent with hormonal therapy alone. Patients who have a Recurrence Score in this range will be randomly assigned to receive chemotherapy plus hormonal therapy (the standard treatment arm) versus hormonal therapy alone (the experimental treatment arm). About 44 percent of patients are estimated to have a Recurrence Score in this range.

What is randomization and why is it necessary?

Randomization is like flipping a coin. The treatment will be assigned by chance. This procedure is commonly used in clinical trials when new treatment approaches are being tested, and when there is uncertainty about the best treatment approach. Patients with a Recurrence Score of 11 to 25 will be randomly assigned to receive, or not to receive, chemotherapy because the benefit of chemotherapy is uncertain in this group, even though chemotherapy would normally be recommended for this group based upon standard characteristics, such as tumor pathology, traditionally used in clinical practice.

Why is randomization not being used for all patients participating in this study?

Patients who have a low Recurrence Score (10 or lower) or high Recurrence Score (26 or higher) will not be randomized. Patients with a low Recurrence Score will be assigned to receive hormonal therapy alone, and patients with a high Recurrence Score will be assigned to receive chemotherapy plus hormonal therapy. Patients in these groups are being directly assigned, rather than randomized, to treatment because researchers already know that chemotherapy is not beneficial or is very unlikely to be beneficial for those who have a low Recurrence Score, and is very likely to be beneficial for those who have a high Recurrence Score.

What treatments will be used in the trial?

All treatments used in this trial, including chemotherapy and hormonal therapy, are commercially available and are not considered experimental. The choice of exactly what type of chemotherapy and hormonal therapy will be used will be left to the discretion of the treating physician.

Hormonal therapies in the trial are assigned based on menopausal status and include tamoxifen and the aromatase inhibitors anastrozole, letrozole, and exemestane. Women on the chemotherapy arm of the trial will receive one of several standard combination chemotherapy regimens considered to be the best available standard care today.

What are some of the side effects caused by these medications?

The most likely side effects of chemotherapy include nausea, vomiting, hair loss, fatigue, anemia, and infection. Some of these side effects can be relieved with medications. Side effects of hormonal therapy include hot flashes, osteoporosis, and vaginal discharge or dryness. If a woman has not entered menopause, some of the treatments may cause premature menopause or sterility.

Will insurance cover the cost of this trial?

The Oncotype DXTM test that is being used in this trial is an established diagnostic test in the United States that was recently approved for coverage by Medicare. The test is commercially available, and the Genomic Health laboratory is certified by federal and state agencies in the United States to perform this test.

The cost of the Oncotype DXTM test will be billed to the patient's insurance company. The treatments and other routine tests done as part of this trial are considered standard care, and also will be billed to the patient's insurance company. Medicare and commercial insurance companies usually cover the routine costs of care required in clinical trials. Coverage may not, however, be the same from plan to plan. Should participants be unsuccessful in receiving reimbursement for all or some of the cost of the Oncotype DXTM test after appealing to their insurance carrier, they will have no financial responsibility for the Oncotype DXTM test.

What treatment would normally be given to someone who did not participate in the trial?

All patients with breast cancer require surgery, or surgery plus radiation therapy. Patients with ER- or PR-positive early-stage breast cancer receive hormonal therapy given for a period of at least five years. There are several types of hormonal therapy, but the treatment usually consists of pills taken once or twice daily. In addition, patients participating in this trial meet standard clinical criteria for administering chemotherapy, which would generally be considered part of standard treatment.

Who is conducting the trial?

This trial is being conducted by the North American Breast Cancer Intergroup, which includes all of the major National Cancer Institute-funded cooperative groups in the United States and Canada. The trial will be coordinated by the Eastern Cooperative Oncology Group (ECOG), which is one of the major groups that are participating in the trial. Other participating groups include the National Surgical Adjuvant Breast and Bowel Project (NSABP), the Cancer and Acute Leukemia Group B (CALGB), the Southwest Oncology Group (SWOG), the North Central Cancer Treatment Group (NCCTG), the National Cancer Institute of Canada (NCIC), and the American College of Surgeons Oncology Group (ACOSOG). These groups include networks of researchers, physicians, and healthcare professionals at public and private institutions across the United States and Canada. They conduct clinical trials on all types of adult cancers. The groups receive funding from the National Cancer Institute and other sources. The goal of these groups is to control, effectively treat, and ultimately cure cancer. These groups provide research results to individuals and the medical community through scientific publications and professional meetings.

Chapter 44

Boost Radiation Beneficial in Early-Stage Breast Cancer

In women with early-stage breast cancer who had been treated with breast-conserving lumpectomy and radiation, an additional "boost" dose of radiation to the original tumor site reduced the risk of cancer coming back in the same breast, though it did not help them live longer.

Source: *Journal of Clinical Oncology*, published online June 18, 2007, and in print Aug. 1, 2007 (J Clin Oncol. 2007 Jun 18; [Epub ahead of print])

Background

Studies have shown that for patients with stage I and stage II breast cancer, long-term survival is similar whether they have a lumpectomy (surgery that removes just the tumor and surrounding tissue) or a mastectomy (removal of the whole breast). Lumpectomy conserves the breast but also leaves open the possibility that cancer could recur there.

Radiation therapy after lumpectomy considerably reduces the risk of a relapse in the same breast. Often such radiation is given to the whole breast. Researchers in Europe decided to test whether a "boost" dose of radiation, given directly to the tumor bed (the site where the tumor had been) after a course of radiation therapy to the whole breast, would further reduce the risk of cancer coming back in the same breast.

"Boost Radiation Beneficial in Early-Stage Breast Cancer," National Cancer Institute (www.cancer.gov), July 11, 2007.

The Study

More than 5,300 women from nine European countries joined this trial between 1989 and 1996. All of the women had had a lumpectomy followed by five weeks of radiation therapy to the whole breast. They were randomly assigned to receive either no additional treatment or a single boost of radiation to the tumor bed.

Preliminary results, published in 2001 after a median follow-up period of five years, showed that women who got the boost dose of radiation had a 41 percent lower risk of cancer coming back in the same breast than women who did not receive a boost dose (see the journal abstract). It was too early to tell, however, whether the boost dose improved patients' long-term survival. The current study updates those findings after a median follow-up period of 10.8 years.

The principal investigator for both studies was Harry Bartelink, M.D., of the Netherlands Cancer Institute in Amsterdam.

Results

Although the boost dose of radiation significantly reduced the risk of cancer coming back in the same breast, it did not help patients live longer overall.

After 10 years of follow-up, 81.7 percent of the women in both groups were still alive. The number of patients who developed second cancers or whose cancer spread to other organs was also the same in both groups.

Moderate to severe scarring of the breast occurred in 28.1 percent of the women who got the boost dose of radiation, compared with 13.2 percent of those who did not.

Of the women who received the boost dose of radiation, 6.2 percent had a recurrence of cancer in the same breast, compared with 10.2 percent of women who did not get the boost dose. As was the case with the earlier report, women who were aged 40 or younger at the time of treatment benefited the most from the boost dose.

Women who had a recurrence of cancer in the same breast were usually treated with mastectomy. Because there were fewer recurrences in the group of patients that received the boost dose of radiation, there was a 41 percent reduction in the number of mastectomies needed in that group.

Comments

Mastectomy may have saved the lives of those women who had a recurrence in the same breast, said the authors, and this may explain why there was no survival difference between women who got the boost dose of radiation and those who did not.

Deborah E. Citrin, M.D., of the National Cancer Institute's Radiation Oncology Branch, agrees, adding that boost radiation for this patient population nonetheless offers some key benefits.

"Preventing a recurrence in the same breast is a very important goal after breast-conserving therapy," she says. The addition of the boost dose of radiation meant that fewer patients needed a mastectomy because of a recurrence in the same breast and thus avoided the adverse physical and psychological effects of losing a breast.

Radiation therapy would not be expected to reduce second cancers or the spread of breast cancer to other organs, says Citrin. The slight increase in the risk of scarring from the additional dose of radiation must be weighed against the lower risk of recurrence and thus of the need for a subsequent mastectomy, Citrin adds.

Chapter 45

Tamoxifen and Recent Research

Chapter Contents

Section 45.1

Questions and Answers about Tamoxifen

"Tamoxifen: Questions and Answers," National Cancer Institute
(www.cancer.gov), March 17, 2008.

What is tamoxifen?

Tamoxifen (Nolvadex®) is a drug, taken orally as a tablet, which interferes with the activity of estrogen, a female hormone. Estrogen can promote the development of cancer in the breast. Tamoxifen is approved by the U.S. Food and Drug Administration (FDA) for the prevention of breast cancer and for the treatment of breast cancer, as well as other types of cancer.

Tamoxifen has been used for more than 30 years to treat breast cancer in women and men. Tamoxifen is used to treat patients with early-stage breast cancer, as well as those with metastatic breast cancer (cancer that has spread to other parts of the body). As adjuvant therapy (treatment given after the primary treatment to increase the chances of a cure), tamoxifen helps prevent the original breast cancer from returning and also helps prevent the development of new cancers in the other breast. As treatment for metastatic breast cancer, the drug slows or stops the growth of cancer cells that are present in the body.

Tamoxifen has been used for almost 10 years to reduce the risk of breast cancer in women who are at increased risk of developing breast cancer. Tamoxifen is also used to treat women with ductal carcinoma in situ (DCIS), a noninvasive condition that sometimes leads to invasive breast cancer.

How does tamoxifen work?

Estrogen can promote the growth of breast cancer cells. Some breast cancers are classified as estrogen receptor-positive (also known as hormone sensitive), which means that they have a protein to which estrogen will bind. These breast cancer cells need estrogen to grow. Tamoxifen works against the effects of estrogen on these cells. It is often called an antiestrogen or a SERM (selective estrogen receptor modulator).

Studies have shown that tamoxifen is only effective in treating estrogen receptor-positive breast cancers. Therefore, the tumor's hormone receptor status should be determined before deciding on treatment options for breast cancer.

Although tamoxifen acts against the effects of estrogen in breast tissue, it acts like estrogen in other tissue. This means that women who take tamoxifen may derive many of the beneficial effects of menopausal estrogen replacement therapy, such as a decreased risk of osteoporosis.

How long should a patient take tamoxifen for the treatment of breast cancer?

Patients with metastatic breast cancer may take tamoxifen for varying lengths of time, depending on the cancer's response to this treatment and other factors. When used as adjuvant therapy for early-stage breast cancer, tamoxifen is generally prescribed for five years. However, the ideal length of treatment with tamoxifen is not known.

Two studies have confirmed the benefit of taking adjuvant tamoxifen daily for five years. When taken for five years, tamoxifen reduces the chance of the original breast cancer coming back in the same breast or elsewhere. It also reduces the risk of developing a second primary cancer in the other breast.

Clinical trials are ongoing to determine whether hormone therapy taken for more than five years is beneficial. These studies usually include aromatase inhibitors (AIs) (another type of antiestrogen). For example, the National Cancer Institute (NCI), a part of the National Institutes of Health, is sponsoring the National Surgical Adjuvant Breast and Bowel Project (NSABP) B-42 trial. This trial is studying the AI letrozole (Femara®) to find out how well it works compared with a placebo in treating postmenopausal women who have received hormone therapy for hormone receptor-positive breast cancer. More information is available in PDQ®, the NCI's comprehensive cancer information database, at http://www.cancer.gov/clinicaltrials/NSABP-B-42 on the internet.

The MA-17R trial, which is being coordinated by the National Cancer Institute of Canada's Clinical Trials Group, is comparing letrozole with placebo in women previously diagnosed with primary breast cancer who participated in another clinical trial of letrozole. Information about the MA-17R trial can be found at https://www.swogstat.org/ROS/ROSBooks/Fall%202006/Intergroup/NCIC%20CTG/JMA17R.pdf on the internet.

What are some of the more common side effects of tamoxifen?

The known, serious side effects of tamoxifen are blood clots, strokes, uterine cancer, and cataracts. Other side effects of tamoxifen are similar to the symptoms of menopause. The most common side effects are hot flashes and vaginal discharge. Some women experience irregular menstrual periods, headaches, fatigue, nausea or vomiting, vaginal dryness or itching, irritation of the skin around the vagina, and skin rash. As with menopause, not all women who take tamoxifen have these symptoms. Men who take tamoxifen may experience headaches, nausea or vomiting, skin rash, impotence, or a decrease in sexual interest.

Does tamoxifen cause blood clots or stroke?

Data from large clinical trials suggest that there is a small increase in the number of blood clots in women taking tamoxifen, particularly in women who are receiving anticancer drugs (chemotherapy) along with tamoxifen. The total number of women who have experienced this side effect is small. The risk of having a blood clot due to tamoxifen is similar to the risk of a blood clot when taking estrogen replacement therapy.

The Breast Cancer Prevention Trial (BCPT), a large research study funded by the NCI, was designed to test the usefulness of tamoxifen in preventing breast cancer in women with an increased risk of developing this disease. This study also found that women who took tamoxifen had an increased chance of developing blood clots and an increased chance of stroke.[1, 2]

Does tamoxifen cause cancers of the uterus?

Tamoxifen increases the risk of two types of cancer that can develop in the uterus: endometrial cancer, which arises in the lining of the uterus, and uterine sarcoma, which arises in the muscular wall of the uterus. Like all cancers, endometrial cancer and uterine sarcoma are potentially life-threatening. Women who have had a hysterectomy (surgery to remove the uterus) and are taking tamoxifen are not at increased risk for these cancers.

- **Endometrial cancer:** Studies have found the risk of developing endometrial cancer to be about two cases per 1,000 women taking tamoxifen each year compared with one case per 1,000 women taking placebo.[1, 2] Most of the endometrial cancers that have occurred in women taking tamoxifen have been found in the early stages, and treatment has usually been effective. However, for some breast cancer patients who developed endometrial cancer while taking tamoxifen, the disease was life-threatening.

- **Uterine sarcoma:** Studies have found the risk of developing uterine sarcoma to be slightly higher in women taking tamoxifen compared with women taking placebo. However, it was less than one case per 1,000 women per year in both groups.[1, 2] Research to date indicates that uterine sarcoma is more likely to be diagnosed at later stages than endometrial cancer, and may therefore be harder to control and more life-threatening than endometrial cancer.

Abnormal vaginal bleeding and lower abdominal (pelvic) pain are symptoms of cancers of the uterus. Women who are taking tamoxifen should talk with their doctor about having regular pelvic examinations and should be checked promptly if they have any abnormal vaginal bleeding or pelvic pain between scheduled exams.

Does tamoxifen cause other types of cancer?

Tamoxifen is not known to cause any types of cancer in humans other than endometrial cancer and uterine sarcoma.

Does tamoxifen cause eye problems?

As women age, they are more likely to develop cataracts (clouding of the lens inside the eye). Women taking tamoxifen appear to be at increased risk for developing cataracts. Other eye problems, such as corneal scarring or retinal changes, have been reported in a few patients.

Should women taking tamoxifen avoid pregnancy?

Yes. Doctors advise women receiving tamoxifen to avoid pregnancy because animal studies have suggested that the use of tamoxifen during pregnancy can cause harm to the fetus. Women who have questions about fertility, birth control, or pregnancy should discuss their concerns with their doctor.

Does tamoxifen cause a woman to begin menopause?

Tamoxifen does not cause a woman to begin menopause, although it can cause some symptoms that are similar to those that may occur during menopause. In most premenopausal women taking tamoxifen, the ovaries continue to act normally and produce estrogen in the same or slightly increased amounts.

Do the benefits of tamoxifen in treating breast cancer outweigh its risks?

The benefits of tamoxifen as a treatment for breast cancer are firmly established and far outweigh the potential risks. Patients who are concerned about the risks and benefits of tamoxifen or any other medications are encouraged to discuss these concerns with their doctor.

Can tamoxifen prevent breast cancer?

Research has shown that when tamoxifen is used as adjuvant therapy for early-stage breast cancer, it reduces the chance that the original breast cancer will come back in the same breast or elsewhere. It also reduces the risk of developing new cancers in the other breast. Based on these findings, the NCI funded the BCPT to determine whether taking tamoxifen for at least five years can prevent breast cancer in women who have never been diagnosed with breast cancer but who are at increased risk of developing the disease. This study found a reduction in diagnoses of invasive breast cancer among women who took tamoxifen for five years. Women who took tamoxifen also had fewer diagnoses of noninvasive breast tumors, such as DCIS or lobular carcinoma in situ (LCIS).[1] After seven years of follow-up, researchers found similar results.[2] The study found that tamoxifen reduced the occurrence of estrogen receptor-positive tumors by 69 percent, but no difference in the occurrence of estrogen receptor-negative tumors was seen.[1] More information about the BCPT is available on the NCI's BCPT home page at http://www.cancer.gov/clinicaltrials/digestpage/BCPT on the internet.

Who should take tamoxifen to reduce breast cancer risk?

The decision to take tamoxifen is an individual one. A woman and her doctor must carefully consider the benefits and risks of therapy. At this time, there is no evidence that tamoxifen has a net benefit for women who do not have an increased risk of developing breast cancer.

What is raloxifene and how does it compare to tamoxifen?

Raloxifene is a drug approved by the FDA for the prevention and treatment of osteoporosis in postmenopausal women. Raloxifene is also approved by the FDA for reducing the risk of invasive breast cancer in postmenopausal women with osteoporosis and in postmenopausal women at high risk for invasive breast cancer.

The NCI funded the Study of Tamoxifen and Raloxifene (STAR), a clinical trial comparing raloxifene (Evista®) with tamoxifen in preventing breast cancer in postmenopausal women who are at an increased risk of developing the disease. The study found that raloxifene and tamoxifen are equally effective in reducing invasive breast cancer risk in postmenopausal women who are at increased risk of the disease. The study also found that women who took raloxifene had fewer uterine cancers and fewer blood clots than the women who took tamoxifen.[3] However, raloxifene did not reduce the risk of noninvasive breast tumors such as DCIS and LCIS.[3] Other side effects associated with raloxifene were similar to tamoxifen and included hot flashes, vaginal dryness, joint pain, and leg cramps. Studies of raloxifene to date have only examined its role in breast cancer prevention, not treatment.

More information about STAR is available in the next section (45.2) and on the NCI's STAR home page at http://www.cancer.gov/star on the internet.

What other hormone therapy may be used for early-stage breast cancer?

Aromatase inhibitors (AIs) are another adjuvant treatment option for some women with early-stage breast cancer. AIs block the action of a protein called aromatase, which helps the body produce estrogen. Most of the estrogen in a woman's body is made in the ovaries, but other tissues can also produce this hormone. AIs are usually used in women who have reached menopause, when the ovaries are no longer producing estrogen.

Although AIs and tamoxifen both help to prevent the growth of estrogen-sensitive breast tumors, they work differently in the body. Tamoxifen blocks the tumor's ability to use estrogen, and AIs reduce the amount of estrogen in the body. Anastrozole (Arimidex®), exemestane (Aromasin®), and letrozole (Femara®) are AIs that have been approved by the FDA.

The American Society of Clinical Oncology (ASCO) recommends that postmenopausal women with hormone-sensitive breast cancer consider one of two adjuvant treatment options:[4]

- Begin treatment with tamoxifen for two to three years or five years, and then switch to an AI for another two to three years or five years.

- Forego tamoxifen entirely and begin adjuvant treatment with an AI for five years.

ASCO concluded that AIs are appropriate as initial treatment for women who should not take tamoxifen and that patients who cannot take AIs should receive tamoxifen.

Whether an individual patient should start therapy with an AI or begin therapy with tamoxifen and then change to an AI is a subject of medical judgment and clinical research. Patients should talk with their doctors about which drug would be best for them given their particular medical situation.

Selected References

1. Fisher B, Costantino JP, Wickerham DL, et al. Tamoxifen for prevention of breast cancer: Report of the National Surgical Adjuvant Breast and Bowel Project P-1 Study. *Journal of the National Cancer Institute* 1998; 90(18):1371–1388.

2. Fisher B, Costantino JP, Wickerham DL, et al. Tamoxifen for the prevention of breast cancer: Current status of the National Surgical Adjuvant Breast and Bowel Project P-1 Study. *Journal of the National Cancer Institute* 2005; 97(22):1652–1662.

3. Vogel VG, Costantino JP, Wickerham DL, et al. Effects of tamoxifen vs raloxifene on the risk of developing invasive breast cancer and other disease outcomes: The NSABP Study of Tamoxifen and Raloxifene (STAR) P-2 Trial. *Journal of the American Medical Association* 2006; 295(23):2727–2741.

4. Winer EP, Hudis C, Burstein HJ, et al. American Society of Clinical Oncology technology assessment on the use of aromatase inhibitors as adjuvant therapy for postmenopausal women with hormone receptor-positive breast cancer: Status report 2004. *Journal of Clinical Oncology* 2005; 23(3):619–629.

Section 45.2

Study of Tamoxifen and Raloxifene (STAR)

Excerpted from "The Study of Tamoxifen and Raloxifene (STAR): Questions and Answers," National Cancer Institute (www.cancer.gov), June 21, 2006.

What is the Study of Tamoxifen and Raloxifene (STAR)?

The Study of Tamoxifen and Raloxifene (STAR) is a clinical trial (a research study conducted with people) comparing the drug raloxifene (Evista®) with the drug tamoxifen (Nolvadex®) in reducing the incidence of breast cancer in postmenopausal women who are at an increased risk of developing the disease. Researchers with the National Surgical Adjuvant Breast and Bowel Project (NSABP) are conducting the study at more than 500 centers across the United States, Canada, and Puerto Rico. The study is funded primarily by the National Cancer Institute (NCI)—part of the National Institutes of Health. NCI is the U.S. Government's main agency for cancer research.

Who participated in STAR?

Women at increased risk of developing breast cancer, who had gone through menopause, and were at least 35 years old took part in STAR. STAR began enrolling participants in 1999. Enrollment was closed on November 4, 2004, with 19,747 women recruited. The ages of women joining STAR were as follows: 35–49, 9.2% (1,815); 50–59, 49.7% (9,821); 60 and older, 41.1% (8,111).

All STAR participants had to have an increased risk of breast cancer equivalent to or greater than that of an average 60- to 64-year-old woman. In that age group, 1.66 percent of women—or about 17 of every 1,000 women—would be expected to develop breast cancer within five years. The average risk of breast cancer in the women who chose to enter STAR was about twice as high as this minimum risk.

What increases a woman's risk of breast cancer? How was it determined that a STAR participant was at increased risk of breast cancer?

A woman's risk of developing breast cancer is determined by many factors. The factors that most affect a woman's risk of the disease are the following:

- Age
- Number of first-degree relatives (mother, daughters, or sisters) diagnosed with breast cancer
- Whether a woman has had any children and her age at her first delivery
- The number of breast biopsies a woman has undergone, especially if the tissue showed a condition known as atypical hyperplasia
- The woman's age at her first menstrual period
- The woman's age when she reached menopause

STAR researchers used the Breast Cancer Risk Assessment Tool, developed by scientists at NCI and NSABP, to estimate a woman's risk of breast cancer using most of the above factors. The tool can be viewed on NCI's website at http://www.cancer.gov/bcrisktool. NSABP also has the tool posted at http://breastcancerprevention.com. From this website, women can also register with the group for information about future breast cancer prevention clinical trials.

In addition, for STAR, women diagnosed as having lobular carcinoma in situ (LCIS), a condition that is not cancer but indicates an increased chance of developing invasive breast cancer, were eligible based on that diagnosis alone, as long as their treatment for the condition was limited to local excision.

What is tamoxifen?

Tamoxifen is a drug, taken by mouth as a pill. It has been used for more than 30 years to treat patients with breast cancer. Tamoxifen works against breast cancer, in part, by interfering with the activity of estrogen, a female hormone that promotes the growth of breast cancer cells. In October 1998, the U.S. Food and Drug Administration (FDA) approved the use of tamoxifen to reduce the incidence of breast cancer in women at increased risk of the disease based on the results of the NSABP Breast Cancer Prevention Trial (BCPT). The BCPT studied

13,388 pre- and postmenopausal women age 35 and older at increased risk of breast cancer who took either tamoxifen or a placebo (an inactive pill that looked like tamoxifen) for up to five years. The BCPT also showed that tamoxifen works like estrogen to preserve bone strength, decreasing fractures of the hip, wrist, and spine in the women who took the drug. Findings from the BCPT were reported in the September 16, 1998, issue of the *Journal of the National Cancer Institute*.

What is raloxifene?

Raloxifene is a drug, taken by mouth as a pill. In December 1997, it was approved by the FDA for the prevention of osteoporosis in postmenopausal women. In October 1999, it was also approved as an osteoporosis treatment. Raloxifene is being studied for breast cancer prevention because large studies testing its effectiveness against osteoporosis have shown that women taking the drug developed fewer breast cancers than women taking a placebo. One of these studies was the Multiple Outcomes of Raloxifene Evaluation (MORE) trial. The MORE trial was designed to study the effects of raloxifene on osteoporosis in postmenopausal women. Researchers also tracked rates of breast cancer and observed a reduction in the incidence of breast cancer among the women who took raloxifene. The results of this study were reported in the June 16, 1999, issue of the *Journal of the American Medical Association* and were updated in the Continuing Outcomes Relevant to Evista (CORE) study published in the *Journal of the National Cancer Institute* on December 1, 2004.

What were the STAR results in terms of reducing breast cancer risk?

The results* of STAR show that raloxifene and tamoxifen are equally effective in reducing breast cancer risk in postmenopausal women at increased risk of the disease. After taking these drugs for an average of almost four years, women in the tamoxifen group and women in the raloxifene group had statistically equivalent numbers of invasive breast cancers (163 cases in 9,726 women in the tamoxifen group versus 167 cases in 9,745 women in the raloxifene group). Tamoxifen is known to be able to reduce breast cancer risk by half, and this study shows that raloxifene can also reduce breast cancer risk by half.

For every 1,000 women similar to those enrolled in STAR, about 40 would be expected to develop breast cancer within five years. The results of STAR show that about 20 of those women would not develop breast cancer if they took tamoxifen or raloxifene for five years.

What are the side effects of tamoxifen and raloxifene?

The known, serious side effects of tamoxifen are uterine cancer, blood clots, strokes, and cataracts. Other side effects of tamoxifen include menopause-like symptoms such as hot flashes and vaginal discharge or bleeding.

Raloxifene has not been studied as long as tamoxifen, and one of the goals of STAR was to better assess the drug's long-term effects. The known, serious side effect of raloxifene is blood clots. Other side effects include menopause-like symptoms such as hot flashes and vaginal dryness as well as joint pain or leg cramps.

How many participants developed uterine cancer?

In STAR, more than half of the women entered the trial having had a hysterectomy. Women without a uterus are not at risk of uterine cancer. For those women in the trial with a uterus, the women in the raloxifene group developed 36 percent fewer uterine cancers during the trial: 36 of 4,732 women in the tamoxifen group developed uterine cancers compared to 23 of the 4,712 women in the raloxifene group. Tamoxifen is known to increase a woman's chance of developing uterine cancer (mostly in the lining of the uterus or endometrium) by two to three times—to a rate of about two cases per 1,000 women per year—compared to a woman who does not use the drug. The rate of uterine cancers in women assigned to take tamoxifen in STAR was similar to this rate.

How many participants developed blood clots?

Both tamoxifen and raloxifene are known to increase a woman's chance of developing blood clots by up to three times that of women who are not taking either drug. In STAR, women in the raloxifene group had 29 percent fewer deep-vein thromboses (blood clots in a major vein) and pulmonary embolisms (blood clots in the lung) than women on tamoxifen: 87 of 9,726 women in the tamoxifen group had a deep-vein thrombosis compared to 65 of 9,745 women in the raloxifene group, and 54 of 9,726 women in the tamoxifen group had a pulmonary embolism compared to 35 of 9,745 women in the raloxifene group.

How many participants developed other cardiovascular problems?

The numbers of myocardial infarctions (heart attacks), strokes, and transient ischemic attacks (strokes that last only a few minutes) were essentially equivalent between the tamoxifen group and the raloxifene group.

The numbers of women who had strokes in the two groups were statistically equivalent with 53 of 9,726 women in the tamoxifen group and 51 of 9,745 women in the raloxifene group having had a stroke during the trial. There were no differences in deaths from strokes with 6 of 9,726 women in the tamoxifen group and 4 of 9,745 women in the raloxifene group dying from this type of event.

Women at increased risk of cardiovascular problems were not eligible to participate in STAR. This includes women who had uncontrolled high blood pressure or uncontrolled diabetes and those with a prior stroke, transient ischemic attack, or atrial fibrillation (a kind of abnormal heart rhythm).

How many women had bone fractures during the trial?

In STAR, women in the tamoxifen group and women in the raloxifene group had similar numbers of bone fractures of the hip, wrist, and spine: 104 of 9,726 women in the tamoxifen group had a bone fracture during the trial compared to 96 of 9,745 women in the raloxifene group. Raloxifene is currently FDA-approved and used for the treatment and prevention of osteoporosis, and data from the BCPT showed that women on tamoxifen have fewer fractures of the hip, wrist, and spine compared to women on placebo. These particular fracture sites were evaluated in the study because they are associated with osteoporosis.

Did raloxifene reduce the incidence of lobular carcinoma in situ or ductal carcinoma in situ?

No. While tamoxifen has been shown to reduce the incidence of lobular carcinoma in situ (LCIS) and ductal carcinoma in situ (DCIS) by half, raloxifene did not have an effect on these diagnoses. (LCIS and DCIS are sometimes called noninvasive or stage 0 breast cancers.) Among the 9,726 women in the tamoxifen group, 57 developed LCIS or DCIS, compared to 81 of 9,745 women in the raloxifene group. This result confirms data reported in 2004 in a large study of raloxifene, the Continued Outcomes Relevant to Evista (or CORE Trial), which showed that raloxifene did not decrease the incidence of LCIS or DCIS in women taking the drug compared to women on a placebo.

Does having taken raloxifene change what a woman could do if she developed LCIS or DCIS?

No. Treatment options for LCIS and DCIS would not change if a woman had been taking raloxifene prior to her diagnosis. For more information on treatment options for LCIS and DCIS, visit NCI's website at: http://www.cancer.gov/cancertopics/pdq/treatment/breast/patient.

How many participants developed a cataract during STAR?

In the BCPT, women in the tamoxifen group had a 14 percent increased risk of developing a cataract. During STAR, 394 of 9,726 women in the tamoxifen group developed a cataract compared to 313 of 9,745 women in the raloxifene group. Based on STAR data and comparing it to data from the BCPT, the risk of cataracts in the raloxifene group does not appear to be elevated over what would expected if these women were not treated with raloxifene.

Did any group of women benefit more from raloxifene than others?

No. Raloxifene reduced breast cancer risk regardless of age, race, family history, or other known breast cancer risk factors.

Should postmenopausal women at increased risk of breast cancer take raloxifene based on these results?

At this time, tamoxifen is the only FDA-approved drug for the reduction of breast cancer risk, and it is approved for both pre- and postmenopausal women. Raloxifene is only FDA-approved for the prevention and treatment of osteoporosis in postmenopausal women and is not approved for use in the reduction of breast cancer risk. Should raloxifene receive FDA approval for this use, postmenopausal women who are at increased risk of breast cancer would be able to consider taking either raloxifene or tamoxifen to reduce their risk. As with any medical procedure or intervention, the decision to take one of these drugs is an individual one in which the benefits and risks of therapy must be considered. The balance of these benefits and risks will vary depending on a woman's personal health history and how she weighs the benefits and risks. Even if a woman is at increased risk of breast cancer, raloxifene or tamoxifen therapy may not be right for her. Women who are considering breast cancer prevention therapy should talk with their health care provider.

What is the average monthly cost of tamoxifen or raloxifene?

On average, a month's supply of raloxifene costs $75 in the United States. A month's supply of generic tamoxifen costs about $100 in the United States.

What can premenopausal women at increased risk of breast cancer do to reduce their risk of breast cancer?

Tamoxifen has already been shown to reduce a premenopausal woman's risk of developing breast cancer by half in the BCPT and the drug is approved by the FDA to reduce breast cancer risk in premenopausal women. In the BCPT, women under age 50 did not have an increased risk of the most serious side effects seen with tamoxifen use: uterine cancer, blood clots, strokes, and cataracts. Premenopausal women at increased risk of breast cancer can discuss tamoxifen therapy as an option with their physicians. Raloxifene is not FDA-approved for use in premenopausal women.

Are there women who should not take raloxifene?

Raloxifene is not approved by the FDA for use in premenopausal women for any indication. It is approved for the prevention and treatment of osteoporosis, and postmenopausal women with a history of blood clots, hypertension, diabetes, and cigarette smoking must also consider that raloxifene increases the risk of serious blood clots.

Selected References

*Vogel VG; Costantino JP; et. al.; for the National Surgical Adjuvant Breast and Bowel Project (NSABP). Effects of Tamoxifen vs Raloxifene on the Risk of Developing Invasive Breast Cancer and Other Disease Outcomes: The NSABP Study of Tamoxifen and Raloxifene (STAR) P-2 Trial. *JAMA*. 2006; 295:2727–2741. Published online June 5, 2006.

Land SR; Wickerham DL; et. al. Patient-Reported Symptoms and Quality of Life During Treatment With Tamoxifen or Raloxifene for Breast Cancer Prevention: The NSABP Study of Tamoxifen and Raloxifene (STAR) P-2 Trial. *JAMA*. 2006; 295:2742–2751. Published online June 5, 2006.

Additional Information

1. Fisher B, Costantino JP, Wickerham DL, et al. Tamoxifen for prevention of breast cancer: Report of the National Surgical Adjuvant Breast and Bowel Project P-1 study. *Journal of the National Cancer Institute* 1998; 90(18):1371–1388.

2. Cummings SR, Eckert S, Krueger KA, et al. The effect of raloxifene on risk of breast cancer in postmenopausal women: Results from the MORE randomized trial. *Journal of the American Medical Association* 1999; 281(23):2189–2197.

3. Martino S, Cauley JA, Barrett-Connor E, et al. Continuing Outcomes Relevant to Evista: Breast Cancer Incidence in Postmenopausal Osteoporotic Women in a Randomized Trial of Raloxifene. *Journal of the National Cancer Institute* 2004; 96(23): 1751–1761.

4. Fisher B, Costantino JP, Wickerham DL, et al. Tamoxifen for the prevention of breast cancer: Current status of the National Surgical Adjuvant Breast and Bowel Project P-1 study. *Journal of the National Cancer Institute* 2005; 97(22): 1652–1662.

Section 45.3

Anastrozole after Tamoxifen Better than Tamoxifen Alone

"Anastrozole after Tamoxifen Better for Early Breast Cancer
than Tamoxifen Alone," National Cancer Institute (www.cancer.gov),
February 12, 2007.

In published reports from two similar clinical trials, researchers show that switching certain breast cancer patients at two years from the standard post-surgery treatment tamoxifen to another drug called anastrozole provides more protection against recurrence. The weight of evidence now favors such an approach for estrogen-receptor positive postmenopausal women with early breast cancer.

Source: Study 1: *The Lancet*, Aug. 6, 2005 (see the journal abstract). Study 2: *Journal of Clinical Oncology*, released online July 11, 2005; published Aug. 1, 2005.

Background

Following surgery for breast cancer, women whose tumors grow in response to the hormone estrogen (estrogen-receptor, or ER, positive) usually receive anti-estrogen therapy to reduce their risk that the disease will recur. Seven in ten breast cancer patients have ER-positive tumors.

Since the 1980s, the adjuvant hormone treatment of choice has been tamoxifen (Nolvadex®), a drug that blocks estrogen from getting to the cancer cells. Tamoxifen has had a major impact on breast cancer, reducing recurrence by about 40 percent in tens of thousands of women participating in hundreds of clinical trials, and has also been used to prevent cancer from occurring in the first place in women who have a higher risk of breast cancer. Tamoxifen's effectiveness comes at a cost, however: a very small number of women on tamoxifen develop endometrial cancer, severe blood clots, and stroke.

A more recently developed class of drugs called aromatase inhibitors (AIs) appears to be equally or even more effective in combating breast tumors that use estrogen to grow. AIs work against the enzyme (aromatase) responsible for turning the small amount of male hormone produced by the adrenal gland into estrogen. AIs don't work in women who have estrogen produced by the ovaries, however, which is why AIs are only effective once the ovaries have shut down—that is, in postmenopausal women.

The newest and most promising AIs are anastrozole (Arimidex®), letrozole (Femara®), and exemestane (Aromasin®). AIs also have some side effects: a reduction in bone density, which can lead to bone fractures; joint pain; and pain in the muscles and bones.

A number of large phase III clinical trials have been undertaken to try to clarify what role the AIs might play in the treatment and prevention of ER-positive breast cancer.

Study 1 (Germany and Austria)

Two separate but coordinated phase III randomized clinical trials were conducted in medical centers across Austria (ABCSG trial 8) and Germany (ARNO 95), to see if anastrozole might be a better hormone treatment than tamoxifen for women who have already had surgery and two years of tamoxifen. Patients were randomly assigned, but they knew which arm of the study they were on: 1,606 took tamoxifen for five years while another 1,616 switched to anastrozole after two years of tamoxifen (the sequential arm) and continued for the rest of the five-year treatment time.

Cancer in all of the women had spread to the lymph nodes, but had spread no further (distant metastasis). Women whose tumors were sensitive to estrogen were enrolled in the trials between January 1996 and August 2003. To date, 55 percent have completed treatment and were included in these results if their surgery was at least two years earlier. They have been followed thus far for a median of 28 months.

The large team including many study groups throughout Austria and Germany was led by Raimund Jakesz, M.D., of the Vienna Medical University and Vienna General Hospital in Vienna, Austria.

Study 1 Results

Of 1,606 women assigned to five years of tamoxifen, 110 (6.8 percent) had a recurrence of their breast cancer compared to 67 of the 1,608 women (4.2 percent) who switched to anastrozole after two years on tamoxifen. Switching to anastrozole therefore reduced the risk by 40 percent.

There were 59 deaths in the tamoxifen-only group, 31 resulting from breast cancer. In the sequential group, 45 women died, 24 from breast cancer.

Three years after switching, there are no statistically significant differences between the two groups in terms of overall survival and death due to breast cancer.

Significantly more women in the tamoxifen-alone group had blood clots (12 compared to 3), and in nine patients they led to a blocked artery, compared to only two in the sequential group. More than twice as many women receiving anastrozole had bone fractures (34 compared to 16) and also nausea (25 compared to 10), both statistically significant, and there was a non-significant trend towards more bone pain, reported by 213 compared to 177 taking tamoxifen alone.

Study 2 (Italy)

In a similar study—the Italian Tamoxifen Arimidex (ITA) trial—a total of 448 postmenopausal women who had been taking tamoxifen for two years or more were randomly assigned either to continue on tamoxifen until five years had elapsed, or to switch to anastrozole for the remainder of that time.

All of the women had had surgery for breast cancer that had spread to the lymph nodes, but no further. All had tumors that were sensitive to estrogen. Women enrolled in the trial between March 1998 and December 2002.

The team of researchers conducting the ITA trial was led by Francesco Boccardo, M.D., of the University and National Cancer Institute in Genoa, Italy. The results were originally presented at the San Antonio Breast Cancer Symposium on December 3, 2003.

Study 2 Results

Of 225 women assigned to continue taking tamoxifen, 32 (14.2 percent) had a recurrence of their breast cancer after a median follow-up period of three years, compared to just 12 of the 223 women taking anastrozole (5.4 percent). Overall, women on anastrozole were 65 percent less likely to suffer a relapse or a new tumor than women on tamoxifen.

There were 10 deaths in the tamoxifen group, seven resulting from breast cancer. In the anastrozole group, four women died, all from breast cancer.

Both treatments caused an array of side effects, ranging from the mild (stomach problems) to the serious (endometrial cancer). Overall, women taking anastrozole experienced more of these adverse events (203 versus 150 in the tamoxifen group). However, more of the adverse events affecting the tamoxifen group were life-threatening or required hospitalization compared to the anastrozole group.

Note: These results were based on the original report's median follow-up period of three years. Updated data from a longer follow-up period of 64 months were subsequently published in the June 2006 *Annals of Oncology*.

Comments

The results from these three clinical trials tip the balance in favor of using anastrozole at some point in the adjuvant therapy for postmenopausal node-positive women. In the United States this is already commonplace.

"I consider aromatase inhibitors for all of my hormone receptor-positive postmenopausal women," said Jo Anne Zujewski, M.D., of the National Cancer Institute's Cancer Therapy Evaluation Program. "Together with other recent results, the data are now strong enough to carve out a role for the aromatase inhibitors, whether following two years of tamoxifen or beginning post-surgical adjuvant therapy."

In an accompanying editorial, Kathleen I. Pritchard of the Toronto Sunnybrook Regional Cancer Center in Ontario, Canada, wrote: "Now, for women nearing completion of five years of tamoxifen, the decision to consider additional years of endocrine therapy with an aromatase inhibitor seems fairly straightforward." Patients should talk to their doctors about which aromatase inhibitor (anastrozole; letrozole; exemestane) might make sense for them, given the different short- and long-term side effects and the patient's own medical history.

Limitations

Nonetheless, caution is warranted, said Zujewski. "This doesn't mean every woman should immediately be switched to anastrozole. Tamoxifen has been a powerful therapy with great results for many years, and may still be appropriate for some women, especially those whose age and bone density put them at elevated risk for fractures."

These findings apply only to postmenopausal women with ER-positive breast cancer; the trial participants were mostly women in their seventies. "We're not any closer with these to treatments for younger women," said Zujewski.

In addition, said Zujewski, "We need longer-term data on how these AI agents interact with one another and with tamoxifen. Resistance to hormone therapy is not clearly understood."

Section 45.4

Trial Results Show Letrozole More Effective Than Tamoxifen in Early Breast Cancer

"Letrozole More Effective Than Tamoxifen in Early Breast Cancer: Results from the BIG 1-98 Trial," National Cancer Institute (www.cancer.gov), November 20, 2007.

In this large international trial of postmenopausal women surgically treated for early-stage, hormone responsive breast cancer, letrozole (Femara®) did better to prevent a recurrence of disease (especially distant metastases) than the commonly prescribed tamoxifen (Nolvadex®).

Source: *The New England Journal of Medicine,* December 29, 2005. (*N Engl J Med.* 2005 Dec 29; 353(26):2747–57)

Background

Women whose early-stage breast tumors grow in response to estrogen usually receive anti-estrogen therapy after surgery to reduce their risk that the disease will recur. Approximately seven in ten breast cancer patients have estrogen receptor (ER) positive tumors and so are candidates for this kind of adjuvant treatment.

Since the 1980s, the anti-estrogen drug tamoxifen has been considered the standard of care. However, women taking tamoxifen face an increased risk of endometrial cancer and blood clot disorders, and the risks start outweighing the benefits after five years on the drug for many women.

An alternative hormone treatment is letrozole (Femara®), which belongs to a class of drugs called aromatase inhibitors (AIs). Letrozole is one of three AIs approved by the U.S. Food and Drug Administration, the other two being anastrazole (Arimidex®) and exemestane (Aromasin®).

While studies have shown letrozole to be effective compared to a placebo, the trial described here was designed to test letrozole and tamoxifen head to head. It is one of a number of large phase III clinical trials undertaken to clarify what role AIs might play in the treatment and prevention of ER-positive breast cancer.

The Study

The Breast International Group (BIG) 1-98 study was a phase III clinical trial designed to compare letrozole and tamoxifen. Between 1998 and 2003, researchers at 27 institutions around the world enrolled 8,010 women who had completed surgery for early, ER-positive breast cancer and who had no evidence of metastasis.

The women were randomly assigned to one of four groups: some women took letrozole and some took tamoxifen for five years (monotherapy); others took letrozole for two years and then switched to tamoxifen while the final group took tamoxifen for two years and then switched to letrozole (sequential therapy).

In the current report, researchers compared 4,007 women in the two tamoxifen groups to 4,003 women in the two letrozole groups. More follow-up is needed before the authors can tell whether the two monotherapy groups (tamoxifen alone; letrozole alone) do any better or worse compared to the two sequential therapy groups (one drug followed by the other).

The study was conducted by the BIG 1-98 Collaborative Group, with Beat Thürlimann, M.D., as the chair of the Writing Committee. Novartis AG supported the trial and also supplied drugs.

Results

After a median follow-up period of just over two years, women in the letrozole groups were 19 percent less likely to have a recurrence. The advantage was even more pronounced when it came to protection against cancer far from the original tumor (distant metastases), with women in the letrozole groups 27 percent less likely to experience a distant recurrence.

Some of the women in the study received chemotherapy after surgery. Among these women, those in the letrozole groups were 30 percent less likely to have a recurrence than those in the tamoxifen groups. Among women whose cancer had spread to their lymph nodes, those in the letrozole groups were 29 percent less likely to have a recurrence than those in the tamoxifen groups.

Researchers also analyzed the data to come up with estimates of how many women would likely be alive and free of disease five years after enrolling in the study, and concluded that this would be true for 84 percent of those in the letrozole groups and 81.4 percent of those in the tamoxifen groups. At the two year mark, there was no difference in overall survival between the letrozole and tamoxifen groups.

As in other trials, side effects such as joint pain and fractures were more common in women who took letrozole, and they were more likely to have heart attacks and other cardiovascular problems. Women who took tamoxifen were more likely to have blood clots, endometrial cancer, and vaginal bleeding.

Note: In a subsequent paper published by the *Journal of Clinical Oncology* online Nov. 12, 2007, in print Dec. 20, 2007, researchers with the trial report a safety analysis of the cardiovascular adverse events in BIG 1-98. The analysis found a low overall incidence of such events.

Comments

The letrozole advantage reported in this trial confirms other results showing the aromatase inhibitors to be generally more effective than tamoxifen, said the study authors, who emphasized the risk reduction in metastasis. Sandra M. Swain, M.D., a senior investigator with the National Cancer Institute's (NCI) Center for Cancer Research, in an accompanying editorial said it was clear that these trials, "with close to 30,000 participants, consistently demonstrate that treatment with an aromatase inhibitor alone or after tamoxifen treatment is beneficial."

Limitations

JoAnne Zujewski, M.D., of NCI's Cancer Therapy Evaluation Program, agreed that letrozole was likely to produce slightly better results than tamoxifen, but emphasized that many women on tamoxifen still do very well, noting that "in this trial more than 80 percent were free of recurrence." The challenge, she said, "is to sort out which patients may be treated with tamoxifen, to avoid the increased risk letrozole poses to bone health."

Section 45.5

Aromatase Inhibitors vs. Tamoxifen

"Aromatase Inhibitors Come of Age," National Cancer Institute
(www.cancer.gov), March 7, 2007.

Aromatase inhibitors (AIs), which interfere with the body's ability
to produce the hormone estrogen, are rapidly changing the standard
of treatment for breast cancer. Researchers have now taken up the challenge of learning how and when to best use these drugs to reduce recurrence for women with hormone-receptor-positive breast cancer.

Two approaches dominate the development of hormone-based
treatments for breast cancer. One approach focuses on preventing
estrogen from binding to its receptor and activating cell-signaling
pathways that accelerate tumor growth. This strategy led to the development of the drug tamoxifen (Nolvadex®), which belongs to a class
of drug called selective estrogen-receptor modulators (SERMs).

Since its approval by the U.S. Food and Drug Administration (FDA)
for the treatment of hormone-receptor-positive breast cancer in 1977,
tamoxifen has become a mainstay of therapy. However, many women
develop resistance to the drug over time, leading to cancer recurrence.
In addition, because tamoxifen binds directly to the estrogen receptor, it
can sometimes activate the signaling pathways it was designed to block.

"We knew that tamoxifen was a partial agonist—a weak estrogen,"
explains Dr. Angela Brodie, professor of pharmacology and experimental therapeutics at the University of Maryland, who has worked on the
development of AIs for more than 35 years. "So we thought it might not
be optimally effective on tumors...and that it could cause side effects. In
fact, it does increase the risk of stroke and endometrial cancer."

A Different Mechanism

AIs take a different approach to hormone therapy—they prevent
the bodies of postmenopausal women from producing estrogen rather
than blocking its activity. AIs accomplish this by interfering with the
enzyme aromatase, which catalyzes the final step in the synthesis of
estrogen from its steroid precursors.

Two different types of AIs are in use in the clinic today. Steroidal AIs, such as exemestane (Aromasin®), bind permanently to aromatase. Nonsteroidal AIs, such as anastrozole (Arimidex®) and letrozole (Femara®), bind reversibly to aromatase and compete with the precursors of estrogen for the enzyme.

Both steroidal and nonsteroidal AIs have been shown in large-scale clinical trials to be superior to tamoxifen in extending survival in women with metastatic disease, and in preventing recurrence when used as primary adjuvant therapy. In addition, treatment with an AI after a full course of tamoxifen continues to improve recurrence-free survival, compared with cessation of hormone therapy.

The challenge remains to determine the best schedule for up-front AI treatment. Studies have shown that five years of an AI alone are more effective at preventing recurrence than five years of tamoxifen alone, and that switching women already taking tamoxifen to an AI after two or three years prevents more recurrences than continuing tamoxifen for a full five years. However, it is not clear yet if sequencing tamoxifen and an AI in women who have not yet been treated with hormone therapy confers a benefit over five years of an AI alone.

Results from trials where women have switched from tamoxifen to an AI cannot be applied to women who have not yet received any hormone therapy. "It's important to understand that while the treatment is the same, the patients are not the same," says Dr. Beat Thürlimann, president of the International Breast Cancer Study Group. "If you have already taken two or three years of tamoxifen and survived disease-free, you belong to a favorable prognostic group."

"When you make a decision about treatment after surgery, you don't know if you belong to this favorable category or not," Dr. Thürlimann continues. "With sequencing trials, you're looking at a broader patient population." The Breast International Group trial BIG 1-98 is comparing sequencing of tamoxifen and letrozole to either tamoxifen or letrozole alone after surgery for early-stage breast cancer. The preliminary results from this part of the trial, expected in 2008, will provide valuable information on sequencing hormone therapies in women who have not yet received hormone therapy.

New Questions

Other questions remain as AIs move to a more prominent position in breast cancer treatment. AIs have side effects of their own, most importantly loss of bone density, which can be especially hazardous for women already at risk for osteoporosis. Therefore, tamoxifen may still provide a more favorable risk/benefit ratio for some subgroups of women, which need to be identified.

In addition, the role of AIs in premenopausal patients remains to be defined. While AIs alone may not have an effect in premenopausal women, because the ovaries can override the inhibition by producing a large amount of aromatase, clinical trials are now testing AIs in premenopausal women in combination with drugs such as goserelin, which suppress ovarian function.

Because AIs have also reduced the occurrence of contralateral breast cancer in several studies, researchers are now testing the compounds as chemopreventive agents. Two large scale trials have begun testing exemestane and anastrozole in women at high risk for developing breast cancer. Although tamoxifen was approved in 1998 for the prevention of breast cancer in high-risk women, fewer women than expected have chosen to take it.

"One reason [healthy] women don't want to take tamoxifen is fear of side effects," explains Dr. Jennifer Eng-Wong, a clinical oncologist in the National Cancer Institute's Center for Cancer Research. If AIs prove to have both efficacy in preventing breast cancer occurrence and acceptable side effects, they and the new generation of SERMs such as raloxifene will provide women at high risk with additional options to help prevent the disease.

Chapter 46

Trastuzumab (Herceptin)

What is Herceptin? How does it work?

Herceptin (trastuzumab) is a monoclonal antibody. Antibodies are substances the body produces to help fight infection or other foreign particles. Monoclonal antibodies are made in the laboratory, and some are designed to attack specific cancer cells.

Herceptin targets cancer cells that "overexpress," or make too much of, a protein called HER2 or erb B2, which is found on the surface of some cancer cells. Herceptin attaches to the HER2-positive cancer cells and slows or stops the growth of the cells. Herceptin is used only to treat breast cancers that are HER2 positive. HER2-positive cancers overexpress the HER2 protein or have amplification (too many copies) of the HER2 gene.

Approximately 20 to 30 percent of breast cancers overexpress HER2. These tumors tend to grow faster and are generally more likely to recur (come back) than tumors that do not overproduce HER2.

How are tumors tested for HER2?

The amount of HER2 protein in the tumor is measured in the laboratory using a test called immunohistochemical (IHC) analysis. The results of the test are measured on a scale from zero (negative) to 3+ (strongly positive). Patients with tumors that are 3+ on the IHC test

"Herceptin® (Trastuzumab): Questions and Answers," National Cancer Institute (www.cancer.gov), June 13, 2006.

are most likely to benefit from Herceptin therapy; those with tumors that are zero or 1+ are unlikely to benefit from this treatment. Patients with tumors that are 2+ often have an additional test, called fluorescence in situ hybridization (FISH), to determine whether the tumor is HER2 positive. FISH measures the number of copies of a gene. Tumors with too many copies of the HER2 gene as determined by the FISH test are considered positive.

How is Herceptin used in the treatment of cancer?

Herceptin is approved by the U.S. Food and Drug Administration (FDA) for the treatment of metastatic breast cancer (breast cancer that has spread to other parts of the body) that is HER2 positive. The FDA approved Herceptin after two clinical trials (research studies) with women whose metastatic breast cancers produced excess amounts of HER2 demonstrated that Herceptin was safe and effective.

In 2005, the results of four clinical trials showed that Herceptin is also effective in the treatment of early-stage breast cancer that overexpresses HER2. In all four studies, women who received Herceptin and chemotherapy lived longer and had significantly less chance of the breast cancer coming back than patients who received chemotherapy alone.

How is Herceptin given? What are some of the common side effects of Herceptin?

Herceptin is given by infusion (a method of putting fluids, including drugs, into the bloodstream). The first dose of Herceptin is usually given over a 90-minute period, and the nurse or doctor watches the patient for signs of side effects. If the patient tolerates this dose well, smaller maintenance doses can be given over a 30-minute period.

Side effects that most commonly occur during the first treatment with Herceptin include fever or chills. Other possible side effects include pain, weakness, nausea, vomiting, diarrhea, headaches, difficulty breathing, and rashes. These side effects generally become less severe after the first treatment with Herceptin.

Patients who receive Herceptin along with chemotherapy may experience side effects that are different from those of patients who take Herceptin by itself. For example, anemia (a condition in which the number of red blood cells is below normal) and infection, primarily mild upper respiratory infection, have been seen more often in patients given Herceptin with chemotherapy compared with those receiving Herceptin alone. Patients should discuss any concerns about the side effects of treatment with their doctor. The doctor may be able to make suggestions for managing side effects.

Can Herceptin cause any serious side effects?

Yes. Herceptin can cause heart muscle damage that can lead to heart failure. Heart failure is a serious condition in which the heart cannot pump enough blood throughout the body. Symptoms of heart failure include shortness of breath, difficulty breathing, and swelling of the feet or lower legs.

Herceptin can also affect the lungs, causing severe or life-threatening breathing problems that require immediate medical attention.

In addition, Herceptin can cause hypersensitivity (allergic) reactions that can be severe or life-threatening. Symptoms of a reaction include a drop in blood pressure, shortness of breath, rashes, and wheezing. Most patients who experience hypersensitivity reactions do so when the drug is being given or within 24 hours after treatment.

Because of these potentially life-threatening side effects, doctors evaluate patients carefully for any heart or lung problems before starting treatment. Doctors and nurses also monitor patients closely during treatment. Patients who develop any problems during or after treatment should call the doctor immediately or go to the nearest emergency care facility.

Is Herceptin still being studied in clinical trials?

Yes. Clinical trials are ongoing to test the safety and effectiveness of Herceptin for breast and other types of cancer. People interested in taking part in a clinical trial should talk with their doctor. Information about clinical trials is available from the National Cancer Institute's (NCI) Cancer Information Service (CIS) at 800-4-CANCER and in the NCI booklet "Taking Part in Clinical Trials: What Cancer Patients Need To Know," which can be found at http://www.cancer.gov/publications on the internet. This booklet describes how research studies are carried out and explains their possible benefits and risks. More information about clinical trials is available at http://www.cancer.gov/clinicaltrials on the NCI's website. The website offers detailed information about specific ongoing studies by linking to PDQ®, the NCI's comprehensive cancer information database.

Chapter 47

New Study of Targeted Therapies for Breast Cancer

Two targeted medications designed to treat an aggressive form of breast cancer are being tested in a new study involving 8,000 participants in 50 countries across six continents—a clinical trial that investigators hope will provide a new model for global cancer research. This trial, dubbed ALTTO (Adjuvant Lapatinib and/or Trastuzumab Treatment Optimization study), will be one of the first global initiatives in which two large, academic breast cancer research networks covering different parts of the world have jointly developed a study in which all care and data collection are standardized, regardless of where patients are treated. The networks are The Breast Cancer Intergroup of North America (TBCI), based in the United States, and the Breast International Group (BIG) in Brussels, Belgium. TBCI consists of six National Cancer Institute (NCI)-funded clinical trials cooperative groups. NCI is part of the National Institutes of Health.

ALTTO is designed to answer the most pressing questions regarding use of two widely used cancer agents: whether one agent is more effective, which agent is safer for patients, and what benefit will be derived by taking the drugs separately, in tandem order, or together? The trial is a randomized, Phase III study, which is considered a gold standard method for proving drug effectiveness.

The two agents tested in ALTTO are drugs designed to treat HER2-positive tumors, which is a particularly aggressive form of cancer that

"New Study of Targeted Therapies for Breast Cancer Establishes Model for Global Clinical Trials," National Cancer Institute (www.cancer.gov), February 29, 2008.

affects approximately 20 percent to 25 percent of breast cancer patients. Both agents, trastuzumab (Herceptin) and lapatinib (Tykerb), have already been approved by the U.S. Food and Drug Administration for use for treatment of HER2-positive breast cancer. ALTTO will provide the first head-to-head comparison of trastuzumab and lapatinib in the earliest, most treatable stages of cancer. It will also be one of the first large-scale studies to evaluate lapatinib's effectiveness in treating early breast cancer.

HER2-positive breast cancer is caused by an excess of HER2 genes or by over-production of its protein, the HER2 cell surface receptor. Trastuzumab consists of large antibodies that once injected into patients, latch on to the portion of the HER2 protein that sits on the outer surface of the cancer cell whereas lapatinib acts by entering a cancer cell and binding to the part of the HER2 protein that lies beneath the surface of the cell.

The trial is unusual in that it has two different designs depending on whether patients with stage I or stage II breast cancer have already been treated with chemotherapy. The study thus will compare four different regimens of targeted therapy administered over a 52-week period. Patients will be randomized to receive either trastuzumab or lapatinib alone, or trastuzumab followed by lapatinib, or the two treatments in combination.

"There have been major improvements in the management of patients with early breast cancer in the last few years, so this new study builds on this knowledge and sets an example of the new era: good science, good worldwide collaboration," said Edith Perez, M.D., an oncologist in the North Central Cancer Treatment Group (NCCTG) at Mayo Clinic in Jacksonville, Florida, who will lead the study for TBCI. "It may be that using two treatments that work in different ways against HER2-positive breast cancer offers a complementary strategy that is more powerful than either drug alone."

ALTTO will be one of the first trials of its scope in which translational research—taking science from bench to bedside—plays a critical role, investigators say. In ALTTO, biological material will be collected from thousands of patients in order to determine a tumor profile that responds best to the drugs—information that could lead to individualized patient care and, possibly, to development of next generation agents.

"The difference between this study and many that came before it is that the collection of biological materials occurs as the trial is being conducted, not as an afterthought. While there are exceptions, not many companies or organizations have been willing to invest in that kind of research before," said Martine J. Piccart, M.D., Ph.D., professor of oncology at the Université Libre de Bruxelles, Belgium, and lead investigator for BIG, which she founded in 1996. "Now we have the chance to optimize therapy with powerful drugs in order to provide the best treatment possible for each of our patients."

Perez and Piccart led the development team of the ALTTO trial and will act as the study's co-principal investigators. On behalf of BIG and TBCI, these two lead investigators have been working toward collaborative clinical studies for a number of years. The ALTTO study, they say, represents a new paradigm that blends the high standards of both systems in order to test the latest breast cancer treatments as efficiently as possible in thousands of women worldwide.

"The NCI greatly appreciates the work that Mayo Clinic, TBCI, and BIG are doing to help advance our understanding of the complex mechanisms that underlie different types of breast cancer," said Jo Anne Zujewski, M.D., a senior investigator in the clinical investigations branch at NCI. "We hope that this model of international collaboration is one which we can build upon in the future."

Lapatinib, in combination with the chemotherapy drug capecitabine, was approved by the U.S. Food and Drug Administration in March 2007 for the treatment of advanced or metastatic HER2-positive breast cancer in patients who had received prior therapy with three agents—an anthracycline, a taxane, and Herceptin. GlaxoSmithKline is providing the study drug, as well as additional financial support for the ALTTO trial. All drugs carry potential side effects, and more information of side effects for lapatinib and trastuzumab can be found in the Q&A at http://www.cancer.gov/newscenter/pressreleases/ALTTOQandA. NCI and GSK also provided comment and input on the design of the study.

NCCTG will act as the treatment base for ALTTO in North America. BIG is a network of 41 non-U.S. research groups from around the world. Its Brussels-based BrEAST Data Center is providing centralized data management for the global study (including the United States). The other members of TBCI include the Eastern Cooperative Oncology Group (ECOG), the Cancer and Leukemia Group B (CALGB), the Southwest Oncology Group (SWOG), the American College of Surgeons Oncology Group (ACOSOG), and the National Cancer Institute of Canada Clinical Trials Group (NCIC CTG).

To date, more than 300 centers around the world have enrolled patients into ALTTO. Full enrollment is expected to involve about 500 centers in the United States and more than 800 centers in Europe and the rest of the world. A complete listing of ALTTO participating sites can be found by searching for ALTTO at http://www.cancer.gov/clinicaltrials/EGF106708.

Chapter 48

Taking Part in Cancer Research

If you have cancer, you may want to think about taking part in a clinical trial. Clinical trials are a treatment option for many people with cancer. This chapter explains cancer treatment clinical trials and gives you some things to think about when deciding whether to take part.

What Are Clinical Trials?

Clinical trials are research studies that involve people. They are the final step in a long process that begins with research in a lab and animal testing. Many treatments used today are the result of past clinical trials. In cancer research, clinical trials are designed to answer questions about new ways to treat cancer, find and diagnose cancer, prevent cancer, and manage symptoms of cancer or its treatment.

This information will focus on cancer treatment studies. These studies are designed to answer questions about new treatments or new ways of using an old treatment and how well they work. These trials test many types of treatments, such as new drugs or vaccines, ways to do surgery or give radiation therapy, and combinations of treatments.

Clinical Trials Take Place in Phases

For a treatment to become part of standard treatment, it must first go through three or four clinical trial phases. You do not have to take

From "Taking Part in Cancer Treatment Research Studies," National Cancer Institute (www.cancer.gov), July 17, 2007; and "How to Find a Cancer Treatment Trial: A 10-Step Guide," NCI, March 21, 2005.

part in all phases. The early phases make sure the treatment is safe. Later phases show if it works better than the standard treatment.

Phase I

- Purpose:
    - To find a safe dose
    - To decide how the new treatment should be given
    - To see how the new treatment affects the human body
- People: 15–30 people

Phase II

- Purpose:
    - To determine if the new treatment has an effect on a certain cancer
    - To see how the new treatment affects the human body
- People: Less than 100 people

Phase III

- Purpose:
    - To compare the new treatment (or new use of a treatment) with the current standard treatment
- People: From 100 to thousands of people

Phase IV

- Purpose:
    - To further assess the long-term safety and effectiveness of a new treatment
- People: Several hundred to several thousand people

Clinical Trials Follow Strict Guidelines

The guidelines that clinical trials follow clearly state who will be able to join the study and the treatment plan. Every trial has a person in charge, usually a doctor, who is called the principal investigator. The principal investigator prepares a plan for the study, called a protocol, which is like a recipe for conducting a clinical trial.

The protocol explains what the trial will do, how the study will be carried out, and why each part of the study is necessary. It includes information on the following:

- The reason for doing the study
- Who can join the study
- How many people are needed for the study
- Any drugs they will take, the dose, and how often
- What medical tests they will have and how often
- What information will be gathered about them

Who Can Join a Clinical Trial?

Based on the questions the research is trying to answer, each clinical trial protocol clearly states who can or cannot join the trial. Common criteria for entering a trial include the following:

- Having a certain type or stage of cancer
- Having received a certain kind of therapy in the past
- Being in a certain age group

Criteria such as these help ensure that people in the trial are as alike as possible. This way doctors can be sure that the results are due to the treatment being studied and not other factors.

These criteria also help ensure safety and accurate and meaningful study results:

- **Safety:** Some people have health problems besides cancer that could be made worse by the treatments in a study. If you are interested in joining a trial, you will receive medical tests to be sure that you are not put at increased risk.
- **Accurate and meaningful study results:** You may not be able to join some clinical trials if you already have had another kind of treatment for your cancer. Otherwise, doctors could not be sure whether your results were due to the treatment being studied or the earlier treatment.

Randomization

Randomization is a process used in some clinical trials to prevent bias. Bias occurs when a trial's results are affected by human choices or other factors not related to the treatments being tested. Randomization helps ensure that unknown factors do not affect trial results.

Randomization is used in all phase III and some phase II trials. These trials are called randomized clinical trials. If you participate in such a trial, you will be assigned by chance to either an investigational group or a control group. Your assignment will be determined with a computer program or table of random numbers.

- If you are assigned to the control group, you will get the most widely accepted treatment (standard treatment) for your cancer.

- If you are assigned to the investigational group, you will get the new treatment being tested.

Comparing these groups to each other often clearly shows which treatment is more effective or has fewer side effects. If you are thinking about joining a randomized clinical trial, you need to understand that you have an equal chance to be assigned to either one of the groups. The doctor does not choose the group for you.

About placebos: A placebo is designed to look like the medicine being tested, but it is not active. Placebos are almost never used in cancer treatment trials. In some cases, a study may compare standard treatment plus a new treatment, to standard treatment plus a placebo. You will be told if the study uses a placebo.

Patient Protection

Federal rules help ensure that clinical trials are run in an ethical manner. Your rights and safety are protected through the following measures:

- Informed consent

- Careful review and approval of the clinical trial protocol by two review panels. These panels include a scientific review panel and an institutional review board (IRB).

- Ongoing monitoring provided during the trial by the IRB, data and Safety Monitoring Boards (DSMBs) for phase III trials, and your research team

Informed Consent

Informed consent is a process through which you learn the purpose, risks, and benefits of a clinical trial before deciding whether to join. It is a critical part of ensuring patient safety in research. During the informed consent process you learn important information about a clinical trial. This information can help you decide whether to join.

The research team, which is made up of doctors and nurses, first explains the trial to you. The team explains the trial's purpose, procedures, and risks and benefits. They will also discuss your rights, including your right to make a decision about participating and leave the study at any time. If you decide to leave the study, your doctor will discuss other treatment options with you.

Before agreeing to take part in a trial, you have the right to the following:

- Learn about all your treatment options

- Learn all that is involved in the trial—including all details about treatment, tests, and possible risks and benefits

- Discuss the trial with the principal investigator and other members of the research team

- Both hear and read the information in language you can understand

After discussing all aspects of the study with you, the team gives you an informed consent form to read. The form includes written details about the information that was discussed and also describes the privacy of your records. If you agree to take part in the study, you sign the form. But even after you sign the consent form, you can leave the study at any time.

Most clinical trials have to go through different types of review that are designed to protect all people who take part. These reviews are conducted by scientific review panels, Institutional Review Boards (IRBs), and Data and Safety Monitoring Boards (DSMBs).

Scientific Review Panels

This panel is made up of experts who review a clinical trial protocol before it starts accepting patients to make sure it is based on sound science. All clinical trials that are funded by the Government must go through this review. Many other clinical trial sponsors, such as drug companies, also seek expert advice on the scientific merit of their trial protocols.

Institutional Review Boards

This board also reviews a clinical trial protocol before it starts accepting patients. The board members make sure the risks involved in the trial are reasonable when compared to the possible benefits. They also closely watch the ongoing progress of the trial from beginning to end.

Federal rules require that each IRB be made up of at least five people. One member must be from outside the institution running the trial. IRBs are usually made up of a mix of medical specialists and members of the community. Many include members from diverse careers and backgrounds. In most cases IRBs are located where the trial is to take place. Many institutions that carry out clinical trials have their own IRBs.

Data and Safety Monitoring Boards (DSMBs)

For phase III trials, DSMBs monitor the trial to help ensure your safety. They may also be appropriate and necessary for certain phase I and II clinical trials. A DSMB is an independent committee made up of statisticians, physicians, and other experts. The Board must ensure that any risks that come from being in the study are reduced as much as possible, ensure that the data are sound, and stop a trial if safety concerns come up or as soon as its objectives have been met.

How to Find a Cancer Treatment Trial: A 10-Step Guide

This information will help you to look for a cancer treatment clinical trial that might benefit you. It is not intended to provide medical advice. You, your health care team, and your loved ones are in the best position to decide whether a clinical trial is right for you.

A Word about Timing: Many treatment trials will only take patients who have not yet been treated for their condition. Researchers conducting these trials are hoping to find an improved "first-line" treatment option for that type of cancer.

- If you are newly diagnosed with cancer, the time to consider joining a clinical trial is before you've had surgery, chemotherapy, radiation, or other forms of treatment (tests to diagnose your cancer are okay). However, don't delay treatment if waiting could harm you. Talk with your doctor about how quickly you need to make a treatment decision.

- If you have received one or more forms of treatment and are looking for a new treatment option, there also are many clinical trial options for you. You may want to look for trials that are testing a new follow-up treatment that may prevent the return of your cancer. Or, if your first treatment failed to work, you may want to look for trials of new "second-line" or even "third-line" treatments.

Before You Start: Steps 1–3

Step 1: Understand Clinical Trials

This section assumes you already know what clinical trials are and why you might want to join one. If you need to, review your understanding of clinical trials before you continue the steps in this guide.

Step 2: Talk with Your Doctor

When considering clinical trials, your best starting point is your doctor and other members of your health care team.

Your primary care physician, cancer doctor (oncologist), surgeon, or other health care provider might know about a clinical trial you should consider. He or she can help you determine whether a clinical trial might be a good option.

Note: In some cases, your doctor may be reluctant to discuss clinical trials as a treatment option for you. Some doctors are unfamiliar with clinical trials, cautious about turning your care over to another medical team, or wary of the extra time that joining a clinical trial might require of them and their staff. If so, you may wish to get a second opinion about your treatment options and clinical trials.

Remember, you do not always need a referral from your doctor to join a clinical trial.

If you are eligible to join a trial, the final decision is up to you. However, be sure to consider the professional opinions of your doctor. He or she may present very specific reasons why a clinical trial may not be beneficial for you right now.

Step 3: Complete the Diagnosis Checklist

Before you begin looking for a clinical trial, you must know certain details about your cancer diagnosis. You will need to compare these details with the eligibility criteria of any trial in which you are interested. Eligibility criteria are the guidelines for who can and cannot participate in a particular study.

To help you gather the details of your diagnosis so you will know which trials you may be eligible to join, complete the Diagnosis Checklist. It asks questions about your diagnosis. Keep this information with you during your search for a clinical trial.

To get the information you need for the form ask a nurse or social worker at your doctor's office for help. Explain to them that you are interested in looking for a clinical trial that may benefit you and that you need these details before starting to look. They will be able to review your medical records and help you fill answer the questions in the checklist.

Diagnosis Checklist

Answer the questions from this Diagnosis Checklist before you start looking for a clinical trial. The checklist will help you know which clinical trials you are eligible to join.

1. *What kind of cancer do you have?* Write down the full medical name.

2. *Where did the cancer first start?* Many cancers spread to the bones, liver, or elsewhere. However, the type of cancer you have is determined by where it first showed up. For example, breast cancer that spreads to the bone is still breast cancer.

3. *What is the cancer's cell type?* This information will be in your pathology report.

4. *If there's a solid tumor, what size is it?*

5. *If there is a solid tumor, where is it located?* If the tumor has spread, list all locations.

6. *What stage is the cancer?* The stage describes the extent of cancer in the body and whether it has spread from the original site. There are different staging systems for different cancers.

7. *Have you had cancer before, different from the one you have now?* If so, answer questions 1–6 for the other cancer, as well.

8. *What is your current performance status?* An assessment from your doctor indicating how well you are able to perform ordinary tasks and carry out daily activities.

9. *If you have not yet had any treatment for cancer, what treatment(s) have been recommended to you?*

10. *If you have had treatment for cancer, please list (for example, type of surgery: chemotherapy, immunotherapy, or radiation).*

11. *Bone marrow function* (blood tests that check whether your blood count is normal):
    - White blood cell count
    - Platelet count
    - Hemoglobin/hematocrit

12. *Liver function* (blood tests that check whether your liver function is normal):
    - Bilirubin
    - Transaminases

13. *Renal function* (blood test that checks whether your kidney function is normal):
    - Serum creatinine

Searching for a Trial: Steps 4–6

You have learned what clinical trials are and how they work, talked with your doctor about your interest in clinical trials, and prepared a checklist of key details about your diagnosis. You are now ready to search for clinical trials.

Note: It is important to understand the possible biases and limitations of any clinical trials website.

Step 4: Search the PDQ® Clinical Trials Database

There are many nonprofit and for-profit resources in the United States that offer lists of cancer clinical trials. Unfortunately, no single list is complete. Clinical trials are run by many different organizations, so it is hard to collect information about all of them in one place.

However, the majority of trials listed in most resources are obtained from the Physician Data Query (PDQ) clinical trials database, which is maintained by the U.S. National Cancer Institute (NCI).

The NCI is the U.S. government's chief agency for cancer research and is part of the National Institutes of Health. The PDQ clinical trials database contains a list of more than 2,000 cancer clinical trials worldwide.

Note: The U.S. National Library of Medicine maintains a database called ClinicalTrials.gov that includes trials for many diseases and conditions, including cancer. The PDQ and ClinicalTrials.gov databases contain the same cancer treatment trial listings. The main difference is in how information is searched and displayed. You may prefer one way over another.

Steps 4 and 5 describe where to look for cancer clinical trials. Whichever resource you use, be sure to get a copy of the protocol summary for each trial you are interested in.

What is a protocol? It is the action plan for the trial. The protocol explains what will be done in the trial, how, and why. The protocol should also list the location(s) where the trial will enroll participants.

Both PDQ and ClinicalTrials.gov provide detailed summaries of the official protocols for each trial listed on their websites. Other resources may or may not provide protocol summaries.

How to Search PDQ

- Search PDQ by telephone. Make a free telephone call—in English or Spanish—within the United States to the National Cancer Institute's Cancer Information Service (CIS) at 800-4-CANCER (800-422-6237). All calls to the CIS are strictly confidential.

  - When you call the CIS, be ready with the details of your Diagnosis Checklist from Step 3.

  - The CIS is staffed with understanding and knowledgeable information specialists who will search PDQ for you. They can send you the search results and protocol summaries by e-mail, fax, or regular mail. The CIS can also provide you with reliable information about your type of cancer and the current standard therapy for treating it.

- Search PDQ through the NCI website. You can look for trials yourself using a PDQ search form on the NCI website. Remember to print out the protocol summaries for each trial you may be interested in.

- The basic search form allows you to search by type of cancer, stage or subtype of cancer, and location of trial (ZIP code).

- The advanced search form lets you create your search using more detailed information, such as the hospital or institution involved, type of treatment, and phase of trial.

- If you would like help searching PDQ while you're online, consider using LiveHelp. Through LiveHelp, you can communicate confidentially and in real time with a CIS information specialist from the National Cancer Institute. The service is available Monday through Friday from 9:00 a.m. to 11:00 p.m. Eastern time.

Step 5: Search Other Resources

While PDQ and ClinicalTrials.gov have the most complete listing of cancer trials, you might want to check a few other resources, as well. Why? Because some may include a few trials not found in the federal databases and you may prefer their way of assisting you in your search.

TrialCheck®: TrialCheck is operated and maintained by the Coalition of Cancer Cooperative Groups (CCCG). The CCCG is made up of groups of doctors and other health professionals that carry out many of the large cancer clinical trials in the United States funded by the National Cancer Institute.

TrialCheck maintains comprehensive data on thousands of cancer clinical trials and contains a copyrighted cancer clinical trials screening questionnaire that will identify trials appropriate for a patient's individual medical condition.

How to search TrialCheck: The TrialCheck Frequently Asked Questions (FAQs) page (available online at http://www.cancertrialshelp.org/trialcheck/default.aspx?intAppMode=11) provides helpful information about how to use TrialCheck.

Third-party clinical trial websites: There are a number of clinical trial websites that are not operated by funders, sponsors, or the organizations carrying out the trials. Some of these websites are operated by private companies—these may be funded through fees that industry sponsors pay to have their trials listed or according to how many participants the website refers to them.

Keep the following points in mind:

- Most third-party clinical trials websites list or link to trials in PDQ or ClinicalTrials.gov.

- They may include a few more trials than you'll find in the federal databases, but they may also include fewer.

- Unlike the federal databases, these sites may not regularly update their content or links.

- Unlike the federal databases, these sites might require you to register to search for trials or to obtain contact information about the trials that interest you.

Here are some possible third-party websites:

- Acurian: https://www.acurian.com

- Cancer411: http://www.cancer411.com

- CancerConsultants: http://www.patient.cancerconsultants.com

- CenterWatch: http://www.centerwatch.com

- ClinicalTrialsSearch.org: http://www.clinicaltrialssearch.org

- EmergingMed: http://www.emergingmed.com

- Veritas Medicine: http://www.veritasmedicine.com

Industry-sponsored cancer trials: Pharmaceutical and biotechnology companies sponsor many of the cancer clinical trials being carried out in the United States. Some of these trials are listed in the federal databases (PDQ and ClinicalTrials.gov), but many are not.

Federal law requires that U.S. researchers submit to ClinicalTrials .gov all phase II, III, and IV trials of therapies for serious or life-threatening illnesses (including cancer) conducted as part of the approval process overseen by the U.S. Food and Drug Administration. However, this law is difficult to enforce and for business reasons, some drug companies have preferred to keep details about their clinical trials from the public.

How to search for industry-sponsored trials: If you are aware of an experimental cancer treatment and know the company that manufactures it, search the internet to find the website of the company. Find the company's customer service telephone number. When you call, ask to speak to the company's clinical trials department. Tell them you are looking for a trial that you might be eligible to join.

Cancer advocacy groups: Cancer advocacy groups work on behalf of people diagnosed with cancer and their loved ones. They provide education, support, financial assistance, and advocacy to help patients and families who are dealing with cancer. These organizations recognize that clinical trials are important to the cancer treatment process and, thus, work to educate and empower people to find information and access to treatment.

Because they work hard to know about the latest research advances in cancer treatment, these groups will sometimes have information about certain key government-sponsored trials, as well as some potentially significant trials sponsored by pharmaceutical companies or cancer care centers.

How to search for trials through a cancer advocacy group: Contact the advocacy group for the type of cancer you are interested in and ask what they can tell you about ongoing clinical trials. The nonprofit Marti Nelson Cancer Foundation maintains a partial list of such groups on its CancerActionNow.org website.

Fee-based private search services: A number of private services will, for a fee, locate clinical trials for you. While having someone search for you may ease your stress, it is important to keep in mind that several of the resources mentioned earlier in this guide provide elements of this kind of service for free. Also, be sure to ask the following questions:

- What list or lists of clinical trials does the service search? Are those lists likely to provide you with an unbiased and largely complete source of options?

- Does the service receive any money for directing patients to certain trials or for including certain trials in their list?

Step 6: Make a List of Potential Trials

At this point you have created a Diagnosis Checklist, identified one or more trials you might be interested in, and obtained a protocol summary for each one.

Now it's time to take a closer look at the protocol summaries you have obtained for the trials you're interested in. You should remove from your list those trials you aren't actually able to join and come up with one or more top possibilities.

What follows are some key questions to consider about each trial. However, don't worry if you cannot answer all of these questions just yet. The idea is to narrow the list if you can, but don't give up on one that you're not sure of.

Note: Ideally, you should consult your doctor during this process, especially if you find the protocol summaries difficult to understand. But you can probably do Step 6 yourself if the protocol summary is relatively complete and easy to understand.

- **Trial objective:** What is the main purpose of the trial? Is it to improve your chances of a cure? To slow the rate at which your cancer may grow or return? To lessen the severity of treatment side effects? To establish whether a new treatment is safe and well tolerated? Read this information carefully to learn whether the trial's main objective matches your goals for treatment.

477

- **Eligibility criteria:** Do your diagnosis and current overall state of health match the eligibility criteria (sometimes referred to as enrollment or entry criteria)? This may tell you whether you could qualify for the trial. If you're not sure, keep the trial on your list for now.

- **Trial location:** Is the location of the clinical trial manageable for you? Some trials are available at more than one site. Look carefully at how often you will need to receive treatment during the course of the trial, and decide how far and how often you are willing to travel. You will also need to ask if the sponsoring organization will provide for some or all of your travel expenses.

- **Study duration:** How long will the study run? Not all protocol summaries list this information. If they do, consider the time commitment and whether it will work for you and your family.

If, after considering these questions, you are still interested in one or more of the clinical trials you have found, then you are ready for Step 7.

After Finding a Trial: Steps 7–10

Now that you have found one or more clinical trials for which you think you are eligible and that may be a good treatment option for you, it is time to make a telephone call to each trial's contact person so you can ask a few more crucial questions. Then, you will be ready to make a final treatment decision.

Step 7: Contact the Clinical Trial Team

There are several ways to contact the Clinical Trial Team.

- Contact the trial team directly. The protocol summary should include the name and telephone number of someone you can contact for more information. You do not need to talk to the lead researcher (called the "protocol chair" or "principal investigator") at this time, even if that is the name that is included with the telephone number. Instead, call the number and ask to speak with the "trial coordinator," the "referral coordinator," or the "protocol assistant." This person can answer questions from potential patients and their doctors. It is also this person's job to determine whether you are likely to be eligible to join the trial. (A final determination would be made only after you had gone in for a first appointment.)

- Ask your doctor or other health care team member to contact the trial team for you. Because the clinical trial coordinator will ask questions related to your diagnosis, you may want to ask your doctor or someone else on your health care team to contact the clinical trial team for you.

- The trial team may contact you. If you have used some a third-party website and identified a trial that interests you, you may have provided your name, phone number, and e-mail address so that the clinical trial team can contact you.

You will need to refer to your Diagnosis Checklist (Step 3) during the conversation, so keep that handy.

Step 8: Ask Questions about the Trial

Whether you or someone from your health care team calls the clinical trial coordinator, this is the time to get answers to questions that will help you decide whether or not to join this particular clinical trial.

It will be helpful if you can talk about your diagnosis in a manner that is brief and to the point. Before you make the call, rehearse with a family member or friend how you will present the key details of your diagnosis (Diagnosis Checklist). This will make you more comfortable when you are talking with the clinical trial coordinator and will enable you to answer his or her questions smoothly.

Questions to Ask the Trial Coordinator

1. *Is the trial still open?* On occasion, clinical trial listings will be out-of-date and will include trials that have actually closed to further enrollment.

2. *Am I eligible for this trial?* The trial coordinator will ask you many, if not all, of the questions listed on your Diagnosis Checklist (Step 3). This is the time to confirm that you are indeed a candidate for this trial, although a final decision will likely await your first appointment with the clinical trial team (Step 10).

3. *Why do researchers think the new treatment might be effective?* Results from earlier clinical trials will highlight the potential effectiveness of the treatment you may receive. The strength of the earlier evidence may influence your decision. You or someone who knows how to read the medical literature may also want to use a web-based service such as PubMed to explore any

previously published evidence related to the trial you're interested in.

4. *What are the risks and benefits associated with the treatments I may receive?* Every treatment has risks. Be sure you understand what risks and side-effects are associated with any of the treatments you might receive as a participant in this trial. Likewise, ask for a detailed description of how the treatments may benefit you.

5. *Who will monitor my care and safety?* Primary responsibility for the care and safety of patients in a cancer clinical trial rests with the clinical trial health care team. In addition, clinical trials are governed by safety and ethical regulations set by the federal government and the institution or organization sponsoring and carrying out the trial, including a group called the Institutional Review Board (IRB). The trial coordinator will be able to give you more information.

6. *May I get a copy of the protocol document?* In some cases, the trial coordinator may be allowed to release the full, detailed protocol document to you. However, the protocol summary and the informed consent document will probably answer most of your questions about the trial's design and intention.

7. *May I get a copy of the informed consent document?* The U.S. Food and Drug Administration requires that potential participants receive complete information about the study. This process is known as "informed consent" and must be in writing. It may be helpful to see a copy of this document before you decide whether or not to join the trial.

8. *Is there a chance I will receive a placebo?* Placebos are rarely used in cancer treatment trials, but be sure you understand what possible treatments you may or may not receive for any trial you are thinking of joining.

9. *Is the trial randomized?* In a randomized clinical trial, participants are assigned, by chance, to separate groups or "arms." Each arm receives a different treatment, and the results are compared. In a randomized trial, you may or may not receive the new treatment.

10. *What is the treatment dose and schedule in each arm of the trial?* You will want to consider this when you are discussing your various treatment options with your health care team.

Does the dose seem reasonable? Is the treatment schedule manageable for you?

11. *What costs will I be responsible for?* In many cases, the research costs are paid by the group sponsoring the trial. Research costs include the treatments under study and any test performed purely for research purposes. However, you or your insurance plan would be responsible for paying "routine patient care costs." These are the costs of medical care (for example, doctor visits, hospital stays, x-rays) that you would receive whether or not you were in a clinical trial. Some insurance plans don't cover these costs once you join a trial. Consult your health plan, if you have one, or go to http://www.cancer.gov/clinicaltrials/ learning/laws-about-clinical-trial-costs to see if your plan must provide such coverage.

12. *If I have to travel, who will pay for travel and lodging?* Some trials may pay for your travel and lodging expenses. Otherwise, you will be responsible for these costs.

13. *Will participation in this trial require more time than if I had elected to receive standard care? Will participation require a hospital stay?* Understanding how much time is involved may influence your decision and help you make plans.

14. *How will participating in the clinical trial affect my everyday life?* A cancer diagnosis can be very disrupting to the routine of everyday life. Many patients seek to keep those routines intact as they deal with their diagnosis and treatment. This information will be useful in evaluating any additional help you may need at home.

Step 9: Discuss Your Options with Your Doctor

To make a final decision, you will want to know the possible risks and benefits of all the various treatment options open to you. You may decide that joining a trial for which you are eligible is your best option, or you may decide not to join a trial. It is your choice.

Step 10: If You Want to Join a Trial, Schedule an Appointment

If you decide to participate in a clinical trial for which you are eligible, schedule an appointment with the trial coordinator you spoke to during Step 8.

You might also want your doctor to contact the study's principal investigator to further discuss your medical history and overall current state of your health. The principal investigator's name should be listed in the protocol summary.

Your doctor might disagree with your decision to participate in a clinical trial. If so, be sure you understand his or her concerns. You also may wish to seek a second opinion about your treatment options at this time. Ultimately, it is up to you to decide what treatment is in your best interest.

Part Seven

Moving Forward

Chapter 49

Your Feelings:
Coping and Support

Cancer Will Change Your Life

Cancer is a major illness, but not everyone who gets cancer will die from it. Close to nine million Americans alive today have a history of cancer. For them, cancer has become a chronic (on-going) health problem, like high blood pressure or diabetes.

Just like anyone with a chronic health problem, people who have cancer must get regular checkups for the rest of their lives, even after cancer treatment ends. But unlike other chronic health problems, if you have cancer you probably will not need to take medicine or eat special foods once you have finished treatment.

If you have cancer, you may notice every ache, pain, or sign of illness. Even little aches may make you worry. While it is normal to think about dying and healthy to explore your feelings about death, it is also important to focus on living. Keep in mind that cancer is not a death sentence. Many people with cancer are treated successfully. Others will live a long time before dying from cancer. So, make the most of each day while living with cancer and its treatment.

Your Feelings: Learning You Have Cancer

You will have many feelings after you learn that you have cancer. These feelings can change from day to day, hour to hour, or even

Excerpted from "Taking Time: Support for People with Cancer," National Cancer Institute (www.cancer.gov), 2006.

minute to minute. Some of the feelings you may go through include the following:

- Denial
- Anger
- Fear
- Stress
- Anxiety
- Depression
- Sadness
- Guilt
- Loneliness

All these feelings are normal.

Feeling hopeful is also normal. No one is cheerful all the time, but while you are dealing with cancer, hope can be an important part of your life.

Denial

When you were first diagnosed, you may have had trouble believing or accepting the fact that you have cancer. This is called denial. Denial can be helpful because it can give you time to adjust to your diagnosis. Denial can also give you time to feel hopeful and better about the future.

Sometimes, denial is a serious problem. If it lasts too long, it can keep you from getting the treatment you need. It can also be a problem when other people deny that you have cancer, even after you have accepted it.

The good news is that most people (those with cancer as well as those they love and care about) work through denial. By the time treatment begins, most people accept the fact that they have cancer.

Anger

Once you accept that you have cancer, you may feel angry and scared. It is normal to ask "Why me?" and be angry.

Anger sometimes comes from feelings that are hard to show—such as fear, panic, frustration, anxiety, or helplessness. If you feel angry, don't pretend that everything is okay. Talk with your family and friends about your anger. Most of the time, talking will help you feel a lot better.

Fear and Worry

It's scary to hear that you have cancer. You may be afraid or worried about being in pain, either from the cancer or the treatment, feeling sick or looking different as a result of your treatment, taking care of your family, paying your bills, keeping your job, or dying.

Your family and close friends may also worry about seeing you upset or in pain, not giving you enough support, love, and understanding, or living without you.

Some fears about cancer are based on stories, rumors, and old information. Most people feel better when they know what to expect. They feel less afraid when they learn about cancer and its treatment.

Stress

Your body may react to the stress and worry of having cancer. You may notice that your heart beats faster; you have headaches or muscle pains; you don't feel like eating; you feel sick to your stomach or have diarrhea; you feel shaky, weak, or dizzy; you have a tight feeling in your throat and chest; or you sleep too much or too little. Stress can also keep your body from fighting disease as well as it should.

You can learn to handle stress in many ways, like exercising; listening to music; reading books, poems, or magazines; getting involved in hobbies such as music or crafts; relaxing or meditating, such as lying down and slowly breathing in and out; or talking about your feelings with family and close friends.

If you are concerned about stress, talk to your doctor or nurse. He or she may be able to help you by referring you to a counselor or support group. You may also join a class that teaches people ways of dealing with stress. The key is to find ways to control stress and not to let it control you.

Pain

Even though almost everyone worries about pain, it may not be a problem for you. Some people do not have any pain. Others have pain only once in a while. Cancer pain can almost always be relieved. If you are in pain, your doctor can suggest ways to help you feel better.

There is no reason for you to be bothered with pain. There are many ways to control pain. Your doctor wants and needs to hear about your pain. As soon as you have pain you should speak up. Dealing with your pain can also help you deal with the feelings discussed in this chapter.

Control and Self-Esteem

When you first learn that you have cancer, you may feel as if your life is out of control.

Even though you may feel out of control, there are ways you can be in charge. For example, you can learn as much as you can about your cancer. You can ask questions. Let your health providers know when you don't understand what they are saying, or when you want more information about something. You can look beyond your cancer. Many people with cancer feel better when they stay busy. You may still go to work, even if you need to adjust your schedule. You can also take part in hobbies such as music, crafts, or reading.

Sadness and Depression

Many people with cancer feel sad or depressed. This is a normal response to any serious illness. When you're depressed, you may have very little energy, feel tired, or not want to eat.

Depression is sometimes a serious problem. If feelings of sadness and despair seem to take over your life, you may have clinical depression. Below are eight common signs of depression. Let your health provider know if you have one or more of these signs almost every day.

Early Signs of Depression

- A feeling that you are helpless and hopeless, or that life has no meaning

- No interest in being with your family or friends

- No interest in the hobbies and activities you used to enjoy

- A loss of appetite, or no interest in food

- Crying for long periods of time, or many times each day

- Sleep problems, either sleeping too much or too little

- Changes in your energy level

- Thoughts of killing yourself. This includes making plans or taking action to kill yourself, as well as frequent thoughts about death and dying.

Depression can be treated. Your doctor may prescribe medication. He or she may also suggest that you talk about your feelings with a counselor or join a support group with others who have cancer.

Guilt

Many people with cancer feel guilty. For example, you may blame yourself for upsetting the people you love. You may worry that you are a burden to others, either emotionally or financially. Or you may envy other people's good health and be ashamed of this feeling. You might even blame yourself for lifestyle choices that could have led to your cancer. For example, that lying out in the sun caused your skin cancer or that smoking cigarettes led to your lung cancer. These feelings are all normal for people with cancer.

Your family and friends may also feel guilty because they are healthy while you are ill, they can't help you as much as they want, or they feel stressed and impatient. They may also want to be perfect and feel guilty when they cannot give you all the care and understanding you need.

Counseling and support groups can help with these feelings of guilt. Let your doctor or nurse know if you, or someone in your family, would like to talk with a counselor or go to a support group.

Loneliness

People with cancer often feel lonely or distant from others. You may find that your friends have a hard time dealing with your cancer and may not visit. Some people might not even be able to call you on the phone. You may feel too sick to take part in the hobbies and activities you used to enjoy. And sometimes, even when you are with people you love and care about, you may feel that no one understands what you are going through.

You may feel less lonely when you meet other people who have cancer. Many people feel better when they join a support group and talk with others who are facing the same challenges.

Not everyone wants or is able to join a support group. Some people prefer to talk with just one person at a time. You may feel better talking to a close friend or family member, someone from your own religion, or a counselor.

Hope

Once people accept that they have cancer, they often feel a sense of hope. There are many reasons to feel hopeful.

- Cancer treatment can be successful. Millions of people who have had cancer are alive today.

- People with cancer can lead active lives, even during treatment.

- Your chances of living with—and living beyond—cancer are better now than they have ever been before. People often live for many years after their cancer treatment is over.

Some doctors think that hope may help your body deal with cancer. Scientists are looking at the question of whether a hopeful outlook and positive attitude helps people feel better.

You may find hope in nature, or your religious or spiritual beliefs. Or you may find hope in stories about people with cancer who are leading active lives.

Sharing Your Feelings about Cancer

Talking about your feelings can help you deal with your cancer. Cancer is too much to handle all by yourself.

Finding a Good Listener

It can be hard to talk about how it feels to have cancer. But talking can help, even though it is hard to do. Many people find that they feel better when they share their thoughts and feelings with their close family and friends.

Friends and family members may not always know what to say to you. Sometimes they can help by just being good listeners. They don't always need to give you advice or tell you what they think. They simply need to show that they care and are concerned about you.

You might find it helpful to talk about your feelings with people who are not family or friends. Instead, you might want to meet in a support group with others who have cancer or talk with a counselor.

Choosing a Good Time to Talk

Some people need time before they can talk about their feelings. If you are not ready, you might say, "I don't feel like talking about my cancer right now." And sometimes when you want to talk, your family and friends may not be ready to listen.

It is hard for other people to know when to talk about cancer. Sometimes people send a signal when they want to talk. They might bring up the subject of cancer; talk about things that have to do with cancer, such as a newspaper story about a new cancer treatment that they just read; spend more time with you; or act nervous or make jokes that aren't very funny.

You can help people feel more comfortable by asking them what they think or how they feel. Sometimes people can't put their feelings into words. Sometimes, they just want to hug each other or cry together.

Expressing Anger

Many people feel angry or frustrated when they deal with cancer. You might find that you get mad or upset with the people you depend on. You may get upset with small things that never bothered you before.

People can't always express their feelings. Anger sometimes shows up as actions instead of words. You may find that you yell a lot at the kids or the dog. You might slam doors.

Try to figure out why you are angry. Maybe you are afraid of the cancer or are worried about money. You might even be angry about your treatment.

Pretending to Be Cheerful

Some people pretend to be cheerful, even when they are not. They think that they will not feel sad or angry when they act cheerful. Your family and friends may not want to upset you and will act as if nothing is bothering them. You may think that by being cheerful, your cancer will go away.

When you have cancer, you have many reasons to be upset. "Down days" are to be expected. Don't pretend to be cheerful when you're not. This can keep you from getting the help you need. Be honest and talk about all your feelings, not just the cheerful ones.

Sharing without Talking

For many, it's hard to talk about being sick. Others feel that cancer is a personal or private matter and find it hard to talk openly about it. If talking is hard for you, think about other ways to share your feelings. For instance, you may find it helpful to write about your feelings. This might be a good time to start a journal or diary if you don't already have one. Writing about your feelings is a good way to sort through them and a good way to begin to deal with them.

Journals can be personal or shared. People can use a journal as a way of 'talking' to each other. If you find it hard to talk to someone near to you about your cancer try starting a shared journal.

If you have e-mail, this can also be a good way to share without talking.

People Helping People

Even though your needs are greater when you have cancer, it can be hard to ask for help to meet those needs. To get the help you need, think about turning to family and friends, others who also have cancer, people you meet in support groups, people from your spiritual or religious community, health care providers, or caregivers.

No one needs to face cancer alone. When people with cancer seek and receive help from others, they often find it easier to cope.

You may find it hard to ask for or accept help. After all, you are used to taking care of yourself. Maybe you think that asking for help is a sign of weakness. Or perhaps you do not want to let others know that some things are hard for you to do. All these feelings are normal.

People feel good when they help others. Your friends may not know what to say or how to act when they are with you. Some people may even avoid you. But they may feel more at ease when you ask them to cook a meal or pick up your children after school. There are many ways that family, friends, other people who have cancer, spiritual or religious leaders, and health care providers can help. In turn, there are also ways you can help and support your caregivers.

Family and Friends

Family and friends can support you in many ways. But, they may wait for you to give them hints or ideas about what to do. Someone who is not sure if you want company may call "just to see how things are going." When someone says, "Let me know if there is anything I can do," tell this person if you need help with an errand or a ride to the doctor's office.

Family members and friends can also keep you company, give you a hug, or hold your hand; listen as you talk about your hopes and fears; help with rides, meals, errands, or household chores; go with you to doctor's visits or treatment sessions; and tell other friends and family members ways they can help.

Other People Who Have Cancer

Even though your family and friends help, you may also want to meet people who have cancer now or have had it in the past. Often, you can talk with them about things you can't discuss with others.

People with cancer understand how you feel and can talk with you about what to expect, tell you how they cope with cancer and live a normal life, help you learn ways to enjoy each day, and give you hope for the future.

Let your doctor or nurse know that you want to meet other people with cancer. You can also meet other people with cancer in the hospital, at your doctor's office, or through a cancer support group.

Support Groups

Cancer support groups are meetings for people with cancer and those touched by cancer. These groups allow you and your loved ones to talk with others facing the same problems. Support groups often have a lecture as well as time to talk. Almost all groups have a leader who runs the meeting. The leader can be someone with cancer or a trained counselor.

You may think that a support group is not right for you. Maybe you think that a group won't help or that you don't want to talk with others about your feelings. Or perhaps you are afraid that the meetings will make you sad or depressed.

It may be good to know that many people find support groups very helpful. People in the groups often talk about what it's like to have cancer; help each other feel better, more hopeful, and not so alone; learn about what's new in cancer treatment; and share tips about ways to cope with cancer.

Spiritual Help

Spirituality means the way you look at the world and make sense of your place in it. Spirituality can include faith or religion, beliefs, values, and "reasons for being."

Most people are spiritual in some way, whether or not they go to a church, temple, or mosque.

Cancer can affect people's spirituality. Some people find that cancer brings a new or deeper meaning to their faith. Others feel that their faith has let them down.

Many people find that their faith is a source of comfort. They find they can cope better with cancer when they pray, read religious books, meditate, or talk with members of their spiritual community.

Many people also find that cancer changes their values. The things you own and your daily duties may seem less important. You may decide to spend more time with loved ones, helping others, doing things in the outdoors, or learning about something new.

People in Health Care

Most cancer patients have a treatment team of health providers who work together to help them. This team may include doctors, nurses, social workers, pharmacists, dietitians, and other people in health care. Chances are that you will never see all these people at the same time. In fact, there may be health providers on your team who you never meet.

Doctors: Most people with cancer have two or more doctors. Chances are you will see one doctor most often. This person is the leader of your team. He or she not only meets with you but also works with all the other people on your treatment team.

Make sure to let your doctor know how you are feeling. Tell him or her when you feel sick, are depressed, or in pain.

Ask your doctor how often he or she will see you, when you will have tests, and how long before you know if the treatment is working.

Nurses: Most likely, you will see nurses more often than other people on your treatment team. If you are in the hospital, nurses will check in on you many times a day. If you are at home, visiting nurses may come to your house and help with your treatment and care. Nurses also work in clinics and doctor offices.

You can talk with nurses about your day-to-day concerns. They can tell you what to expect, such as if a certain drug is likely to make you feel sick. You can also talk with nurses about what worries you. They can offer hope, support, and suggest ways to talk with family and friends about your feelings.

Nurses work with all the other health providers on your treatment team. Let them know if you need or want more help.

Pharmacists: Pharmacists not only fill prescriptions but also can teach you about the drugs you are taking. They can help you by talking with you about how your drugs work; telling you how often to take your drugs; teaching you about side effects and how to deal with them; warning you about the danger of mixing drugs together; and letting you know about foods you shouldn't eat or things you shouldn't do, like being in the sun for too long.

Dietitians: People with cancer often have trouble eating or digesting food. Eating problems can be a side effect from cancer drugs or treatments. They can also happen when people are so upset that they lose their appetite and don't feel like eating.

Dietitians can help by teaching you about foods that are healthy, taste good, and are easy to eat. They can also suggest ways to make eating easier, such as using plastic forks or spoons so food doesn't taste like metal when you are having chemo. Ask your doctor or nurse to refer you to a dietitian who knows about the special needs of cancer patients.

Social Workers: Social workers assist patients and families with meeting their daily needs such as the following tasks:

- Finding support groups near where you live
- Dealing with money matters, like paying the bills
- Talking about your cancer with your boss
- Filling out paperwork, such as advance directives or living wills
- Talking about your cancer with your family and other loved ones
- Dealing with your feelings such as depression, sadness, or grief
- Coping with stress and learning new ways to relax
- Learning about health insurance, such as what your policy covers and what it does not
- Finding rides to the hospital, clinic, or doctor's office
- Setting up visits from home health nurses

Patient educators: Patient or health educators can help you learn more about your cancer. They can find information that fits your needs. Patient educators are also experts in explaining things that may be hard to understand. Many hospitals and treatment centers have resource centers run by health educators. These centers contain books, videos, computers, and other tools to help you and your family. These tools can help you understand your type of cancer, your treatment choices, side effects, and tips for living with and beyond your cancer. Ask your doctor or nurse about talking to a patient educator.

Psychologists: Most people are very upset when they face a serious illness such as cancer. Psychologists can help by talking with you and your family about your worries. They can not only help you figure out what upsets you but also teach you ways to cope with these feelings and concerns.

Let your doctor or nurse know if you want to talk with a psychologist who is trained to help people with cancer.

Psychiatrists: Sometimes people with cancer are depressed or have other psychiatric (mental health) disorders. Psychiatrists are medical doctors who can prescribe drugs for these disorders. They can also talk with you about your feelings and help you find the mental health services you need.

Let your doctor know if you feel like you need to meet with a psychiatrist.

Licensed counselors and other mental health professionals: Licensed counselors, pastoral care professionals, spiritual leaders, nurse practitioners, and other mental health professionals also help people deal with their feelings, worries, and concerns. Talk with your doctor or contact your local cancer center to find mental health professionals near you.

People in the Hospital

Many hospitals have people on staff to help make your stay a little easier.

Patient advocates can help when you have a problem or concern that you don't feel you can discuss with your doctor, nurse, or social worker. They can act as a bridge between you and your health care team.

Discharge planners work with you and your family to help you get ready to leave the hospital. The discharge planner helps with tasks like making follow-up appointments and making sure you have things you need at home.

Volunteers often visit with patients in the hospital and offer comfort and support. They may also bring books, puzzles, or other things to do. Many volunteers have had cancer themselves. Let a hospital staff member know if you want to meet with a volunteer.

Caregivers

Caregivers are the people who help with your daily tasks such as bathing, getting dressed, or eating. Caregivers are often family members or close friends. Just like you, your caregivers need help and support. There are several ways to help your caregiver:

- **Building a team:** Build a team of caregivers so that you don't have to depend on just one person.

- **Keeping your caregivers informed:** Make sure your caregivers know about your treatment and care. Ask your doctor or nurse to talk with the person who helps you the most.

- **Finding extra help:** Many towns have community volunteers. These people offer help to others near where they live or work. Some towns also have services such as respite care, home care, and hospice.

- **Doing what you can to help your caregiver:** Encourage your caregivers to take time off so they can do errands, enjoy hobbies, or simply have a rest.

- **Showing your caregiver that you care:** Remember to say "thank you." Let your caregivers know that you value their help, support, and love.

Chapter 50

Talking with Family, Friends, and Children about Breast Cancer

Talking with Family and Friends

Telling people you have cancer will relieve you of the burden of inventing explanations, or being on guard against discovery of your illness. You may find unexpected sources of support and understanding from others, including people who have struggled with a life-threatening illness.

Here are ten suggestions on communicating with your friends and family:

- Be honest and direct. Give clear guidelines about what others can do to help you.

- Don't assume people know what you need, or what the "right" thing to do is.

- If you don't feel like company, say that you appreciate their concern but would much rather they visit you at another time, when you feel better.

- Some people are better at coping with a crisis than others. Most people truly care, but don't know what to say or do. Accept their limitations.

"Talking with Family and Friends" and "How to Talk with Your Children," © 2008 Breast Cancer Network of Strength. Reprinted with permission. For additional information about Breast Cancer Network of Strength, visit www.networkofstrength.org.

- If you just need to be with someone or want them to just listen to you, tell them so. Explain to them that you don't expect answers or solutions; you just want them to listen to your concerns.

- Coping with breast cancer may reveal long-standing problems in a relationship, like poor communication or lack of trust—problems clearly not caused by cancer. Recognizing this may allow you to let go of old behaviors and patterns while identifying ongoing stressful relationships.

- Even thoughtful family and friends may be impatient for you to "get over" your experience. You have survived an ordeal—do not let their expectations pressure you to ignore your feelings.

- Give yourself permission to explore ways to enhance your health and self-esteem. Focus on building a stronger sense of self and purpose to survive your treatments.

- You can become preoccupied with the cancer so much that certain feelings linger and you may become stuck in the process of emotional healing. Get assistance from a support group or therapist to help you move forward.

- While it is not your responsibility to take care of others' feelings, understand that they, too, are trying to cope.

How to Talk to Your Children

Parents find it very difficult to tell their children about cancer. There are a couple of basic guidelines that can help parents discuss their cancer diagnosis with their children. However, the type of discussion you have with your children will depend on their ages.

Children of any age can sense when something is wrong and they usually imagine the worst possible problem. Telling them what is going on can actually alleviate some anxiety and fear that they may be feeling. It is important to answer only the questions your children ask and nothing more. Children, especially between the ages of six to 10, can only handle little bits of information at a time. As they ask for more detail you can provide it to them, but try to focus on what their concerns are for the moment.

Answer your children's questions as honestly as possible. An environment of honesty and openness can help children deal with the crisis that results when a parent is diagnosed with cancer.

Up to Two Years Old

For small children, their biggest concern comes from the disruption of their daily routine. They do not understand the concept of cancer, but will be disturbed if their parent is away for several days, or is too tired to play. Establish a new routine as soon as possible, one that can accommodate your recovery and treatment needs. Ask for help from friends and family to give them extra attention and love.

Ages Two to Seven Years

For younger children, it is very common that they assume they might be responsible for you getting cancer. For instance, they may think that because they got in trouble at school you got cancer. Use simple terms to explain your illness, like "good" and "bad" cells. Remind your children often that cancer is not something you catch and that they did not do anything to cause your cancer.

Try to explain the treatments and procedures that you will have in terms of how it will affect them and their routine. For instance, "I will be having chemotherapy next week, and it will make me very tired. I won't be able to drive you to school then, but Susie's mother will come to our house to pick you up at your regular time." Or, "When I have the medicine that will remove my cancer cells, my hair will fall out and you will see me without any hair. Sometimes I will wear a hat or a wig to keep me warm and comfortable. My hair will grow back."

Ages Seven to 12 Years

School-aged children will understand more about the causes and effects of a serious illness, but you should still keep your explanations simple. They may hesitate to bring up a concern or a fear they have because they are afraid of burdening the parent who is facing cancer. It is good to ask them once a week how things are going and how they are feeling. By encouraging them to verbalize their concerns, you are teaching them how to handle crisis in a positive way, and you will also have a sense of how your child is coping.

Be sure to watch for changes in school performance, as well as eating and sleeping patterns. Any changes may be an indicator that your child is worried and unable to verbalize his or her feelings.

Ages 12 and Older

Children at this age can understand most aspects of breast cancer causes and treatments. You should spend time listening to their concerns and trying to help them get the best information to answer their questions. Older teenagers may want to know detailed information about breast cancer and may want to do their own research about the illness. Others may want to rely only on what you tell them.

Each child may respond differently to their parent's illness. Some may get angry and distant. Others may feel insecure and scared. If they are having a hard time talking to you, encourage them to talk with other members of the family, or to a teacher or friend.

Just like you, children will have to react to the wide-range of emotions that occur when cancer invades a family. Fear, sadness, insecurity, anger, and curiosity are just some of the feelings they will have. Keep talking to and with them. Try to plan activities for the whole family on a regular basis. Most importantly, try to give them extra love and attention—it will benefit everyone.

Chapter 51

Questions Women with Breast Cancer Frequently Ask about Health Insurance

From past experience myself as well as having talked with many breast cancer patients, there are some key questions that arise related to health insurance coverage that might be helpful for you to know. Concerns about what your health insurance does and doesn't cover can add unnecessary anxiety and worry to you at a time that you don't need it. By being proactive you can contact your insurance company and get information up front about what they do and don't cover. This information below will also help advise you how to optimize the coverage you do have.

Will my insurance company cover my mastectomy/ lumpectomy surgery if I am an inpatient?

Most insurance companies, including managed care organizations, will cover an overnight stay. However there has been a trend toward outpatient surgery unless you are having reconstruction done at the same time or you have other medical conditions warranting hospitalization.

"Questions Women with Breast Cancer Frequently Ask about Health Insurance Benefits," by Lillie Shockney, RN, BS, MAS, University Distinguished Service Assistant Professor of Breast Cancer, Administrative Director, Johns Hopkins Breast Center, Assistant Professor, Department of Surgery and Department of Obstetrics and Gynecology, Johns Hopkins University School of Medicine. © 2008 Johns Hopkins Avon Foundation Breast Center (www .hopkinsbreastcenter.org). All rights reserved. Reprinted with permission.

Depending in what state you live, there might be specific legislature related to ensuring coverage for overnight stays as well. The need to be an inpatient or an ambulatory surgery patient should be decided by you with input from your surgeon. Discuss this with your surgeon first then talk with your insurance company if you are planning to be hospitalized. (Johns Hopkins makes it the patient's choice to be an inpatient or outpatient for mastectomy surgery without reconstruction based on input from her surgeon. We are strong advocates that only hospitals who have developed comprehensive patient education programs which are conducted in advance of the patient's surgery should be performing mastectomies on an outpatient basis. We know from experience however that patients prefer going home the day of surgery 71% of the time and do very well. They score us high on patient satisfaction surveys and feel confident that they made the right choice in electing to have their surgery performed on an outpatient basis. It requires a commitment of time, effort, and resources to develop a program that works well however. Not many facilities have invested this time and energy unfortunately. So ask your doctor how many patients have been done on an outpatient basis if he is considering recommending to you to have your surgery done in this way. Pressure from insurance carriers should not dictate whether you are done on an inpatient or outpatient basis. Decisions about this must rest with you and your doctor.)

I don't know if I want to have reconstruction yet. Will it still be covered if I choose to wait until a later time, or is it only covered if done as part of my breast cancer surgery now? Will my insurance cover any type of reconstruction, such as tram flap, saline implant, or dorsal flap?

Most insurance companies will cover reconstruction of all types, but check to see if they place a time limit when you can have it done. There is active legislature now (September 1997 [see Chapter 30 for more information about your rights under the Women's Health and Cancer Rights Act of 1998]) which, if passed, will require that all insurance companies cover reconstruction of all types for an unlimited length of time after the initial mastectomy surgery. Presently, there are some insurance companies who require that the reconstruction be done within one year of the initial mastectomy surgery, if it is to be a covered benefit.

I've decided not to have reconstruction. I'd prefer to wear a breast prosthesis. How expensive are they, and how much will my insurance cover?

This is a tricky question. Breast prostheses range in price from $50 (made of cloth with tiny pillows for fillers inside) to $1400 (made of silicone and created from a mold of the other breast), with the standard prosthesis costing about $350. Silicone prostheses usually come with a two year warranty. There are also breast prostheses designed for swimming; these range in price from $15 to $40. If an insurance company only covers one prosthesis, make sure you submit the sales receipt of the permanent silicone breast prosthesis to your insurance company, not the receipt of the swimmer's prosthesis or a less expensive model such as the cloth prosthesis. Since the insurance company will only cover one you need to submit the more expensive one to them, otherwise you will be stuck with a large bill and they will have technically paid for a prosthesis even if it is a swimmer's model or cloth model. This can result in serious financial hardship which is avoidable if you know how to submit your insurance bills up front. Also make sure you get a prescription from your surgeon ordering that you be fitted for a breast prosthesis as well as mastectomy bra. Without the prescription you will probably have trouble getting fitted and definitely trouble getting your insurance company to pay the bill. Most insurance companies pay 80%–100% of the bill for prostheses. Some companies are rigid and only cover the purchase of one prosthesis for a lifetime. This is an important benefit to ask about. Other companies will cover reimbursement for a prosthesis every two years.

What happens if my body changes in size and my prosthesis no longer fits properly? Can I get a replacement, and is it covered by my insurance?

Most insurance companies will cover replacements for this reason, provided there is a prescription from a doctor stating the reason for the replacement.

Can I go anywhere to get a breast prosthesis, or are there only certain locations approved for me to go?

Most insurance companies will let a patient go anywhere she chooses. It is wise to choose a store that employs certified fitters who are specially trained to fit women for breast prostheses. Being fitted for a mastectomy bra and/or breast prosthesis is very intimidating, and can be degrading if not done by a highly professional staff dedicated to making the experience a nonstressful one. Ask the health care professionals if they have a list of stores who they recommend and who have certified fitters there. You will probably find that many of the mastectomy supply shops are owned by women who have had breast cancer themselves. These women have chosen to help others like you and I. These women know how you feel because they've been there themselves. Feel free to ask when you call to make a fitting appointment if any of the fitters are breast cancer survivors.

Are mastectomy bras covered by my insurance, and if so, how many will they cover per year?

There is some variance among insurance companies about this particular benefit. Most insurers will cover two bras a year, provided they are accompanied with a prescription from a doctor. During the month of October, National Breast Cancer Awareness Month, many mastectomy supply shops have sales on their mastectomy supply items. This is especially important if your insurance company doesn't cover reimbursement for mastectomy bras beyond the initial coverage of two bras. Bras are expensive and take advantage of sales! (Mastectomy bathing suits, by the way, are not covered by insurance companies. These items are almost always on sale around Labor Day.)

I've been told I might need chemotherapy. Is it covered by my insurance? What if I choose to participate in a clinical trial? What drugs are and aren't covered?

This varies from company to company. Call and ask them specific questions. It is best to also ask the oncologist if a research grant will cover any drug and treatment costs if you do participate in a clinical trial. There is a positive trend developing now, which is good news, of insurance companies covering health expenses related to clinical trial participation.

I might need radiation therapy. Is this covered by my insurance?

Check to see what sites are covered for radiation therapy. Sometimes patients assume they will receive all medical care at the place they were diagnosed and initially treated, and are later surprised to discover that the site for radiation treatment is in a different location and will be provided by health care professionals who are not part of the patient's original treatment team. If this is the case, you need to know up front to prevent anxiety about it later.

Based on my understanding of the type of chemotherapy I'll be receiving, I might lose my hair. Will my insurance company cover the cost of a wig? How soon can I get one? Does my hair have to be completely gone in order to get one?

Many companies do cover this expense. However, it might require sending a letter to the insurance company from your doctor. If they don't cover it, check with the American Cancer Society or with the breast center where you are being treated; they might have access to wigs for you if this is a financial burden for you. There are various organizations and hospitals who have a supply for "recycling" to newly diagnosed patients who are in need of such an item. It is advisable to be fitted for a wig before you begin to lose your hair. This way, the wig will be easily matched to your hair color and hair style.

My doctor plans to do my procedure (mastectomy or lumpectomy with axillary node removal) as an outpatient procedure. Arrangements are going to be made by the breast center for a home health nurse to come to my home the night of my surgery and the next day. Is this expense covered by insurance?

Most insurance companies do cover home health care following this type of surgery. They usually cover two visits and there must be extenuating medical circumstances to warrant approval of additional visits. There are special forms that the doctor or nurse fill out for the insurance company and for the home health nurse to help assist with ensuring coverage. Insurance companies usually contract with specific home health care agencies too. Ideally the home health nurse caring for you is familiar with out patient mastectomy care. (Johns Hopkins has trained home health care nurses specifically for this purpose to ensure they know what is expected of them when conducting a home health visit. This better ensures continuity of care for you.)

I might be switching insurance companies in the middle of my treatment. Will my new insurance company cover the continuation of my current cancer treatments?

If at all possible it is best not to switch insurance companies in the midst of treatment. There can be serious problems with insurance coverage for continuation of your breast cancer care. If you are leaving your present place of employment you might want to strongly consider continuing your current insurance coverage by paying the monthly premiums yourself at least until your treatments are completed. You should also check with your new insurance company about their policies regarding "pre-existing conditions." Some companies picking you up as a new member will continue your coverage for breast cancer treatment and others may not for a specified period of time.

What can I do to influence changes in insurance coverage if I think that my insurance company is being unreasonable about my treatment benefits?

First talk with the member relations manager for your insurance company to see if you can come to some agreement about what is reasonable coverage and what is not. If you are unsuccessful in getting satisfactory help, you may need your doctor to write a letter on your behalf explaining the medical need for certain treatments and such. If the problem is one related to your insurance company not providing a specific benefit at all or a limited benefit (for example, one prosthesis for a life time) you may want to write to your insurance commissioner or even contact your local congressman or senator who may be able to promote legislation requiring certain types of coverage for all women unrelated to the type of insurance they have.

Chapter 52

I'm Done with My Treatment: Now What?

Being diagnosed with breast cancer is a life altering experience. Though your surgical and medical treatment may be over, the effects of having been diagnosed and treated may continue for some time. After treatment your body is different. You have lost part or all of your breast(s). You've undergone lymph node surgery. You may have had chemotherapy, radiation, or both. Each phase of treatment unto itself is unique and how your body and mind coped with it during and after care is equally unique. It is common to have remaining concerns about your health and how to best move forward after treatment ends. There are some similarities about how women feel after treatment too and learning about these common reactions can help to prepare you for life after treatment. Your doctors, nurses, and other breast center team members want to see you well again. Defining wellness for each patient can be different. It is rare that anyone having had breast cancer feels physically or psychologically as they did before their diagnosis but all patients should look forward to being healthy again.

All breast cancer survivors live with concern about recurrence of breast cancer. This fear is usually the biggest worry of all. Women feel that their body has betrayed them and therefore it takes time to trust

"I'm Done with My Treatment: Now What?" by Lillie Shockney, RN, BS, MAS, University Distinguished Service Assistant Professor of Breast Cancer, Administrative Director, Johns Hopkins Breast Center, Assistant Professor, Department of Surgery and Department of Obstetrics and Gynecology, Johns Hopkins University School of Medicine. © 2008 Johns Hopkins Avon Foundation Breast Center (www.hopkinsbreastcenter.org). All rights reserved. Reprinted with permission.

it again. Learning how to cope with fears of recurrence is important so that you can make the most of your life and what it has to offer you and you offer to it. And though your body has gone through many changes as a result of the cancer diagnosis and treatment, you will more than likely find yourself healthy, strong, and optimistic once again.

Your body has been through physical changes. You may have a different silhouette than you had before. Depending on the type of breast surgery performed, you may have some potential physical restrictions related to reconstructive surgery or to having lymph nodes removed or both. You may be experiencing skin or breast changes as a result of radiation therapy. As a result of chemotherapy your hair may still be gone or just now starting to grow back. You may also be experiencing symptoms of menopause.

So why are family and friends saying to you now that you should be getting your life back to normal? Partly because they desperately want to see things in your life (and theirs) back to the way it was before your diagnosis of breast cancer. And perhaps so would you.

We can't rewind the clock however. This life altering experience can't be erased. So let's see how to begin a new life with a new definition of "normal" for you. It is not uncommon for women who have experienced breast cancer to find that this experience in the long run has made their life better and helped them to learn some valuable things about themselves and make their new life after treatment more fulfilling. Priorities are set differently going forward, relationships are strengthened, and what is important in life takes on a different meaning.

This section contains information to help you and your family adjust to your "new normal" and define how to cope with symptoms that linger after treatment, deal with fear of recurrence, and learn ways to adjust to other changes that your body may experience in the future, like menopause. We want to help you achieve that "new normal" so that you can enjoy living and feel confident again in trusting your body, making the most of each day, and gaining insight into how this breast cancer experience can result in a new beginning for you.

Recurrence and Follow-Up

Once the treatment for breast cancer is completed, patients enter a period of follow-up which remains ongoing for the rest of their lives. During follow-up, the major concern of patients and their doctors is further problems with breast cancer. You will also be watched for any long-term side effects from the treatment you received. These problems can take two forms. The original breast cancer can recur or a patient can develop a new breast cancer. It is important to distinguish these two because the prognosis is very different for each. The most serious form of recurrence is metastasis that develops when breast cancer spreads to other sites in the body. A second type of recurrence, which has a more favorable prognosis, is when breast cancer is detected at or near the original site in the breast in a patient who has had breast-conserving therapy.

Patients who have had one breast cancer are at higher-than-average risk for developing another breast cancer. The new breast cancer can develop in remaining breast tissue, including the conserved breast in a patient who has had breast-conserving therapy, or in the opposite breast.

Studies show that about 80% of breast cancer recurrences are detected by the patient herself either because she developed symptoms or she detected some physical abnormality. The second most common way in which recurrences are detected is by physical exam performed by a physician or other care provider or by mammogram at the time of the patient's annual breast x-ray. Only uncommonly do laboratory or radiology tests detect metastases in the absence of symptoms or physical abnormalities.

All breast cancer survivors are highly attuned to their bodies. They notice everything. Moreover, it is the norm for patients to worry that any symptom or physical abnormality is related to breast cancer. This is not the case. However, the anxiety about recurrence is so pervasive that it is hard for patients not to assume that symptoms or physical abnormalities are related to breast cancer. This anxiety tends to be greatest soon after diagnosis and initial treatment. It gradually subsides, but never fully goes away.

It's important to remember that breast cancer survivors are not immune to everyday aches and pains. However, breast cancer patients don't think of aches and pains as everyday. Symptoms that breast cancer patients would have ignored before their diagnosis are now taken ever so seriously. While it is important to pay attention to symptoms, it is also important not to assume the worst. Unless symptoms are very clearly in need of medical attention immediately, it is best to give them a week or two to see if they will go away on their own. Most symptoms and physical abnormalities go away on their own. Most will never be explained. Symptoms that are related to cancer do not go away. They may come and go initially, but eventually cancer-related symptoms persist and worse symptoms that wax and wane or come and go without worsening are very unlikely to related to cancer. If symptoms or physical findings do not go away or if they become more persistent or severe, it is suggested that they be brought to the attention of the physician.

Follow-up after diagnosis and initial treatment should include regularly scheduled visits with breast cancer doctors, special gynecologists, as well as mammography. It is important to point out that the recommendation against screening tests for distant recurrences does not apply to screening for new breast cancers or for a recurrence in the same breast following breast conservation treatment. Screening for new breast cancers is done by mammography. Screening mammography has been shown to improve survival. In other words screening mammograms can pick up cancers early enough that effective treatment can be instituted. Therefore, during post treatment follow-up, breast cancer survivors are encouraged to have routine screening mammography. Typically the uninvolved breast should be screened annually while a conserved breast should be screened every six months for the first one to two years and then annually.

Screening tests for metastases have not been shown to improve the outcome of patients. Therefore, they are not recommended. In other words, blood tests, including tumor or cancer markers, x-rays, and scans are not recommended on a routine basis in the absence of symptoms or abnormal physical findings. On the other hand, some or all of these tests are warranted in an attempt to explain symptoms or abnormal physical findings.

Patients are typically perplexed that blood tests, x-rays, and scans to search for asymptomatic metastases are not recommended. It is quite natural to believe that the outcome of treatment of metastases will be better if they are detected as early as possible. Unfortunately, this is currently not the case. Typically, screening tests for metastases will only pick up abnormalities a few weeks or months before they would cause symptoms and be otherwise detected. However, your chances of responding or benefiting from breast cancer treatment once it has metastasized are essentially the same regardless of when treatment is started. Two large clinical trials have shown that patients who have screening laboratory work for metastases do not have any better outcome or quality of life than patients who do not have these tests.

Research into more accurate ways to detect metastases is ongoing. At the same time, there is enormous effort underway to develop better treatments for metastatic breast cancer. It is hoped and expected that in the future there will be more effective screening tests and treatments for metastases. At that time, screening for metastases may become routine. Until then however, it is not recommended. More detailed information on follow-up recommendations after your initial diagnosis and treatment is available in the public area of the American Society of Clinical Oncology website (www.asco.org).

With regards to physician follow-up, it is important that patients follow-up with all of the physicians involved in their treatment. However, this follow-up should be done sequentially rather than in parallel. It is suggested that patients see one of their breast cancer doctors every three to six months during the first three years after diagnosis, then six to 12 months for the next two years, then annually. Your breast cancer team will help you in making these follow up appointments at the appropriate intervals. Thereafter, follow-up visits can be every six to 12 months. While patients will always need breast screening, they may not always need to have follow-up with the physicians who treated their breast cancer. After five or more years of follow-up, patients may be able to be followed by an internist, gynecologist, or primary care physician knowledgeable about the health issues of breast cancer survivors.

Coping with the Years That Lay Ahead

"There have certainly been times when I have felt greater uncertainty about my long-term survival than I have at other times. In each of the last three autumns, I have wondered whether to plant the tulip and daffodil bulbs for the spring bloom or not to bother. Now again this past spring, a glory of living color rewarded me, and once again I survive," *A Cancer Survivor's Almanac.*

The emotional response following the completion of treatment is demanding, just as it was during diagnosis and treatment. The most prevalent challenges include learning to live with uncertainty, fear of recurrence, sexuality concerns, and the impact on the family.

When someone is diagnosed with breast cancer they realize that life will never be the same and the expectations of the future are unknown. For most, this is a new realization of one's mortality and vulnerability. There may be feelings of anger, resentment frustration, and grief about the uncertainty. There is also the pervasive fear of a new cancer diagnosis and the worry that is created when experiencing a new symptom. Doctor's appointments and medical procedures may become anxiety-provoking events and adversely, patients also feel less secure when the need for medical observation and staff support diminishes.

There are skills patients can utilize to manage these fears. Use techniques to lower anxiety such as exercise, meditation, and/or relaxation. Educate yourself about available resources that deal with survivorship. Re-establish goals to live life one day at a time. Try and focus on the simple pleasures before taking on the big tasks. Allow

513

yourself to appreciate day to day accomplishments. Take this opportunity to deepen meaningful relationships. Give yourself permission to feel a range of emotions—it is ok to feel sad even after your treatment is over! Bring someone with you to future appointments... not only is it reassuring to have company but if you are anxious they will be able to hear information that you won't. Prepare your questions for your doctor or nurse before you come to the appointment. If you haven't already, join a support group. There's nothing more life affirming than meeting women who battled cancer years ago and are still having meaningful lives! If you need extra help don't be afraid to ask for professional counseling and/or spiritual guidance. Recovery takes different forms for everyone and sometimes people need assistance to get to their "new normal."

Many women experience loss of sense of self due to physical changes and energy level. It is quite normal for women to experience diminished sexual desire. You may have difficulty reestablishing intimacy with your partner and communicating your needs. This can be due to many factors including alterations to appearance, side effects of hormonal therapy, and fatigue. Don't be afraid to discuss sexual concerns with your medical team. They can give you information about resolving many problems such as loss of sexual desire and vaginal dryness. Your health care team can also assist you in seeing specialists who can help, if needed. It is also very important to communicate with your partner not only about your physical needs and changes but your emotional feelings about yourself.

You are probably not the only one experiencing new fears and concerns. Your family is also trying to adjust to your "new normal." There may be conflict between you and your loved ones as you continue to cope with the emotional impact of having cancer and they want you to move on. There may be new expectations and responsibilities for members of your family. They may stop talking about the cancer experience in an effort to move forward and protect you. There may also be a new fear for daughters and other family members regarding the genetic legacy of breast cancer.

It is important to communicate these common fears with the entire family as well as acknowledge that there will be differences in adjustment styles. Discuss your expectations and needs and let them discuss their needs as well. Communication is key for a healthy recovery. Discuss with your physicians the potential benefits of genetic counseling and/or medical follow-up, whenever appropriate, for your immediate relatives (siblings and children).

Try to recognize that there are positive influences from the cancer experience. You may experience a change in priorities and values towards a more meaningful life. Many have a growth in personal philosophy and spirituality. You have learned new coping skills to combat fear and uncertainty. It is important to remember that the personal triumph in survivorship requires approaching life in a day to day, week to week, and year to year process. This individual journey will help reestablish a sense of hope and certainty for your future.

Breast Cancer Survivors—The Other Medical Issues

Because most women will survive breast cancer, other aspects of their general medical care including immunizations, preventative medicine, and, especially, non-breast cancer screening are of utmost importance for their future health. While the different "consensus groups" (American College of Physicians, American Cancer Society, U.S. Preventative Service Task Force, etc.) may vary on the recommended age and frequency for cancer screening in the general population, there are some general guidelines to follow. Some women with a history of breast cancer are at slightly increased risk for colon, ovarian, or endometrial cancer and the minimum cancer screening for a breast cancer survivor should be very conservative. Because these are only guidelines, every woman should discuss her situation with her doctor.

Colon Cancer Screening

- Fecal occult blood testing done annually beginning at age fifty
- Baseline colonoscopy at age 50, then sigmoidoscopy every three to five years
- If high risk for colon cancer (familial syndromes), consider begin screening at an earlier age

Cervical Cancer Screening/Gynecologic Evaluation

- Papanicolaou (Pap) testing and pelvic exam should be performed yearly
- Any abnormal vaginal bleeding should be reported to your physician

Skin Cancer Screening/Prevention

- Regular skin self-examinations as instructed by the physician
- After age forty, annual skin exams by a physician

- Routine use of sunscreens and avoidance of excessive amounts of sun

Vaccinations and Other Concerns

In addition to cancer screening, every woman should remain updated on her vaccinations. Besides the childhood primary immunizations the following should be maintained:

- Tetanus toxoid: A booster shot every 10 years for all adults

- Pneumococcal vaccine: All adults over sixty-five or those that are immunocompromised

- Influenza vaccine: Given yearly

- Hepatitis B vaccination: Given to adults considered high risk (consult a physician)

- Varicella (chicken pox) vaccine: For adults with no history of chicken pox (not for the immunocompromised)

Finally, as part of the yearly visit to the physician, attention should be given to the following areas:

- Blood pressure, height, and weight checks

- Glucose (blood sugar) screening

- Cholesterol screening—beginning age 45

- Tobacco cessation (if applicable)

- Regular exercise (at least 30 minutes of aerobic exercise three or four times per week)

- Adequate calcium intake for osteoporosis prevention (calcium supplements will likely be needed if your diet is not rich in calcium)

- Maintain a low fat diet and limit consumption of red meat

Again, these are basic guidelines and every woman should discuss her past, present, and future health issues with her physician to tailor them to her individual needs.

Managing Fatigue: A Guide for Individuals with Cancer

Fatigue is an unpleasant feeling of weariness, tiredness, or lack of energy that interferes with everyday activities.

Everyone feels tired at certain times. However, individuals with cancer may feel excessively tired or fatigued any time during the day, even upon awakening, and it may not disappear with rest or sleep. Fatigue is the most common problem that occurs during cancer treatment and after treatment.

The cause of cancer treatment-related fatigue is not entirely clear. However, problems such as anemia, stress, insufficient diet, sleep disruption, as well as cancer treatments, and other factors are some of the causes. Treatments are available for anemia, nausea, vomiting, pain, depression, and other side effects from cancer. It is important to discuss your fatigue and other symptoms with your nurse or doctor.

You are not alone! Remember, it is normal and expected that persons with cancer will feel fatigued at some time. Although you should expect fatigue, you can learn to manage it, reduce your stress and feel more positive about your life!

Guidelines for Managing Fatigue

Conserving energy: You can do more be spreading your activities throughout the day. Take rest breaks between activities. Do not do more than you can manage and avoid heavy lifting. Save energy for the things you want to do. Let other people help. It will make your life easier and it will make others feel good.

Working outside the home: Talk to your supervisor and selected coworkers about your fatigue so that they can understand. If possible do some of your work at home so that you can pace yourself. Schedule the tasks that require attention and detail for energized times of the day. Trade duties if certain tasks are too fatiguing. Take a "sick day" from work when you are especially fatigued. Ease yourself back into work gradually when returning from sick leave.

Sleeping and resting: Create a soothing, restful setting for sleep. Set up regular bedtime and waking routines. Plan rest periods or short naps to restore your energy during the day. Arrange relaxing or enjoyable activities when you are trying to rest. If these suggestions are not helpful, please talk with your doctor or nurse about medications that can help you sleep better.

Keeping active: Include light exercise in your daily routine (but not too close to meals or bedtime). While getting enough rest is important, not enough activity can make you feel more tired! Plan periods of activity each day along with some rest periods. Include other people in your daily plans. A simple exercise program may help you feel better. For more information about beginning or continuing an exercise program, talk to your doctor or nurse. Remember some days are going to be easier than others. Pushing too hard and ignoring fatigue may slow the healing process.

Eating well: Eating a balanced diet during your treatment and recovery period will help you feel stronger. Eat small meals throughout the day instead of large meals. Choose foods high in protein and low in fat. Pay attention to your body. If nausea makes certain foods unappealing, then ask about appropriate food substitutes. Ask your doctor for a referral to a dietitian. Get help with food shopping and meal preparation.

Reducing stress: Many activities can reduce your level of stress and increase your ability to relax. Crafts, hobbies, and reading serve to relax and distract you from more stressful thoughts. Do fun things with your friends. Stay involved in some social activities. Music or warm baths can be soothing and relaxing. Commune with nature. A friend or family member may perform body message. Join a support group. Try relaxation tapes from the local library or bookstore. Meditation can lead to feelings of peacefulness. Keep a journal. Thinking positively by focusing on healing and recovery. Be patient with yourself. Reward yourself. Make long-term goals.

In summary: Remember, although fatigue is a common and expected problem for people with cancer... you can do something about it! If you need help, consult your doctor or nurse.

Chapter 53

Managing Holidays and Milestones after Breast Cancer

Kathi Hansen, a 51-year-old retired teacher from Wrightstown, Wisconsin, never felt much like celebrating her birthdays—until she was diagnosed with breast cancer in March 2003.

"While I never minded growing older and being reminded of that, it was not an event that I relished either," she recalls. "But after having cancer, my attitude toward my birthday became much more positive. I love the idea that I am here to celebrate another year of my life, and I am so pleased and proud of the fact. No black balloons or 'over the hill' banners for me!"

Lori Flagg, also 51, from Glendale, California, who was diagnosed with inflammatory breast cancer in April 2002, has a very different perspective.

"I used to feel like my birthday was very special," she says. "I looked forward to celebrating it for weeks ahead of time. Now I would rather it not be acknowledged. I just don't want a big to-do over it. I kind of feel that if I celebrate it, I'm jinxing myself."

Kathi and Lori's attitudes couldn't be more different. Yet they represent a trend among women who find that after a breast cancer diagnosis, birthdays and holidays take on new meanings, attitudes shift and in many cases new milestones emerge.

"Times to Celebrate, Times to Remember: Managing Milestones after Breast Cancer," by Debbie Lerman, reprinted with permission from the Winter 2005 issue of *Insight*, the quarterly newsletter of Living Beyond Breast Cancer, lbbc.org. All rights reserved.

Discussing this topic with women and healthcare professionals, a wide range of attitudes can be heard and much advice can be gathered for getting through the holidays—and other major life events—with your sanity intact, and perhaps a new appreciation of what is most meaningful to you.

Milestones during Treatment

For many women in treatment, milestones are understandably pushed aside in favor of the more urgent needs of getting through it all.

Cindi Gibbs, a 36-year-old elementary school teacher and administrator from Silver Spring, Maryland, looks forward to celebrating her birthday in March. "Last year, I was in the thick of treatment," she recalls, "so I didn't celebrate at all."

Not celebrating, or scaling back on elaborate, time-consuming preparations, is not necessarily a bad thing. But it can be hard to let go and accept help.

Lori used to have specific dates by which certain tasks had to be completed during the winter holidays. "Before I was diagnosed, I did this huge elaborate yard display," she says. "My house had to be the best in the neighborhood, and inside it had to be perfect."

Even when she was going through chemotherapy treatment, Lori forced herself to stick to that rigorous timetable: "I was very anxious because I wanted everyone to think I was normal, even though I didn't look or feel normal."

It took Lori several years to realize not only that she could let go, but also that she could enjoy not doing everything.

"At some point I had an epiphany and realized there's so much more to the celebrating than the gifts and lights and decorations," she says. "That epiphany relieved me of the nit-picky obsessiveness, and that's really, really nice. Now I know I am here to celebrate and be with my family, and that is the important part."

Lori's epiphany came several years after her diagnosis. According to Mary Jane Massie, MD, a psychiatrist at Memorial Sloan-Kettering Cancer Center, it takes most women a few years to let go of anxieties arising from diagnosis and find new ways of celebrating.

Linda Abrams, PhD, a psychologist from the Philadelphia area who had breast cancer, agrees. She says she finds that "sometimes it's after getting through treatment and the side effects of treatment that people really let themselves deal with the emotional piece of having had cancer—the exhaustion, the heightened awareness of mortality."

Important points to remember about holidays and other life events:

- Your thoughts and feelings around holidays and other milestones have probably changed since diagnosis.

- There is no right or wrong way to feel, and no two women feel exactly the same.

- How your attitudes evolve can depend on when you were diagnosed, how far along you are in or out of treatment, your type of breast cancer, your feelings about milestones before diagnosis, your family and support networks, and your general outlook on life.

- If approaching holidays or milestones make you feel anxious, upset, or totally stressed out, there are ways to manage the stress and find new joy and meaning in these special events.

Milestones after Treatment

One important step to gaining a new appreciation is dealing with milestones directly related to diagnosis and treatment.

Dr. Massie says she tries to "help women extinguish a lot of the memories of certain dates—dates of breast removal, diagnosis" and other potentially traumatic events.

"My perspective has always been that we celebrate presidents' birthdays, not their death days," Dr. Massie says. She gives her clients this example in working with them to transform—or transcend—fears and anxieties about death and find the things they can enjoy in life.

Dr. Abrams says her clients often report feeling anxious or depressed without knowing why. Upon further discussion, they find there's an anniversary of diagnosis or treatment looming in the very near future.

"The anniversaries are triggers that remind people of their vulnerability," says Dr. Abrams. "The first birthday, or Christmas, or Jewish high holidays after diagnosis can also be a strong trigger."

In dealing with milestone-related triggers, Drs. Abrams and Massie help women talk about their fears and move beyond them.

"Women work so hard during treatment. Everybody's terrified, but there comes a point—depending on a woman's stage of disease—when it's time to put the hospital and cancer office behind and get on with the more pleasurable parts of life," Dr. Massie says. "In fact, many of my patients feel that life is more precious after they've survived cancer."

This feeling seems to be shared by many women, of many different ages and stages of disease.

"I hold my diagnosis date sacred," says Cindi. "Not because it was the day when my world collapsed, but I consider it my day of 'rebirth,' when I began to see life through different eyes."

Lori, who still lives with inflammatory breast cancer, shares these sentiments. "Every time I have a birthday I think that's another year of my life," she explains. "We celebrate April 23rd—the date I discovered my giant swollen breast. Every year I live past that I feel gifted. I don't mourn my diagnosis day. I count it as every year I become more victorious."

Managing Holiday-Related Stress

It's normal to feel stressed and anxious about upcoming events. But remember also that there are ways to lower the stress and increase your enjoyment.

Make a list of people you can depend on for help: a friend or neighbor who's good at listening, a partner or child who's a good household helper. Then ask for the help you need.

Professional counselors and mental health workers can offer much-needed support. Ask your oncology team for recommendations, or check with a local hospital or clinic.

Talk to a woman affected by breast cancer on Living Beyond Breast Cancer's (LBBC) toll-free Survivors' Helpline at 888-753-LBBC (5222). Helpline volunteers offer guidance, information, and hope in a confidential setting.

Pamper yourself. In the past you may have spent all your energy making the holidays special for everyone else, and then collapsing in utter exhaustion. This year, buy yourself a present. Get a massage or a facial. Treat yourself and a loved one to a special dinner (without cooking it!).

Try to focus on the things that make the holidays special for you: spending time with loved ones, getting in touch with a long-lost friend, spending quiet time by yourself.

Instead of worrying about creating the perfect yard display or baking the best holiday cookies, spend time creating memories to cherish throughout the year.

Celebrations Small and Large

If you are living with advanced disease, it can be much more difficult to achieve the transformations described here. Dr. Abrams tries to help women living with metastatic disease manage the unknown.

"One way to do that is to enumerate where you are in control and how you can take control," she says. "For example, a patient might say she wants to lose weight. That's something she can take control of and celebrate when she succeeds."

Kathi experienced this when she lost 90 pounds several years after her diagnosis. "I'm 4'11" and I weighed 200 pounds," she recalls. "So I became a Weight Watcher leader, and now, every day I get on the scale and haven't gained weight is a milestone."

That sense of gratitude for daily accomplishments, and wonder at seasonal events, marks many women's experiences.

"I have learned to appreciate small events just as much as big ones," Lori says. "The first day of spring, a thunderstorm, fall." She has also found a new sense of wonder and joy in family celebrations.

"My new milestones are now my grandsons' birthdays," Lori says. "I look forward to my youngest getting married and seeing her raise her family (soon, I hope). And I look toward the day when I can afford to travel. I have been saving money for my 5-year 're-birthday.' I would love to go to Fiji."

Creating Memories

One of the most important realizations in managing cancer-related and other anxieties around milestones is an awareness of family and loved ones and a renewed appreciation of times spent together.

Debbie Osborne, a 49-year-old former nurse from Oley, Pennsylvania, was diagnosed with metastatic breast cancer the day after Thanksgiving four years ago. Ever since, Thanksgiving has been a time of "heightened awareness" for her. At first, it was mostly painful, but now she looks at it differently.

"Before I would shut down the week before Thanksgiving. I couldn't wait for it to be over," she recalls. "Now, every holiday, every Thanksgiving, is like: Wow! I'm still here to celebrate."

Once she started celebrating Thanksgiving again, Debbie discovered joy in many other occasions. "Milestones are a thousand-fold different for me now," she says. "When my son graduated from high school, you would have thought he got married, had a baby, and was king of the universe!"

Debbie's fiftieth birthday is coming up and she's planning to spend it with her husband and three sons. "I told my husband I don't want any party or anything, just to be with my family. We decided to do a family vacation," she says. "This is giving me such happiness, hope, and strength, to think now about a vacation in a few months' time.

It's creating memories, and memories can give you a lot of strength in low times."

Cindi echoes these sentiments. "My thoughts go much deeper than just the date," she says. "I spend my time now remembering my nephews' great smiles and the way they strutted proudly off the football field after helping their team win their game this fall. I recall how sweet my other nephew smelled when he snuggled into me for a hug on that cold Christmas morning at my parents'. I remember how warm I felt inside that Thanksgiving Day when my entire family was together giving thanks for everything good that God has given us, knowing that Mom's macaroni and cheese was just about to be served—one of the few dishes I continued to eat throughout chemo."

"I really try to think about what makes those milestones significant," Cindi concludes, "and that makes all the difference."

Chapter 54

Intimacy and Sexuality after Breast Cancer Treatment

A Candid Conversation on Sexuality, Intimacy, and Fertility

Although concerns about sexuality, physical intimacy, and fertility may not take center stage when you are first diagnosed with breast cancer—whether you are single or engaged in an intimate relationship—you may find yourself dealing with these issues at some point during your cancer experience.

Sexuality and Body Image

While current research suggests that approximately 50 percent of women who have been treated for breast cancer experience long-term sexual dysfunction, other studies indicate that many women who undergo breast conservation procedures or mastectomy do not experience persistent sexual difficulties. In fact, many researchers and health care professionals concur that the primary predictors of good sexual health after breast cancer may have more to do with a positive body image and satisfaction with sex and relationships prior to the cancer diagnosis.

Body image concerns for all breast cancer survivors are prevalent, though several findings suggest that women who undergo breast conservation surgery have more positive feelings about their bodies and appearing in the nude. Other studies indicate that women who had mastectomies did not demonstrate any significant problems with sexual and emotional adjustment. What is important to emphasize is that every breast cancer experience is unique, and can have a distressing impact on you and your feelings of attractiveness and desirability, even if you don't display the physical manifestations associated with cancer and ensuing therapies.

Why and Where Did My Libido Go?

Treatments for breast cancer—including chemotherapy and radiotherapy—and side effects like nausea, fatigue, pain, and hair loss may affect your body image, lower your sex drive, or cause discomfort during sex. Moreover, chemotherapy can propel some women into early menopause, generating the sudden onset of symptoms that are supposed to appear gradually during a transitional phase of the life cycle.

In addition, if you are receiving hormone replacement therapy (HRT) to alleviate menopausal symptoms, you usually need to stop HRT after a breast cancer diagnosis, particularly if your cancer is sensitive to estrogen and/or progesterone.

Treatment protocols for breast cancer also use hormonal therapies. For example, the effect of tamoxifen on sexual functioning remains inconclusive though recent studies conducted by Mortimer and colleagues suggests that tamoxifen, whether taken alone or concurrently with chemotherapy, may negatively impact sexual intercourse. Again, it's important to reiterate that each experience is unique and many women can and do regain improved sexual functioning anywhere from six months to one year after breast cancer treatment.

Medicines given to treat symptoms can also lead to a loss of interest in sex, as well as difficulties in attaining an orgasm. "Some of the medicine used to treat depression greatly affect sexual function, as do pain medications," says Judith Paice, Ph.D., R.N., a pain management specialist with Northwestern University Medical School in Chicago. "The opioids can cause suppression of testosterone and other hormones which then causes problems with sexual function—all of these work hand in hand." Dr. Paice judiciously includes questions about physical intimacy in her assessment process and notes that people are appreciative when she brings it up, but she also states that many health care professionals are hesitant to broach the subject for fear of offending, upsetting, or embarrassing their patients.

The Emotional Rollercoaster

You and your partner may confront immediate or subsequent worries about body image and sexual relations. A series of questions will likely surface for both of you—Will treatment disfigure me? How will I cope with losing my breast from surgery or my hair from chemo? Will I still want sex and will I still be sexually attractive? Will she still want sex? Can I touch her? Will I hurt her more if she's already in pain? All too often assumptions are made and direct communication avoided when it is most needed to clarify respective feelings and needs.

If you are single and dating, you may be even more keenly aware of subsequent alterations in your appearance and how if will affect potential relationships.

Resetting the Biological Clock

If you are a woman of childbearing age, you may be concerned about your ability to conceive. Chemotherapy and radiation treatment may cause damage to the ovaries and can result in menstrual irregularities, temporary, or permanent infertility. Nonetheless, many women do regain reproductive capacity after treatment has been completed, although research has suggested that older women have a higher risk of developing complete ovarian failure.

The good news is that fertility preservation options do exist for breast cancer survivors and can be initiated prior to the start of chemotherapy. In addition to the widely accepted medical practice of embryo freezing, experimental methods include egg and ovarian tissue freezing, as well as the promising development of alternative hormone stimulation protocols utilizing tamoxifen and aromatase inhibitors to minimize estrogen levels.

Lindsay Nohr Beck is founder and executive director of Fertile Hope, a national nonprofit organization dedicated to providing the latest research and information on fertility and preservation options for cancer survivors and their families. She stresses that there is a lot people can do to preserve fertility.

"Many people think that if they didn't bank eggs or freeze embryos, they've missed the boat, especially if they experience premature menopause," she says. "But there are a lot of options before, during, and after treatment." Lindsay also draws a clear distinction between infertility and premature ovarian failure—damage sustained to eggs and ovaries can still cause difficulty conceiving even if your menstrual flow resumes and appears normal years later. Thus, immediate and appropriate family planning is important.

Moving Towards Intimacy

As breast cancer survivorship rates continue to increase, many patients, their loved ones, and their healthcare teams are focusing on these important quality of life issues. So what can you and your partner do now to adapt to the changes in your body and create an environment where physical and emotional intimacy can flourish?

Les Gallo-Silver, an oncology social worker and Director of Clinical Programs for CancerCare in New York, suggests that partners need to cultivate their listening skills. "You must listen to what is said and what is not said. Sometimes the woman you love with breast cancer is going to want to be alone, leave her alone. Sometimes the woman you love will want to be with you, be with her. If you don't know which time, ask." He also offers some very practical tips for women: seek a cosmetologist evaluation to help you adjust your makeup, if you wear it, to changes in skin texture and hair loss; take control of your hair loss—if you can't bear to have a short haircut or hair removed suddenly, shop for a wig before your hair is gone to match texture and color; throw away your long T-shirt and wear something colorful—something that makes you feel beautiful—to bed; and keep a personal diary or journal to help you begin to articulate your inner feelings.

Dr. Paice also stresses the importance of communication. If you can't discuss your feelings with your partner, talk to your physician, nurse, or seek the assistance of a sex therapist. Many breast cancer survivors find support groups to be an invaluable source of support and shared information. The Breast Cancer Network of Strength Hotline (800-221-2141) and Men's/Partner's Match program also provide a confidential outlet to discuss your feelings about intimacy-related issues.

During or after breast cancer, intimacy may take on an entirely new dimension. Learn to touch, hold hands, experiment, be together, and simply try to relax. You may rediscover yourself—and romance and sex—in very different and fulfilling ways.

Chapter 55

Considering Pregnancy after Breast Cancer Treatment

Is it safe to become pregnant after completing treatment for breast cancer?

For women who are planning on having a child but have yet to give birth, a breast cancer diagnosis can raise a number of questions. Among them are, "Will the hormones of pregnancy increase the risk of my cancer coming back?" and, "How long must I wait after completing treatment to have a child?" According to breast cancer surgeon Jeanne Petrek, M.D., it is important for a woman to allow herself enough time to regain the nutritional and metabolic health she needs to meet the demands of a pregnancy. Dr. Petrek, who serves as director of the Evelyn H. Lauder Breast Cancer Center at Memorial Sloan-Kettering Cancer Center, says that a key consideration is making sure that any aggressive disease that may have been underestimated does not come back.

Although there is no guarantee that the patient will remain cancer free, this is why doctors suggest waiting two or more years before becoming pregnant. It would be even better to wait five years, she says, if indeed a woman has that kind of time available. Often she does not. Dr. Petrek suggests that a woman consider those factors that govern her long-term health when considering a pregnancy. For instance, what was the stage of her cancer when it was diagnosed? Were her lymph nodes free of cancer at that time? What is her prognosis now? Another concern is that doctors don't know exactly whether there is anything unique about one breast cancer versus another. Dr. Petrek explains that a woman may have had chemotherapy, but maybe the treatment merely damaged the cancer cells. Could they, perhaps, be dormant and come to grow again from the pregnancy?

What is unknown at this time is how to identify women in whom pregnancy is safe and women in whom it is not safe. "At present, there is no way to know," she says. Dr. Petrek says that these concerns are theoretical because many pre-menopausal women—perhaps the large majority—do go on to safely become pregnant after breast cancer. The problem is that no long-term prospective studies have been completed at this time to provide solid answers for women. All past studies are retrospective and, she believes, scientifically weak. She has little confidence in these findings.

Meanwhile, a study led by epidemiologist Beth Mueller, Ph.D., a member of the Public Health Sciences Division at the Fred Hutchinson Cancer Research Center, and published in the journal *Cancer* in 2003 (Vol. 98, No. 6; pages 1131–1140), appears encouraging. This study retrospectively followed 438 women in Seattle, Detroit, and Los Angeles. The women were younger than 45 years of age with primary invasive breast cancer, who gave birth after diagnosis. In addition, 2,775 comparison women, matched on the basis of a number of criteria, were identified with breast cancer—but without births after diagnosis. "The results of this study may provide some reassurance to young women with breast carcinoma in that subsequent childbearing is unlikely to increase their risk of dying," says Dr. Mueller. "I can assure women that we conducted the study as carefully as possible, using the tools and data available at that time.

"It is reassuring that we did not observe an increased risk of mortality and that our results appear to be consistent with those from many other studies—including some studies using other designs," continued Dr. Mueller. Although Dr. Mueller did not observe an increased risk for women who had births 10 months or more after their breast cancer diagnosis, relative to the control group who did not have children since diagnosis, she cautions readers to be careful not to over-interpret the results. She says that their finding of a decreased risk of dying may be due to what she calls a "healthy woman bias." She explains that women who are healthier, or have a better prognosis, may be more likely to attempt pregnancies after diagnosis. "Although we attempted to control for this by using the data available about the severity of the women's disease at diagnosis, we had limited knowledge about their health status afterwards," she says.

Both researchers look forward to large population-based prospective studies in the years ahead, which would provide the best assessment of the question of an individual woman's safety to proceed with pregnancy. Dr. Petrek, in fact, is currently recruiting women for two such trials to shed light on these and other quality-of-life questions, but her studies are just beginning and her findings a long way off. In the meantime, Dr. Petrek suggests that a woman who wishes to have a child confer with her family as well as with her health care providers—particularly a medical oncologist and a high-risk obstetrician. Dr. Mueller agrees and adds that each woman has a different situation regarding her own health status, social support, and desire for offspring. "One's decision may incorporate several factors including family cancer history, the presence of a supportive family and/or partner, and whether or not she already has children," she says. "Ultimately, every woman faced with this scenario makes a personal decision based on her own situation." "If there is any question," Dr. Petrek adds, "adoption is a great way to go."

Chapter 56

Breast Cancer Survivors and Osteoporosis

What Breast Cancer Survivors Need to Know about Osteoporosis

The Impact of Breast Cancer

The National Cancer Institute reports that one in eight women in the United States (approximately 13 percent) will develop breast cancer in her lifetime. In fact, next to skin cancer, breast cancer is the most common type of cancer among U.S. women.

While the exact cause of breast cancer is not known, the risk of developing it increases with age. The risk is particularly high in women over the age of 60. Because of their age, these women are already at increased risk for osteoporosis. Given the rising incidence of breast cancer and the improvement of long-term survival rates, bone health and fracture prevention have become important health issues among breast cancer survivors.

Facts about Osteoporosis

Osteoporosis is a condition in which the bones become less dense and more likely to fracture. Fractures from osteoporosis can result in

This chapter includes text from "What Breast Cancer Survivors Need to Know About Osteoporosis," National Institute of Arthritis and Musculoskeletal and Skin Diseases, August 2005; and, "Study Confirms Risk of Bone Loss for Patients Taking Exemestane," National Cancer Institute, February 14, 2007.

significant pain and disability. It is a major health threat for an estimated 44 million Americans, 68 percent of whom are women.

Risk factors for developing osteoporosis include the following:

• Being thin or having a small frame

• Having a family history of the disease

• For women, being postmenopausal, having an early menopause, or not having menstrual periods (amenorrhea)

• Using certain medications, such as glucocorticoids

• Not getting enough calcium

• Not getting enough physical activity

• Smoking

• Drinking too much alcohol

Osteoporosis is a silent disease that can often be prevented. However, if undetected, it can progress for many years without symptoms until a fracture occurs. It has been called "a pediatric disease with geriatric consequences" because building healthy bones in one's youth is important to help prevent osteoporosis and fractures later in life.

The Breast Cancer—Osteoporosis Link

Women who have had breast cancer treatment may be at increased risk for osteoporosis and fracture for several reasons. First, estrogen has a protective effect on bone, and reduced levels of the hormone trigger bone loss. Because of chemotherapy or surgery, many breast cancer survivors experience a loss of ovarian function, and consequently, a drop in estrogen levels. Women who were premenopausal prior to their cancer treatment tend to go through menopause earlier than those who have not had the disease.

Studies also suggest that chemotherapy may have a direct negative effect on bone. In addition, the breast cancer itself may stimulate the production of osteoclasts, the cells that break down bone.

Osteoporosis Management Strategies

Several strategies can reduce one's risk for osteoporosis or lessen the effects of the disease in women who have already been diagnosed.

Nutrition: Some studies have found a link between diet and breast cancer. However, it is not yet clear which foods or supplements may play a role in reducing breast cancer risk. As far as bone health is concerned, a well-balanced diet rich in calcium and vitamin D is important. Good sources of calcium include low-fat dairy products; dark green, leafy vegetables; and calcium-fortified foods and beverages. Also, supplements can help ensure that the calcium requirement is met each day. The Institute of Medicine recommends a daily calcium intake of 1,000 mg (milligrams) for men and women between the ages of 19 and 50, increasing to 1,200 mg for those over 50.

Vitamin D plays an important role in calcium absorption and bone health. It is synthesized in the skin through exposure to sunlight. Some individuals may require vitamin D supplements in order to achieve the recommended intake of 400 to 800 IU (International Units) each day.

Exercise: Like muscle, bone is living tissue that responds to exercise by becoming stronger. The best exercise for bones is weight-bearing exercise that forces you to work against gravity. Some examples include walking, climbing stairs, lifting weights, and dancing. Regular exercise such as walking may help prevent bone loss and provide many other health benefits. Recent research suggests that exercise may also reduce breast cancer risk in younger women.

Healthy lifestyle: Smoking is bad for bones as well as the heart and lungs. In addition, smokers may absorb less calcium from their diets. Some studies have found a slightly higher risk of breast cancer in women who drink alcohol, and evidence also suggests that alcohol can negatively affect bone health. Those who drink heavily are more prone to bone loss and fracture, because of both poor nutrition and an increased risk of falling.

Bone density test: Specialized tests known as bone mineral density (BMD) tests measure bone density at various sites of the body. These tests can detect osteoporosis before a fracture occurs and predict one's chances of fracturing in the future. A woman recovering from breast cancer should ask her doctor whether she might be a candidate for a bone density test.

Medication: There is no cure for osteoporosis. However, medications are available to prevent and treat this disease. Bisphosphonates, a class of osteoporosis treatment medications, are being studied and have demonstrated some success in their ability to treat breast cancers that have spread to bone.

Another osteoporosis treatment medication, raloxifene, is currently being evaluated for its ability to decrease breast cancer risk. Raloxifene is a selective estrogen receptor modulator (SERM) that has been shown to reduce the risk of breast cancer in women with osteoporosis. The National Institutes of Health is currently sponsoring the Study of Tamoxifen and Raloxifene, known by the acronym STAR. The study compares the effectiveness of raloxifene with that of tamoxifen in preventing breast cancer in postmenopausal women who have a high risk of developing the disease.

Study Confirms Risk of Bone Loss for Patients Taking Exemestane

Women who switched to the drug exemestane (Aromasin®) after taking tamoxifen (Nolvadex®) to prevent a breast cancer relapse lost more bone density and had a higher risk of bone fractures than women who continued taking tamoxifen, an international study has concluded.

Source: *The Lancet Oncology*, published online Jan. 26, 2007; in print February 2007 (see the journal abstract). (*Lancet Oncol*. 2007 Feb; 8(2):119–27)

Background

Many breast tumors are "estrogen sensitive," meaning the hormone estrogen helps them to grow. Women whose tumors are estrogen sensitive are advised to take anti-estrogen drugs for five years to reduce the risk of a relapse after their initial treatment. Tamoxifen was the first anti-estrogen drug shown to lower the risk of a breast cancer recurrence.

However, several large clinical trials have now shown that drugs called aromatase inhibitors (AIs) are more effective than tamoxifen at preventing the recurrence of estrogen-sensitive breast cancer. AIs also carry a lower risk of blood clots and endometrial cancer, both of which are possible side effects of tamoxifen.

AIs have their own side effects, however. Studies of two AIs, anastrozole (Arimidex®) and letrozole (Femara®), have shown that these drugs cause a loss of bone density and increase the risk of bone fractures. One of estrogen's effects on the body is to protect bones from thinning. Tamoxifen, because of the way it works in the body, actually has a protective effect on bone. AIs, by contrast, block the production of estrogen, reducing the amount of the hormone in the body. The absence of estrogen leads to accelerated loss of bone density.

In 2006 a large international clinical trial showed that women who switched after two or three years of tamoxifen to an AI called exemestane lived longer and had a lower risk of breast cancer relapse than women who stayed on tamoxifen for five years (see the related story). Now researchers have published data from a subgroup of the women on that trial showing exemestane's effect on bone density and fracture risk.

The Study

In the original trial, 4,724 postmenopausal women with early breast cancer who had been taking tamoxifen for two or three years were assigned at random either to remain on tamoxifen or to switch to exemestane until they had completed five years of treatment.

A subgroup of 206 patients took part in the bone density study. Roughly half of them had been assigned to stay on tamoxifen, the other half to switch to exemestane. Their bone density (in the lumbar spine and in the hip) was measured when they entered the study and again after six months, one year, and two years. The researchers also collected blood and urine samples to measure markers of bone loss. In addition, the researchers kept a record of all patients in the main trial who suffered bone fractures.

The principal investigator for the bone study was Robert E. Coleman, M.D., of Weston Park Hospital in Sheffield in the United Kingdom.

Results

At the two-year mark, the loss of bone density in the lumbar spine experienced by women who had switched to exemestane was 4.0 percent, compared to just 0.6 percent among women who stayed on tamoxifen. In the exemestane group, most of the bone loss occurred in the first six months.

Among women who had normal bone density when they entered the study, a higher percentage of those on exemestane were diagnosed with low bone mass, or osteopenia, after two years, compared with those on tamoxifen. The difference was statistically significant. No one in either group whose bone density was normal at the start of the study later developed osteoporosis, a disease characterized by brittle bones that break easily.

Among those women who were already showing signs of bone loss at the start of the study, five of those on exemestane developed osteoporosis by the two-year mark, compared to none of those taking tamoxifen.

Researchers have followed the 4,724 participants from the original trial for nearly five years and report that 162 women in the exemestane group (7 percent) had fractures, compared with 115 (5 percent) of those in the tamoxifen group.

Comments

"These results indicate that the increase in survival shown previously with [the switch from tamoxifen to exemestane] is achieved at the expense of some detriment to [bone] health," Coleman and his coauthors write. They note that the rate of bone loss is about the same for patients on letrozole and anastrozole, two other AIs previously studied.

Jennifer Eng-Wong, M.D., a clinical oncologist at the National Cancer Institute's Center for Cancer Research, agrees that this study confirms earlier research showing that AIs reduce bone density and increase the risk of fractures. In the United States, patients taking AIs should receive bone density tests every 12 to 18 months as part of standard care, she adds.

The researchers recommend that all women switching from tamoxifen to exemestane have a bone density test around the time they make the switch. Those with normal bone density, they say, may not need further testing but should be counseled about lifestyle changes that can protect them from bone loss (such as consuming adequate calcium and vitamin D and getting regular weight-bearing exercise).

The risks and benefits of AI therapy for a woman with low bone mass or osteoporosis should be considered individually, Eng-Wong says, weighing the risk of breast cancer recurrence against the risk of further loss of bone density. "If a woman has already had an osteoporotic fracture, she would not be a good candidate for AI therapy," she says.

Part Eight

Additional Help and Information

Chapter 57

A Glossary of Breast Cancer Terms

acupuncture: A technique of inserting thin needles through the skin at specific points on the body to control pain and side effects. It is a type of complementary and alternative medicine.

adjuvant chemotherapy: Chemotherapy used to kill cancer cells after surgery or radiation therapy.

alopecia: The lack or loss of hair from areas of the body where hair is usually found. Alopecia can be a side effect of chemotherapy.

anemia: A problem in which the number of red blood cells is below normal.

antiemetic: A drug that prevents or controls nausea and vomiting. Also called antinausea.

antiestrogen: A substance that blocks the activity of estrogens, the family of hormones that promote the development and maintenance of female sex characteristics.

antinausea: A drug that prevents or controls nausea and vomiting. Also called antiemetic.

anxiety: Feelings of fear, dread, and uneasiness that may occur as a reaction to stress. A person with anxiety may sweat, feel restless and

---

This glossary includes terms excerpted from several documents produced by the National Cancer Institute (www.cancer.gov).

541

tense, and have a rapid heart beat. Extreme anxiety that happens often over time may be a sign of an anxiety disorder.

applicator: A large device used to place brachytherapy in the body.

aromatase inhibitor: A drug that prevents the formation of estradiol, a female hormone, by interfering with an aromatase enzyme. Aromatase inhibitors are used as a type of hormone therapy for postmenopausal women who have hormone-dependent breast cancer.

axilla: The underarm or armpit.

biological therapy: Treatment to stimulate or restore the ability of the immune system to fight cancer, infections, and other diseases. Also used to lessen certain side effects that may be caused by some cancer treatments.

biopsy: The removal of cells or tissues for examination by a pathologist. The pathologist may study the tissue under a microscope or perform other tests on the cells or tissue. There are many different types of biopsy procedures. The most common types include: (1) incisional biopsy, in which only a sample of tissue is removed; (2) excisional biopsy, in which an entire lump or suspicious area is removed; and (3) needle biopsy, in which a sample of tissue or fluid is removed with a needle. When a wide needle is used, the procedure is called a core biopsy. When a thin needle is used, the procedure is called a fine-needle aspiration biopsy.

blood cell count: The number of red blood cells, white blood cells, and platelets in a sample of blood. This is also called a complete blood count (CBC).

blood clot: A mass of blood that forms when blood platelets, proteins, and cells stick together. When a blood clot is attached to the wall of a blood vessel, it is called a thrombus. When it moves through the bloodstream and blocks the flow of blood in another part of the body, it is called an embolus.

blood vessel: A tube through which the blood circulates in the body. Blood vessels include a network of arteries, arterioles, capillaries, venules, and veins.

bone density: A measure of the amount of minerals (mostly calcium and phosphorous) contained in a certain volume of bone. Bone density measurements are used to diagnose osteoporosis (a condition marked by decreased bone mass), to see how well osteoporosis treatments are working, and to predict how likely the bones are to break.

Low bone density can occur in patients treated for cancer. Also called bone mineral density, BMD, and bone mass.

bone marrow: The soft, sponge-like tissue in the center of most bones. It produces white blood cells, red blood cells, and platelets.

brachytherapy: Treatment in which a solid radioactive substance is implanted inside your body, near or next to the cancer cells.

BRCA1: A gene on chromosome 17 that normally helps to suppress cell growth. A person who inherits a mutated (changed) BRCA1 gene has a higher risk of getting breast, ovarian, or prostate cancer.

BRCA2: A gene on chromosome 13 that normally helps to suppress cell growth. A person who inherits a mutated (changed) BRCA2 gene has a higher risk of getting breast, ovarian, or prostate cancer.

breast cancer: Cancer that forms in tissues of the breast, usually the ducts (tubes that carry milk to the nipple) and lobules (glands that make milk). It occurs in both men and women, although male breast cancer is rare.

cancer clinical trials: Type of research study that tests how well new medical approaches work in people. These studies test new methods of screening, prevention, diagnosis, or treatment of a disease. Also called a clinical study or research study.

cataract: A condition in which the lens of the eye becomes cloudy. Symptoms include blurred, cloudy, or double vision; sensitivity to light; and difficulty seeing at night. Without treatment, cataracts can cause blindness. There are many different types and causes of cataracts. They may occur in people of all ages, but are most common in the elderly.

catheter: A flexible tube through which fluids enter or leave the body.

chemotherapy: Treatment with drugs that kill cancer cells.

cholesterol: A waxy, fat-like substance made in the liver, and found in the blood and in all cells of the body. Cholesterol is important for good health and is needed for making cell walls, tissues, hormones, vitamin D, and bile acid. Cholesterol also comes from eating foods taken from animals such as egg yolks, meat, and whole-milk dairy products. Too much cholesterol in the blood may build up in blood vessel walls, block blood flow to tissues and organs, and increase the risk of developing heart disease and stroke.

complementary and alternative medicine (CAM): Forms of treatment that are used in addition to (complementary) or instead of (alternative) standard treatments. These practices generally are not considered standard medical approaches. Standard treatments go through a long and careful research process to prove they are safe and effective, but less is known about most types of CAM. CAM may include dietary supplements, megadose vitamins, herbal preparations, special teas, acupuncture, massage therapy, magnet therapy, spiritual healing, and meditation.

computed tomography (CT) scan: A series of detailed pictures of areas inside the body, taken from different angles; the pictures are created by a computer linked to an x-ray machine.

constipation: When bowel movements become less frequent, and stools are hard, dry, and difficult to pass.

course of treatment: All of your radiation therapy sessions.

cystitis: Inflammation in your urinary tract.

depression: A mental condition marked by ongoing feelings of sadness, despair, loss of energy, and difficulty dealing with normal daily life. Other symptoms of depression include feelings of worthlessness and hopelessness, loss of pleasure in activities, changes in eating or sleeping habits, and thoughts of death or suicide. Depression can affect anyone, and can be successfully treated. Depression affects 15–25% of cancer patients.

diarrhea: Frequent bowel movements that may be soft, loose, or watery.

dilator: A device that gently stretches the tissues of the vagina.

disorder: In medicine, a disturbance of normal functioning of the mind or body. Disorders may be caused by genetic factors, disease, or trauma.

dose: The amount of medicine taken, or radiation given, at one time.

drug: Any substance, other than food, that is used to prevent, diagnose, treat or relieve symptoms of a disease or abnormal condition. Also refers to a substance that alters mood or body function, or that can be habit-forming or addictive, especially a narcotic.

dry heaves: A problem that occurs when your body tries to vomit even though your stomach is empty.

duct: In medicine, a tube or vessel of the body through which fluids pass.

early menopause: A condition in which the ovaries stop working before age 40. Symptoms include hot flashes, mood swings, night sweats, vaginal dryness, and infertility. Some cancer treatments, such as chemotherapy, radiation therapy, and surgery can cause early menopause. This may be temporary or permanent and may be treated with hormone replacement therapy. Also called premature ovarian failure or primary ovarian insufficiency.

endogenous: Produced inside an organism or cell. The opposite is external (exogenous) production.

endometrial cancer: Cancer that forms in the tissue lining the uterus (the small, hollow, pear-shaped organ in a woman's pelvis in which a baby grows). Most endometrial cancers are adenocarcinomas (cancers that begin in cells that make and release mucus and other fluids).

enzyme: A protein that speeds up chemical reactions in the body.

esophagitis: Inflammation of the esophagus (the tube that carries food from the mouth to the stomach).

estrogen: A type of hormone made by the body that helps develop and maintain female sex characteristics and the growth of long bones. Estrogens can also be made in the laboratory. They may be used as a type of birth control and to treat symptoms of menopause, menstrual disorders, osteoporosis, and other conditions.

exemestane: A drug used to treat advanced breast cancer and to prevent recurrent breast cancer in postmenopausal women who have already been treated with tamoxifen. It is also being studied in the treatment of other types of cancer. Exemestane causes a decrease in the amount of estrogen made by the body. It is a type of aromatase inhibitor. Also called Aromasin.

external beam radiation therapy: Treatment in which a radiation source from outside your body aims radiation at your cancer cells.

fatigue: A problem of extreme tiredness and inability to function due lack of energy.

fenretinide: A substance being studied in the treatment and prevention of some types of cancer. Fenretinide may cause ceramide (a wax-like substance) to build up in tumor cells and kill them. It is a type of retinoid, which are substances related to vitamin A.

fetus: The developing offspring from seven to eight weeks after conception until birth.

gene: The functional and physical unit of heredity passed from parent to offspring. Genes are pieces of DNA, and most genes contain the information for making a specific protein.

genome: The complete genetic material of an organism.

genomic profile: Information about all the genes in an organism, including variations, gene expression, and the way those genes interact with each other and with the environment. A genomic profile may be used to discover why some people get certain diseases while other people do not, or why people respond differently to the same drug.

hormone: One of many chemicals made by glands in the body. Hormones circulate in the bloodstream and control the actions of certain cells or organs. Some hormones can also be made in the laboratory.

hormone replacement therapy (HRT): Hormones (estrogen, progesterone, or both) given to women after menopause to replace the hormones no longer produced by the ovaries. Also called HRT and menopausal hormone therapy.

hot flash: A sudden, temporary onset of body warmth, flushing, and sweating (often associated with menopause).

hyperfractionated radiation therapy: Treatment in which radiation is given in smaller doses twice a day.

hysterectomy: Surgery to remove the uterus and, sometimes, the cervix. When the uterus and part or all of the cervix are removed, it is called a total hysterectomy. When only the uterus is removed, it is called a partial hysterectomy.

imaging tests: Tests that produce pictures of areas inside the body.

implant: A substance or object that is put in the body as a prosthesis, or for treatment or diagnosis.

incontinence: A problem in which you cannot control the flow of urine from your bladder.

infertility: For women, it means that you may not be able to get pregnant. For men, it means that you may not be able to get a woman pregnant.

inflammation: Redness, swelling, pain, and/or a feeling of heat in an area of the body.

infection: Invasion and multiplication of germs in the body. Infections can occur in any part of the body and can spread throughout the body. The germs may be bacteria, viruses, yeast, or fungi. They can cause a fever and other problems, depending on where the infection occurs. When the body's natural defense system is strong, it can often fight the germs and prevent infection. Some cancer treatments can weaken the natural defense system.

inherited: Transmitted through genes that have been passed from parents to their offspring (children).

intensity-modulated radiation therapy (IMRT): A technique that uses a computer to deliver precise radiation doses to a cancer tumor or specific areas within the tumor.

internal radiation therapy: Treatment in which a radioactive substance is put inside your body.

intra-arterial: Within an artery. Also called IA.

intraoperative radiation: Radiation treatment aimed directly at cancer during surgery.

intraperitoneal: Within the peritoneal cavity. Also called IP.

intravenous: Within a blood vessel. Also called IV.

late side effects: Side effects that first occur six or more months after radiation therapy is finished.

lobe: A portion of an organ, such as the liver, lung, breast, thyroid, or brain.

lobule: A small lobe or a subdivision of a lobe.

local treatment: Radiation is aimed at only the part of your body with cancer.

long-term side effects: Problems from chemotherapy that do not go away.

lumpectomy: Surgery to remove the tumor and a small amount of normal tissue around it.

lymph: The clear fluid that travels through the lymphatic system and carries cells that help fight infections and other diseases. Also called lymphatic fluid.

lymph node: A rounded mass of lymphatic tissue that is surrounded by a capsule of connective tissue. Lymph nodes filter lymph (lymphatic fluid), and they store lymphocytes (white blood cells). They are located along lymphatic vessels. Also called lymph gland.

lymph vessel: A thin tube that carries lymph (lymphatic fluid) and white blood cells through the lymphatic system. Also called lymphatic vessel.

lymphedema: A problem in which excess fluid collects in tissue and causes swelling. It may occur in the arm or leg after lymph vessels or lymph nodes in the underarm or groin are removed by surgery or treated with radiation.

magnetic resonance imaging (MRI): A procedure in which radio waves and a powerful magnet linked to a computer are used to create detailed pictures of areas inside the body.

menopause: The time of life when a woman's menstrual periods stop. A woman is in menopause when she hasn't had a period for 12 months in a row. Also called change of life.

menstrual cycle: The monthly cycle of hormonal changes from the beginning of one menstrual period to the beginning of the next.

menstruation: Periodic discharge of blood and tissue from the uterus. From puberty until menopause, menstruation occurs about every 28 days when a woman is not pregnant.

metastatic: The spread of cancer from one part of the body to another.

National Cancer Institute (NCI): Part of the National Institutes of Health of the United States Department of Health and Human Services, it is the Federal Government's principal agency for cancer research. It conducts, coordinates, and funds cancer research, training, health information dissemination, and other programs with respect to the cause, diagnosis, prevention, and treatment of cancer.

nausea: When you have an upset stomach or queasy feeling and feel like you are going to throw up.

neoadjuvant chemotherapy: When chemotherapy is used to shrink a tumor before surgery or radiation therapy.

neutropenia: An abnormal decrease in the number of neutrophils, a type of white blood cell.

neutrophil: A type of white blood cell.

obesity: A condition marked by an abnormally high, unhealthy amount of body fat.

oral contraceptive pill: A pill used to prevent pregnancy. It contains hormones that block the release of eggs from the ovaries. Most oral contraceptives include estrogen and progestin. Also called birth control pill.

osteoporosis: A condition that is marked by a decrease in bone mass and density, causing bones to become fragile.

outpatient: A patient who visits a health care facility for diagnosis or treatment without spending the night.

ovarian ablation: Surgery, radiation therapy, or a drug treatment to stop the functioning of the ovaries. Also called ovarian suppression.

ovary: One of a pair of female reproductive glands in which the ova, or eggs, are formed. The ovaries are located in the pelvis, one on each side of the uterus.

palliative care: Care given to improve the quality of life of patients with serious or life-threatening diseases.

peritoneal cavity: The space within the abdomen that contains the intestines, stomach, liver, ovaries, and other organs.

Physician Data Query (PDQ): PDQ is an online database developed and maintained by the National Cancer Institute. Designed to make the most current, credible, and accurate cancer information available to health professionals and the public, PDQ contains peer-reviewed summaries on cancer treatment, screening, prevention, genetics, complementary and alternative medicine, and supportive care; a registry of cancer clinical trials from around the world; and directories of physicians, professionals who provide genetics services, and organizations that provide cancer care.

platelet: A type of blood cell that helps prevent bleeding by causing blood clots to form.

port: An implanted device through which blood may be drawn and drugs may be given without repeated needle sticks.

positron emission tomography (PET) scan: A procedure in which a small amount of radioactive glucose (sugar) is injected into a vein, and a scanner is used to make detailed, computerized pictures of areas inside the body where the glucose is used. Because cancer cells often use more glucose than normal cells, the pictures can be used to find cancer cells in the body.

precancerous: A term used to describe a condition that may (or is likely to) become cancer. Also called premalignant.

premenopausal: Having to do with the time before menopause. Menopause ("change of life") is the time of life when a woman's menstrual periods stop permanently.

prevention: In medicine, action taken to decrease the chance of getting a disease or condition. For example, cancer prevention includes avoiding risk factors (such as smoking, obesity, lack of exercise, and radiation exposure) and increasing protective factors (such as getting regular physical activity, staying at a healthy weight, and having a healthy diet).

progesterone: A type of hormone made by the body that plays a role in the menstrual cycle and pregnancy. Progesterone can also be made in the laboratory. It may be used as a type of birth control and to treat menstrual disorders, infertility, symptoms of menopause, and other conditions.

progestin: Any natural or laboratory-made substance that has some or all of the biologic effects of progesterone, a female hormone.

prophylactic mastectomy: Surgery to reduce the risk of developing breast cancer by removing one or both breasts before disease develops. Also called preventive mastectomy.

prophylactic oophorectomy: Surgery intended to reduce the risk of ovarian cancer by removing the ovaries before disease develops.

protective factor: Something that may decrease the chance of getting a certain disease. Some examples of protective factors for cancer are getting regular physical activity, staying at a healthy weight, and having a healthy diet.

pruritus: Severe itching.

pump: A device that is used to deliver a precise amount of a drug at a specific rate.

psychostimulants: Medicines that can help decrease fatigue, give a sense of well-being, and increase appetite.

puberty: The time of life when a child experiences physical and hormonal changes that mark a transition into adulthood. The child develops secondary sexual characteristics and becomes able to have children. Secondary sexual characteristics include growth of pubic, armpit, and leg hair; breast enlargement; and increased hip width in girls. In boys, they include growth of pubic, face, chest and armpit hair; voice changes; penis and testicle growth; and increased shoulder width.

radiation: Energy released in the form of particles or electromagnetic waves. Common sources of radiation include radon gas, cosmic rays from outer space, and medical x-rays.

radiation oncologist: A doctor who specializes in using radiation to treat cancer.

radiation therapy: The use of high-energy radiation from x-rays, gamma rays, neutrons, protons, and other sources to kill cancer cells and shrink tumors. Radiation may come from a machine outside the body (external-beam radiation therapy), or it may come from radioactive material placed in the body near cancer cells (internal radiation therapy). Systemic radiation therapy uses a radioactive substance, such as a radiolabeled monoclonal antibody, that travels in the blood to tissues throughout the body. Also called radiotherapy and irradiation.

radiotherapy: Another word for radiation therapy.

raloxifene: A drug used to reduce the risk of invasive breast cancer in postmenopausal women who are at a high risk of developing the disease or who have osteoporosis. It is also used to prevent and treat osteoporosis in postmenopausal women and is being studied in the prevention and treatment of other conditions. Raloxifene blocks the effects of the hormone estrogen in the breast and increases the amount of calcium in bone. It is a type of selective estrogen receptor modulator (SERM). Also called raloxifene hydrochloride and Evista.

recurrent: Cancer that returns after not being detected for a period of time.

red blood cells: Cells that carry oxygen to all parts of the body. Also called RBC.

retinoid: Vitamin A or a vitamin A-like compound.

risk factor: Something that may increase the chance of developing a disease. Some examples of risk factors for cancer include age, a family history of certain cancers, use of tobacco products, certain eating habits, obesity, lack of exercise, exposure to radiation or other cancer-causing agents, and certain genetic changes.

screening: Checking for disease when there are no symptoms.

secondhand smoke: Smoke that comes from the burning of a tobacco product and smoke that is exhaled by smokers. Inhaling secondhand smoke is called involuntary or passive smoking. Also called environmental tobacco smoke and ETS.

selective estrogen receptor modulator: A drug that acts like estrogen on some tissues but blocks the effect of estrogen on other tissues. Tamoxifen and raloxifene are selective estrogen receptor modulators. Also called SERM.

side effect: A problem that occurs when treatment affects healthy tissues or organs.

simulation: A process used to plan radiation therapy so that the target area is precisely located and marked.

sitz bath: A warm-water bath taken in a sitting position that covers only the hips and buttocks.

skin breakdown: A side effect from radiation therapy in which the skin in the treatment area peels off faster than it can grow back.

skin cancer: Cancer that forms in tissues of the skin. There are several types of skin cancer. Skin cancer that forms in melanocytes (skin cells that make pigment) is called melanoma. Skin cancer that forms in basal cells (small, round cells in the base of the outer layer of skin) is called basal cell carcinoma. Skin cancer that forms in squamous cells (flat cells that form the surface of the skin) is called squamous cell carcinoma. Skin cancer that forms in neuroendocrine cells (cells that release hormones in response to signals from the nervous system) is called neuroendocrine carcinoma of the skin. Most skin cancers form in older people on parts of the body exposed to the sun or in people who have weakened immune systems.

standard treatment: Treatment that experts agree is appropriate, accepted, and widely used.

statin: Any of a group of drugs that lower the amount of cholesterol and certain fats in the blood. Statins inhibit a key enzyme that helps make cholesterol. Statin drugs are being studied in the prevention and treatment of cancer.

stroke: In medicine, a loss of blood flow to part of the brain, which damages brain tissue. Strokes are caused by blood clots and broken blood vessels in the brain. Symptoms include dizziness, numbness, weakness on one side of the body, and problems with talking, writing, or understanding language. The risk of stroke is increased by high blood pressure, older age, smoking, diabetes, high cholesterol, heart disease, atherosclerosis (a build-up of fatty material and plaque inside the coronary arteries), and a family history of stroke.

supplementation: Adding nutrients to the diet.

support groups: Meetings for people who share the same problems, such as cancer.

tamoxifen: A drug used to treat certain types of breast cancer in women and men. It is also used to prevent breast cancer in women who have had ductal carcinoma in situ (abnormal cells in the ducts of the breast) and are at a high risk of developing breast cancer. Tamoxifen is also being studied in the treatment of other types of cancer. It blocks the effects of the hormone estrogen in the breast. Tamoxifen is a type of antiestrogen. Also called tamoxifen citrate and Nolvadex.

treatment field: One or more places on your body where the radiation will be aimed. Also called treatment port.

treatment port: One or more places on your body where the radiation will be aimed. Also called treatment field.

3-D conformal radiation therapy: Uses a computer to create a 3-D picture of a cancer tumor. This allows doctors to give the highest possible dose of radiation to the tumor, while sparing the normal tissue as much as possible.

thrombocytopenia: A decrease in the number of platelets in the blood that may result in easy bruising and excessive bleeding from wounds or bleeding in mucous membranes and other tissues.

tissue: A group or layer of cells that work together to perform a specific function.

vaginal: Having to do with the vagina (the birth canal).

vaginal stenosis: A problem in which the vagina narrows and gets smaller.

vitamin A: A family of nutrients needed by the body for vision, bone growth, reproduction, cell division, and cell differentiation. Vitamin A also helps the immune system protect the body against many types of infections. Foods with vitamin A include animal foods, such as liver, whole eggs and milk, and plant foods such as carrots, cantaloupes, sweet potatoes, and spinach. Vitamin A is being studied in the prevention and treatment of some types of cancer.

white blood cell: Refers to a blood cell that does not contain hemoglobin. White blood cells include lymphocytes, neutrophils, eosinophils, macrophages, and mast cells. These cells are made by bone marrow and help the body fight infections and other diseases. Also called WBC.

xerostomia: Dry mouth.

x-ray: A type of high-energy radiation. In low doses, x-rays are used to diagnose diseases by making pictures of the inside of the body. In high doses, x-rays are used to treat cancer.

Chapter 58

National Breast Cancer Organizations and Sources of Support

Breast Cancer Toll-Free Helplines

American Cancer Society
Phone: 800-ACS-2345

CancerCare
Phone: 800-813-HOPE (4673);
212-302-2400 (outside North
America)

Cancer Information and Counseling Line (CICL)
Phone: 800-525-3777

Cancer Research Foundations of America
Phone: 800-227-2732

Komen (Susan G.) Breast Cancer Foundation
Phone: 800-I'M-AWARE
(462-9273)

Living Beyond Breast Cancer
Phone: 888-753-LBBC (5222)

Medicare Hotline
Phone: 800-MEDICARE
(633-42273)

National Cancer Institute's Cancer Information Service
Phone: 800-4-CANCER
(422-6237)

Information in this chapter was compiled from resources listed in *Breast Cancer: A Resource Guide for Minority Women*, Office of Minority Health, U.S. Department of Health and Human Services, 2005, as well as information from the National Cancer Institute and other sources deemed reliable. All contact information was updated and verified in June 2008.

National Patient Travel Center (NPTC)
Phone: 800-296-1217

SHARE: Self Help for Women with Breast or Ovarian Cancer
Phone: 866-891-2392

Informational Organizations

AMC Cancer Research Center
1600 Pierce Street
Denver, CO 80214
Toll-Free: 800-321-1557
Phone: 303-233-6501
Fax: 303-129-3400
Website: http://www.amc.org
E-mail: contactus@amc.org

American Cancer Society
250 Williams Street, NW
Atlanta, GA 30303
Phone: 800-227-2345
Website: http://www.cancer.org

American Society of Plastic Surgeons (ASPS)
444 East Algonquin Road
Arlington Heights, IL 60005
Phone: 888-475-2784
Website: http://www.plasticsurgery.org

Asian American Network for Cancer Awareness, Research, and Training
University of California, Davis
Cancer Center/EPM
4501 X Street, Suite 3011
Sacramento, CA 95817
Phone: 916-734-5105
Website: http://www.aancart.org

Breast and Cervical Cancer Early Detection Program
Centers for Disease Control and Prevention (CDC)
Phone: 888-842-6355
Website: http://www.cdc.gov/cancer/NBCCEDP

Breast and Cervical Cancer Prevention and Treatment (BCCPTA)
Centers of Medicare and Medicaid
7500 Security Blvd.
Baltimore, MD 21244
Toll-Free: 877-267-2323
Phone: 410-786-3000 (Local)
TTY Toll-Free: 866-226-1819
TTY Local: 410-786-0727
Website: http://www.cms.hhs.gov/MedicaidSpecialCovCond/02_BreastandCervicalCancer_PreventionandTreatment.asp

Breast Cancer Fund
1388 Sutter Street, Suite 400
San Francisco, CA 94109-5400
Toll-Free: 866-760-8223
Phone: 415-346-8223
Fax: 415-346-2975
Website: http://
www.breastcancerfund.org
E-mail:
info@breastcancerfund.org

Cancer and Careers.org
c/o Cosmetic Executive Women,
Inc.
286 Madison Avenue, 19th Floor
New York, NY 10017
Phone: 212-685-5955 (ext. 22)
Website: http://
www.cancerandcareers.org

Cancer Consultants, Inc.
491 North Main Street, Suite 200
P.O. Box 724
Ketchum, ID 83340
Website: http://
patient.cancerconsultants.com
E-mail:
Info@cancerconsultants.com

Center for Drug Evaluation and Research's Approved Oncology Drugs
Division of Drug Information
Food and Drug Administration
10903 New Hampshire Avenue,
WO51-2201
Silver Spring, MD 20993-0002
Toll-Free: 888-INFO-FDA
(463-6332)
Website: http://www.fda.gov/
cder/cancer/approved.htm

Division of Cancer Prevention and Control
National Center for Chronic
Disease Prevention and Health
Promotion
Centers for Disease Control and
Prevention
4770 Buford Highway, NE
MS K-64
Atlanta, GA 30341-3717
Phone: 770-488-4751
Fax: 770-488-4760
Website: http://www.cdc.gov/
cancer

Food and Drug Administration Mammography Program
Toll-Free: 888-INFO-FDA
(463-6332)
Website: http://www.fda.gov/
cdrh/mammography
E-mail:
MQSAhotline@hcmsllec.com

Health Disparities: Minority Cancer Awareness
Centers for Disease Control and
Prevention
Division of Cancer Prevention
and Control
4770 Buford Hwy., NE, MS K-64
Atlanta, GA 30341-3717
Phone: 800-CDC-INFO
(232-4636)
TTY: 888-232-6348
Fax: 770-488-4760
Website: http://www.cdc.gov/
cancer/minorityawareness/
index.htm
E-mail: cdcinfo@cdc.gov

Health Resources and Services Administration

U.S. Department of Health and Human Services
5600 Fishers Lane, Room 1445
Rockville, MD 20857
Toll-Free Information Center:
888-ASK-HRSA (275-4772)
Phone: 301-443-3376
Website: http://www.hrsa.gov

Imaginis Corporation

P.O. Box 8398
Greenville, SC 29604
Phone: 864-335-1139
Website: http://www.imaginis.com

Intercultural Cancer Council

1709 Dryden Road, Suite 1025
Houston, TX 77030-3411
Phone: 713-798-4617
Fax: 713-798-6222
Website: http://iccnetwork.org
E-mail: icc@bcm.edu

Johns Hopkins Breast Cancer Center

601 North Caroline Street
Room 4161
Baltimore, MD 21287
Phone: 443-287-BRST (2778)
Fax: 410-614-1947
Website: http://
www.hopkinsbreastcenter.org

Living Beyond Breast Cancer (LBBC)

354 West Lancaster Avenue
Suite 224
Haverford, PA 19041
Phone: 610-645-4567;
484-708-1550
Survivors' Helpline:
888-753-LBBC (5222)
Fax: 610-645-4573
Website: http://www.lbbc.org
E-mail: mail@lbbc.org

Mayors' Campaign Against Breast Cancer

U.S. Conference of Mayors
1620 Eye Street, NW, 3rd Floor
Washington, DC 20006
Phone: 202-293-7330
Fax: 202-293-2352
Website: http://
www.usmayors.org/cancer
E-mail: info@usmayors.org

National Asian Women's Health Organization

One Embarcadero Center
Suite 500
San Francisco, CA 94111
Phone: 415-773-2838
Fax: 415-773-2872
Website: http://www.nawho.org

National Breast Cancer Awareness Month

P.O. Box 15437
Wilmington, DE 19850-5437
Phone: 877-88-NBCAM
(886-2226)
Website: http://www.nbcam.org

National Breast Cancer Coalition

1101 17th Street, NW
Suite 1300
Washington, DC 20036
Phone: 800-622-2838
Fax: 202-265-6854
Website: http://
www.stopbreastcancer.org

National Breast and Ovarian Cancer Centre

Phone (Australia): 02-9357-9400
Fax (Australia): 02-9357-9477
International Phone:
+61-2-9357-9400
International Fax:
+61-2-9357-9477
Website: http://www.nbocc.org.au
E-mail: directorate@nbocc.org.au

National Cancer Institute

3035A, MSC 8322
6116 Executive Blvd.
Bethesda MD 20892
Phone: 800-4-CANCER
(422-6237)
Website: http://cancer.gov

National Comprehensive Cancer Network

275 Commerce Drive
Suite 300
Fort Washington, PA 19034
Phone: 215-690-0300
Fax: 215-690-0280
Website: http://www.nccn.org

National Indian Women's Health Resource Center

228 South Muskogee Avenue
Tahlequah, OK 74464
Phone: 918-456-6094
Fax: 918-456-8128
Website: http://www.niwhrc.org
E-mail: peiron@niwhrc.org

National Library of Medicine

8600 Rockville Pike
Bethesda, MD 20894
Toll Free: 888-FIND-NLM
(346-3656)
Phone: 301-594-5983
Fax: 301-402-1384
Website: http://www.nlm.nih.gov
E-mail: custserv@nlm.nih.gov

National Women's Health Information Center

Office on Women's Health
200 Independence Ave., SW
Room 712E
Washington, DC 20201
Toll-Free: 800-994-9662
Toll-Free TDD: 888-220-5446
Phone: 202-690-7650
Fax: 202-205-2631
Website: http://www.4woman.gov

National Women's Health Network

514 10th Street, NW, Suite 400
Washington, DC 20004
Phone: 202-628-7814;
202-347-1140
Fax: 202-347-1168
Website: http://
www.womenshealthnetwork.org
E-mail: nwhn@nwhn.org

Native American Cancer Research
393 South Harlan 125
Lakewoood CO 80226
Phone: 303-838-9359
Fax: 303-838-7629
Website: http://natamcancer.org

Native American Women's Health Education Resource Center
Native American Community Board
P.O. Box 572
Lake Andes, SD 57356
Phone: 605-487-7072
Fax: 605-487-7964
Website: http://www.nativeshop.org/nawherc.html

Native C.I.R.C.L.E.
Charlton 6, Room 282
200 First Street, SW
Rochester, MN 55905
Phone: 877-372-1617
Fax: 507-538-0504
Website: http://cancercenter.mayo.edu/native_circle.cfm

Office of Minority Health Resource Center
U.S. Department of Health and Human Services
Phone: 800-444-6472
Website: http://www.omhrc.gov

Office on Women's Health
U.S. Department of Health and Human Services
200 Independence Avenue, SW
Room 712E
Washington, DC 20201
Phone: 202-690-7650
Website: http://www.4woman.gov/owh

OncoLink
Abramson Cancer Center of the University of Pennsylvania
3400 Spruce Street - 2 Donner
Philadelphia, PA 19104-4283
Fax: 215-349-5445
Website: http://www.oncolink.org

Prevent Cancer Foundation
1600 Duke Street, Suite 500
Alexandria, VA 22314
Toll-Free: 800-227-2732
Phone: 703-836-4412
Fax: 703-836-4413
Website: http://www.preventcancer.org

Program on Breast Cancer and Environmental Risk Factors
Cornell University
College of Veterinary Medicine
Vet Box 31
Ithaca, NY 14853-6401
Phone: 607-254-2893
Fax: 607-254-4730
Website: http://envirocancer.cornell.edu
E-mail: breastcancer@cornell.edu

Redes En Acción
Chronic Disease Prevention
and Control Research Center
Baylor College of Medicine
8207 Callaghan Road
Suite 353
San Antonio, TX 78230
Phone: 210-562-6500
Fax: 210-348-0554
Website: http://redesenaccion.org
E-mail:
redesenaccion@uthscsa.edu

**Salud En Acción: National
Hispanic/Latino Health
Communication Research**
Chronic Disease Prevention
and Control Research Center
Baylor College of Medicine
8207 Callaghan Road
Suite 353
San Antonio, TX 78230
Phone: 210-562-6500
Fax: 210-348-0554
Website: http://saludenaccion.org
E-mail:
saludenaccion@uthscsa.edu

**Society of Surgical
Oncology**
85 West Algonquin Road
Suite 550
Arlington Heights, IL 60005
Phone: 847-427-1400
Fax: 847-427-9656
Website: http://www.surgonc.org
E-mail: webmaster@surgonc.org

**Southeast Asian Health
Program**
Family Health and Social
Service Center
26 Queen Street
Worcester, MA 01610
Phone: 508-860-7700
Fax: 508-860-7792
Website: http://www.fhcw.org/
seap.htm

Support Groups and Organizations

**African American Breast
Cancer Alliance**
P.O. Box 8981
Minneapolis, MN 55408
Phone: 612-825-3675
Fax: 612-827-2977
Website: http://
www.geocities.com/aabcainc

**American Breast Cancer
Foundation**
1220 B East Joppa Road
Suite 332
Baltimore, MD 21286
Toll-free: 877-Key-2-Life
(539-2543)
Phone: 410-825-9388
Fax: 410-825-4395
Website: http://www.abcf.org
E-mail: contactABCF@abcf.org

Asian American Pacific Islander Cancer Survivors Capacity Building Project

c/o Asian & Pacific Islander American Health Forum
450 Sutter Street, Suite 600
San Francisco, CA 94108
Phone: 415-954-9988
Fax: 415-954-9999
Website: http://www.apiahf.org/programs/ncsn

Avon Breast Cancer Crusade

Avon Foundation
1345 Avenue of the Americas
New York, NY 10105
Phone: 212-282-5000
Website: http://www.avoncompany.com/women/avoncrusade

Black Women's Health Imperative

1420 K Street, NW,
Suite 1000, 10th Floor
Washington, DC 20005
Phone: 202-548-4000
Fax: 202-543-9743
Website: http://www.blackwomenshealth.org
E-mail: Info@BlackWomensHealth.org

Breast Cancer Network of Strength™

212 West Van Buren Street
Suite 1000
Chicago, IL 60607
Toll-Free: 800-221-2141 (English);
800-986-9505 (Spanish)
Phone: 312-986-8338
Fax: 312-294-8597
Website: http://www.networkofstrength.org

CancerCare

275 Seventh Avenue, Floor 22
New York, NY 10001
Toll-Free: 800-813-HOPE (4673)
Phone: 212-712-8400
Fax: 212-712-8495
Website: http://www.cancercare.org
E-mail: info@cancercare.org

Cancer Hope Network

2 North Road, Suite A
Chester, NJ 07930
Toll-Free: 877-HOPENET
(877-467-3638)
Phone: 908-879-4039 (Local)
Fax: 908-879-6518
Website: http://www.cancerhopenetwork.org
E-mail: info@cancerhopenetwork.org

Celebrating Life Foundation

12100 Ford Road, Suite 100
Dallas, TX 75234
Phone: 800-207-0992
Website: http://
www.celebratinglife.org/
Foundation_Profile.htm
E-mail: info@celebratinglife.org

Gilda's Club® Worldwide

322 Eight Avenue, Suite 1402
New York, NY 10001
Phone: 888-GILDA-4-U
(888-445-3248)
Website: http://
www.gildasclub.org
E-mail: info@gildasclub.org

Hospice Education Institute

3 Unity Square
P.O. Box 98
Machiasport, ME 04655
Toll-Free: 800-331-1620
Phone: 207-255-8800
Website: http://
www.hospiceworld.org
E-mail: info@hospiceworld.org

Look Good...Feel Better

c/o CTFA Foundation
American Cancer Society
Toll-Free: 800-395-LOOK (5665);
800-ACS-2345 (227-2345)
Phone: 202-331-1770
Website: http://
www.lookgoodfeelbetter.org

Mautner Project for Lesbians with Cancer

1875 Connecticut Avenue, NW
Washington, DC 20009
Toll-Free: 866-MAUTNER
(628-8637)
Phone: 202-332-5536
Fax: 202-332-0662
Website: http://
www.mautnerproject.org

Men Against Breast Cancer

P.O. Box 150
Adamstown, MD 21710-0150
Phone: 866-547-MABC (6222)
Fax: 301-874-8657
Website: http://
www.menagainstbreastcancer.org
E-mail:
info@menagainstbreastcancer.org

National Breast Cancer Foundation

2600 Network Blvd., Suite 300
Frisco, TX 75034
Website: http://
www.nationalbreastcancer.org

National Coalition for Cancer Survivorship

1010 Wayne Avenue, Suite 770
Silver Spring, MD 20910
Toll-Free: 888-650-9127
Phone: 301-650-9127
Fax: 301-565-9670
Website: http://
www.canceradvocacy.org
E-mail: info@canceradvocacy.org

National Hospice and Palliative Care Organization (NHPCO)
1700 Diagonal Road
Suite 625
Alexandria, VA 22314
Toll-Free: 800-658-8898
(helpline); 877-658-8896
(Spanish-speaking families)
Phone: 703-837-1500
Website:
http://www.nhpco.org
E-mail:
nhpco_info@nhpco.org

People Living with Cancer
American Society of Clinical
Oncology
2318 Mill Road
Alexandria, VA 22314
Toll-Free: 888-651-3038
Phone: 703-797-1914
Fax: 703-299-1044
Website: http://www.plwc.org

Reach to Recovery
American Cancer Society
Phone: 800-ACS-2345
(800-227-2345)
Website: http://www.cancer.org/
docroot/ESN/content/
ESN_3_1x_Reach_to_Recovery_5
.asp

Sisters Network
8787 Woodway Drive
Suite 4206
Houston, TX 77063
Phone: 713-781-0255
Fax: 713-780-8998
Website: http://
www.sistersnetworkinc.org

"TLC" Tender Loving Care®
American Cancer Society
P.O. Box 395
Louisiana, MO 63353
Phone: 800-850-9445
Website: http://www.tlcdirect.org
E-mail:
customerservice@tlccatalog.org

Vital Options®
International TeleSupport®
Cancer Network
4419 Coldwater Canyon Avenue
Suite I
Studio City, CA 91604
Toll-Free: 800-GRP-ROOM
(800-477-7666)
Phone: 818-508-5657
Fax: 818-788-5260
Website: http://
www.vitaloptions.org
E-mail: info@vitaloptions.org

Wellness Community®
919 18th Street, NW, Suite 54
Washington, DC 20006
Toll-Free: 888-793-WELL
(888-793-9355)
Phone: 202-659-9709
Website: http://
www.thewellnesscommunity.org
E-mail:
help@thewellnesscommunity.org

Young Survival Coalition
61 Broadway, Suite 2235
New York, NY 10006
Toll-Free 877-YSC-1011 (972-1011)
Phone: 646-257-3000
Fax: 646-257-3030
Website: www.youngsurvival.org
E-mail: info@youngsurvival.org

Chapter 59

National Breast and Cervical Cancer Early Detection Program: State Contacts

About the Program

The Centers for Disease Control and Prevention provides low-income, uninsured, and underserved women access to timely, high-quality screening and diagnostic services, to detect breast and cervical cancer at the earliest stages, through the National Breast and Cervical Cancer Early Detection Program (NBCCEDP).

An estimated 8–11% of U.S. women of screening age are eligible to receive NBCCEDP services. Federal guidelines establish an eligibility baseline to direct services to uninsured and underinsured women at or below 250% of federal poverty level; ages 18–64 for cervical screening; ages 40–64 for breast screening.

This chapter includes information from "National Breast and Cervical Cancer Early Detection Program," Centers for Disease Control and Prevention (CDC), August 29, 2007; and "State, U.S. Territory, and Organization Program Contacts," CDC. All contact information was updated and verified in June 2008.

State, U.S. Territory, and Organization Program Contacts

Alabama

Breast and Cervical Cancer
Early Detection Program
Bureau of Health Promotion and
Chronic Disease
Alabama Department of Public
Health
RSA Tower, 201 Monroe Street
Suite 1364
Montgomery, AL 36104
P.O. Box 303017
Montgomery, AL 36130-3017
Phone: 334-206-5851
Fax: 334-206-2950

Alaska

Breast and Cervical Health
Check
Division of Public Health
Section of Women's, Children's,
and Family Health
4701 Business Park Blvd.
Building J, Suite 20
Anchorage, AK 99503-7123
Phone: 800-410-6266 (in state);
907-269-3491 (outside of state)
Fax: 907-269-3414

American Samoa

Breast and Cervical Cancer
Early Detection Program
Department of Health
American Samoa Government
Territory of American Samoa
Pago Pago, AS 96799
Phone: 011-684-633-2135
Fax: 011-684-633-2136

Arizona

Well Woman Healthcheck
Program
Office of Nutrition and Chronic
Disease Prevention Services
Arizona Department of Health
Services
150 North 18th Avenue, Suite 310
Phoenix, AZ 85007
Phone: 888-257-8502
Fax: 602-542-7520

Arkansas

BreastCare Program
Arkansas Department of Health
4815 West Markham Street
Slot 11
Little Rock, AR 72205
Phone: 501-661-2273
Enrollment Number:
877-670-2273
Fax: 501-280-4049
Website: http://
www.arbreastcare.com/core.html

California

Cancer Detection Programs:
Every Woman Counts
Cancer Detection Section
California Department of
Health Services
1616 Capitol Avenue, MS-7203,
Suite 74.421
P.O. Box 997377
Sacramento, CA 95814
Phone: 916-449-5300
Fax: 916-440-5184

Colorado

Colorado Women's Cancer
Control Initiative
Colorado Department of Public
Health and Environment
PSD-CWCCI-A5
4300 Cherry Creek Drive South
Denver, CO 80246-1530
Phone: 303-692-2480;
303-692-2600 (in state)
Enrollment Number:
866-951-9355
Fax: 303-691-7900

Commonwealth of Northern Mariana Islands

Breast and Cervical Cancer
Screening Program
Department of Public Health
P.O. Box 500409
Saipan, MP 96950
Phone: 670-236-8703
Fax: 670-236-8700

Connecticut

Breast and Cervical Cancer
Program
Connecticut Department of
Public Health
410 Capitol Avenue, MS-11CCSS
Hartford, CT 06106
Phone: 860-509-8309
Enrollment Number:
860-509-7804
Fax: 860-509-7855

Delaware

Screening for Life
Division of Public Health
Delaware Department of Health
and Social Services
Blue Hen Corporate Center
540 South Dupont Highway
Suite 11
Thomas Colons Building
Dover, DE 19904
Toll-Free: 800-464-4357
Phone: 302-741-8600
Fax: 302-741-8601

District of Columbia

Breast and Cervical Cancer
Early Detection Program
District of Columbia
Department of Health
825 North Capitol Street, NE
3rd Floor
Washington, DC 20002
Phone: 202-442-5900;
202-442-9128 (Spanish)
Fax: 202-442-4825

Florida

Breast and Cervical Cancer
Early Detection Program
Bureau of Chronic Disease
Prevention
Florida Department of Health
4052 Bald Cypress Way
Bin #A-18
Tallahassee, FL 32399-1744
Phone: 850-245-4444
Enrollment Number:
800-451-2229
Fax: 850-414-6625

Georgia

Breast and Cervical Cancer
Program
Georgia Cancer Control Section,
Division of Public Health
Georgia Department of Human
Resources
2 Peachtree Street, NW
13th Floor
Atlanta, GA 30303-3142
Phone: 404-657-3156
Fax: 404-657-1463

Guam

Breast and Cervical Cancer
Early Detection Program
Division of Public Health
Department of Public Health
and Social Services
123 Chalan Kareta, Route 10
Mangilao, GU 96913
Phone: 671-735-7174
Enrollment Number:
850-245-4455; 617-735-7174
Fax: 671-735-7103

Hawaii

Hawaii Breast and Cervical
Cancer Program
Breast and Cervical Cancer
Control Program
Hawaii State Department of
Health
601 Kamokila Boulevard #344
Kapolei, HI 96707
Phone: 808-586-4609
Enrollment Number:
808-692-7460
Fax: 808-587-5340

Idaho

Women's Health Check
Division of Health
Idaho Department of Health
and Welfare
450 W. State Street, 4th Floor
P.O. Box 83720
Boise, ID 83720-0036
Phone: 208-334-5805
Enrollment Number:
800-926-2588
Fax: 208-334-0657
Website:
www.healthandwelfare.idaho.gov

Illinois

Illinois Breast and Cervical
Cancer Program
Office of Women's Health
Services
Illinois Department of Public
Health
535 West Jefferson Street
1st Floor
Springfield, IL 62761-0001
Phone: 217-785-1050
Enrollment Number:
888-522-1282
Fax: 217-557-3326

Indiana

Breast and Cervical Cancer
Early Detection Program
Indiana State Department of
Health
2 North Meridian Street
Mailstop 6B-F4
Indianapolis, IN 46204
Toll-Free: 800-433-0746
Phone: 317-234-1356
Fax: 317-234-2699

Iowa

Care for Yourself
Iowa Breast and Cervical
Cancer Early Detection Program
Iowa Department of Public
Health
321 East 12th Street
Des Moines, IA 50319-0075
Phone: 515-242-6067
Enrollment Number:
800-369-2229
Fax: 515-281-6475

Kansas

Early Detection Works
Office of Health Promotion
Kansas Department of Health
and Environment
State Office Building
1000 Southwest Jackson
Suite 230
Topeka, KS 66612-1274
Phone: 877-277-1368
Fax: 785-368-7287

Kentucky

Kentucky Women's Cancer
Screening Program
Chronic Disease Prevention and
Control Branch
Kentucky Department of Public
Health
275 East Main Street, HS2GW-A
Frankfort, KY 40621-0001
Phone: 502-564-2154 Ext. 3821
Fax: 502-564-8389

Louisiana

Louisiana Breast and Cervical
Health Program
Louisiana State University
Health Sciences Center
School of Public Health
P.O. Box 2018
Mandeville, LA 70112
Phone: 888-599-1073
Enrollment Number:
888-599-1073
Fax: 504-218-2324

Maine

Breast and Cervical Health
Program
Maine Bureau of Health
11 State House Station
Key Bank Plaza
286 Water Street, 4th Floor
Augusta, ME 04333-0011
Phone: 207-287-8068
Enrollment Number:
800-350-5180 (in state)
Fax: 207-287-4100

Maryland

Breast and Cervical Cancer
Screening Program
Center for Cancer Surveillance
and Control
Maryland Department of Health
and Mental Hygiene
201 West Preston Street
3rd Floor
Baltimore, MD 21201
Phone: 410-767-6728
Enrollment Number:
800-477-9774
Fax: 410-333-7279

Massachusetts

Women's Health Network
Massachusetts Department of
Health
250 Washington Street, 4th Floor
Boston, MA 02108-4619
Phone: 617-624-5434
Enrollment Number:
877-414-4447
Fax: 617-624-5055

Michigan

Breast and Cervical Cancer
Control Program
Cancer Prevention and Control
Section
Michigan Department of
Community Health
Washington Square Building
5th Floor
109 Michigan Avenue
Lansing, MI 48913
Phone: 517-335-8049
Enrollment Number:
800-922-MAMM (6266)
Fax: 517-335-9397

Minnesota

SAGE Screening Program
Minnesota Department of
Health
85 East 7th Place
P.O. Box 64882
St. Paul, MN 55164-0882
Phone: 651-201-5618
Enrollment Number:
888-643-2584
Fax: 651-201-5601

Mississippi

Mississippi Breast and Cervical
Cancer Early Detection Program
Mississippi Department of Health
570 East Woodrow Wilson
P.O. Box 1700
Jackson, MS 39215-1700
Phone: 601-576-7466
Enrollment Number:
800-721-7222
Fax: 601-576-8030

Missouri

Show Me Healthy Women
Program
Cancer Control Unit
Missouri Department of Health
and Senior Services
920 Wildwood Drive
P.O. Box 570
Jefferson City, MO 65102-0570
Phone: 573-522-2845
Fax: 573-522-2899

Montana

Breast and Cervical Health
Program
Montana Department of Public
Health and Human Services
Cogswell Building
1400 Broadway, C-317
P.O. Box 202951
Helena, MT 59620-2951
Phone: 406-444-0063
Enrollment Number:
888-803-9343 (in state)
Fax: 406-444-7465

Nebraska

Every Woman Matters Program
Office of Women's Health
Nebraska Health and Human
Services
301 Centennial Mall South
3rd Floor
P.O. Box 94817
Lincoln, NE 68509-4817
Phone: 402-471-0314
Enrollment Number:
402-471-0929 (in Lincoln);
800-532-2227 (outside Lincoln)
Fax: 402-471-0913

Nevada

Women's Health Connection
Nevada State Health Division
4150 Technology Way, Suite 101
Carson City, NV 89706
Phone: 775-684-5926
Enrollment Number:
888-463-8942 (in state);
775-684-5936 (outside of state)
Fax: 775-684-4031

New Hampshire

Breast and Cervical Cancer
Program
Division of Public Health Services
New Hampshire Department of
Health and Human Services
29 Hazen Drive
Concord, NH 03301-4604
Toll-Free: 800-852-3345 (in state)
Phone: 603-271-4886
Fax: 603-271-0539

New Jersey

Cancer Education and Early
Detection Program
New Jersey Department of
Health and Senior Services
50 East State Street, 6th Floor
P.O. Box 364
Trenton, NJ 08625-0364
Phone: 609-292-8540
Enrollment Number:
800-328-3838
Fax: 609-292-3580

New Mexico

Breast and Cervical Cancer
Early Detection Program
New Mexico Department of
Health
5301 Central Avenue NE
Suite 800
Albuquerque, NM 87108
Phone: 505-841-5847;
877-852-2585
Fax: 505-22-8608

New York

Cancer Services Program
Bureau of Chronic Disease
Services
New York State Department of
Health
150 Broadway, 3rd Floor West
Room 350
Albany, NY 12204
Phone: 518-474-1222
Enrollment Number:
866-442-CANCER; 866-442-2262
Fax: 518-473-0642

North Carolina

Breast and Cervical Cancer
Control Program
Division of Public Health
North Carolina Department of
Health and Human Services
1922 Mail Service Center
Raleigh, NC 27699-1922
Shipping Address:
5505 Six Forks Road, 1st Floor
Room B11
Raleigh, NC 27609
Phone: 919-707-5300
Enrollment Number:
800-4-CANCER (in state);
919-715-0111 (outside of state)
Fax: 919-870-4812

North Dakota

Women's Way Program
Division of Cancer Prevention
and Control
North Dakota Department of
Health
600 East Boulevard Avenue
Department 301
Bismarck, ND 58505-0200
Phone: 701-328-2472
Enrollment Number:
800-449-6636 (in state);
701-328-2333 (outside of state)
Fax: 701-328-2036

Ohio

Breast and Cervical Cancer
Project
Ohio Department of Health
246 North High Street
Columbus, OH 43215
Phone: 614-387-0537
Enrollment Number:
800-4-CANCER
Fax: 614-564-2409

Oklahoma

Breast and Cervical Cancer
Early Detection Program
Oklahoma State Department of
Health
1000 Northeast 10th Street
Oklahoma City, OK 73117-1299
Phone: 405-271-4072
Enrollment Number:
888-669-5934
Fax: 405-271-6315

Oregon

Breast and Cervical Cancer
Program
Health Promotion and Chronic
Disease Prevention
Oregon Department of Human
Services
800 NE Oregon Street
Suite 360
Portland, OR 97232-2162
Toll-Free: 877-255-7070
Phone: 971-673-0581
Enrollment Number:
971-673-0984
Fax: 971-673-0997

Pennsylvania

Breast and Cervical Cancer
Early Detection Program
Division of Chronic Disease
Intervention
Pennsylvania Department of
Health
Health and Welfare Building
Room 1011
P.O. Box 90
Harrisburg, PA 17120
Delivery Address: Health and
Welfare Bldg., Room 1011
Commonwealth and Forster
Harrisburg, PA 17120
Phone: 717-783-1457
Enrollment Number:
800-4-CANCER (422-6237)
Fax: 717-772-0608

Puerto Rico

Breast and Cervical Cancer
Early Detection Program
University of Puerto Rico
Office of Sponsored Research
Medical Sciences Campus
P.O. Box 365067
San Juan, PR 00936
Phone: 787-766-1240
Fax: 787-767-8008

Republic of Palau

Breast and Cervical Cancer
Early Detection Program
Republic of Palau Ministry of
Health
P.O. Box 6027
Koror, PW 96940
Phone: 011-680-488-4612
Fax: 011-680-488-1211

Rhode Island

Women's Cancer Screening
Program
Rhode Island Cancer Control
Program
Rhode Island Department of
Health
3 Capitol Hill, Room 408
Providence, RI 02908
Phone: 401-222-1161
Fax: 401-222-4895

South Carolina

Breast and Cervical Cancer
Early Detection Program
Division of Cancer Prevention
and Control
Bureau of Chronic Disease
Prevention, DHEC
1777 St. Julian Place
Columbia, SC 29204
Phone: 803-545-4145
Enrollment Number:
800-227-2345
Fax: 803-545-4445

South Dakota

All Women Count!
South Dakota Department of
Health
615 East 4th Street
Pierre, SD 57501-1700
Phone: 605-773-5728
Enrollment Number:
800-738-2301(in state)
Fax: 605-773-5509

Tennessee

Breast and Cervical Cancer
Early Detection Program
Tennessee Department of
Health
Cordell Hull Building, 6th Floor
425 5th Avenue North
Nashville, TN 37247-5262
Phone: 615-532-8494
Fax: 615-741-3806

Texas

Breast and Cervical Cancer
Control Program
Texas Department of State
Health Services
Preventive and Primary
Care Unit
1100 West 49th Street
Mail Code 1923
Austin, TX 78756-3199
Phone: 512-458-7796
Fax: 512-458-7650

Utah

Utah Cancer Control Program
Utah Department of Health
288 North 1460 Street
P.O. Box 142107
Salt Lake City, UT 84114-2107
Phone: 801-538-6233
Fax: 801-538-9495

Vermont

Ladies First
Chronic Disease Program
Vermont Department of Health
108 Cherry Street
P.O. Box 70
Burlington, VT 05402-0070
Enrollment Number:
800-508-2222
TTD: 800-319-3141
Fax: 802-657-4208

Virginia

Breast and Cervical Cancer
Early Detection Program
Virginia Department of Health
109 Governor Street, 8th Floor
Richmond, VA 23219
Phone: 804-864-7756
Enrollment Number:
866-EWL-4-YOU (866-395-4968)
(in state); 804-864-7761 (outside
of state)
Fax: 804-864-7763

Washington

Washington Breast and Cervical
Health Program
Washington State Department
of Health
Cancer Prevention and Control
Unit
P.O. Box 47855
Olympia, WA 98504-7855
111 Israel Road SE
Tumwater, WA 98501
Enrollment Number:
888-438-2247
Fax: 360-664-2619

West Virginia

Breast and Cervical Cancer
Screening Program
West Virginia Department of
Health and Human Resources
350 Capital Street, Room 427
Charleston, WV 25301-3714
Phone: 304-558-7180
Enrollment Number:
800-4-CANCER (422-6237)
Fax: 304-558-7164

Wisconsin

Well Woman Program
Division of Public Health
Wisconsin Department of
Health and Family Services
One West Wilson Street
Room 218
P.O. Box 2659
Madison, WI 53701-2659
Phone: 608-261-6872
Fax: 608-261-8625

Wyoming

Breast and Cervical Cancer
Early Detection Program
Preventive Health and Safety
Division
Wyoming Department of Health
6101 Yellowstone Road
Room 259A
Cheyenne, WY 82002
Enrollment Number:
800-264-1296
Fax: 307-777-3765

American Indian/Alaska Native Organizations and Program Contacts

Arctic Slope Native Association Limited

Breast and Cervical Cancer Early Detection Program
Department of Health and Social Services
P.O. Box 69
Barrow, AK 99723
Phone: 907-852-5880
Fax: 907-852-5882

Cherokee Nation

Breast and Cervical Cancer Early Detection Program
P.O. Box 948
Tahlequah, OK 74465
Overnight Address:
1200 West 4th Street, Suite C
Tahlequah, OK 74464
Phone: 918-458-4491
Fax: 918-458-6267

Cheyenne River Sioux Tribe

Breast and Cervical Cancer Early Detection Program
312 Main Street
P.O. Box 590
Overnight Address: Field Health, Main Street
Eagle Butte, SD 57625
Phone: 605-964-8917
Fax: 605-964-1176

Hopi Tribe

Breast and Cervical Cancer Early Detection Program
P.O. Box 123
Kykotsmovi, AZ 86039
Phone: 928-734-1150
Fax: 928-734-1158

Kaw Nation of Oklahoma

Kaw Nation Programs and Services
Kanza Health Clinic
P.O. Box 474
Newkirk, OK 74647
FedEx Address: 3151 East River Road
Newkirk, OK 74647-0474
Phone: 580-362-1039 Ext. 228
Fax: 580-362-2988
Website: http://www.kawnation.com/Programs/proghome.html

Native American Rehabilitation Association of the Northwest, Inc.

Women's Wellness Program
15 N. Morris Street
Portland, OR 97227
Phone: 503-230-9875 Ext. 250
Fax: 503-230-9877

Navajo Nation

Breast and Cervical Cancer
Early Detection Program
P.O. Box 1390
Window Rock, AZ 86515
Overnight Address:
Window Rock Boulevard
Administration Building 2
Window Rock, AZ 86515
Phone: 928-871-6249
Ext. 23
Fax: 928-871-6255

Poarch Band of Creek Indians

Breast and Cervical Cancer
Early Detection Program
5811 Jack Springs Road
Atmore, AL 36502
Phone: 850-476-5128
Fax: 850-478-0832

South East Alaska Regional Health Consortium

Breast and Cervical Cancer
Early Detection Program
222 Tongass Drive
Sitka, AK 99835
Phone: 888-388-8782

South Puget Intertribal Planning Agency

Breast and Cervical Cancer
Early Detection Program
3104 Old Olympic Highway, SE
Shelton, WA 98581
Phone: 360-462-3222
Fax: 360-427-1625

Southcentral Foundation

Breast and Cervical Cancer
Early Detection Program
4320 Diplomacy Drive
Suite 2630
Anchorage, AK 99508
Phone: 907-729-8891
Fax: 907-729-3265

Yukon-Kuskokwim Health Corporation

Breast and Cervical Cancer
Early Detection Program
700 Chief Eddy Hoffman
Highway
P.O. Box 287, Pouch 3000
Bethel, AK 99559
Overnight Address: P.O. Box 287
Bethel, AK 99559
Phone: 907-543-6996
Fax: 907-543-6561

Index

Index

Page numbers followed by 'n' indicate a footnote. Page numbers in *italics* indicate a table or illustration.

Health Reference Series
COMPLETE CATALOG
List price $87 per volume. **School and library price $78 per volume.**

Adolescent Health Sourcebook, 2nd Edition

Basic Consumer Health Information about the Physical, Mental, and Emotional Growth and Development of Adolescents, Including Medical Care, Nutritional and Physical Activity Requirements, Puberty, Sexual Activity, Acne, Tanning, Body Piercing, Common Physical Illnesses and Disorders, Eating Disorders, Attention Deficit Hyperactivity Disorder, Depression, Bullying, Hazing, and Adolescent Injuries Related to Sports, Driving, and Work

Along with Substance Abuse Information about Nicotine, Alcohol, and Drug Use, a Glossary, and Directory of Additional Resources

Edited by Joyce Brennfleck Shannon. 683 pages. 2006. 978-0-7808-0943-7.

"It is written in clear, nontechnical language aimed at general readers. . . . Recommended for public libraries, community colleges, and other agencies serving health care consumers."
— *American Reference Books Annual, 2003*

"Recommended for school and public libraries. Parents and professionals dealing with teens will appreciate the easy-to-follow format and the clearly written text. This could become a 'must have' for every high school teacher." — *E-Streams, Jan '03*

"A good starting point for information related to common medical, mental, and emotional concerns of adolescents." — *School Library Journal, Nov '02*

"This book provides accurate information in an easy to access format. It addresses topics that parents and caregivers might not be aware of and provides practical, useable information."
— *Doody's Health Sciences Book Review Journal, Sep-Oct '02*

"Recommended reference source."
— *Booklist, American Library Association, Sep '02*

AIDS Sourcebook, 3rd Edition

Basic Consumer Health Information about Acquired Immune Deficiency Syndrome (AIDS) and Human Immunodeficiency Virus (HIV) Infection, Including Facts about Transmission, Prevention, Diagnosis, Treatment, Opportunistic Infections, and Other Complications, with a Section for Women and Children, Including Details about Associated Gynecological Concerns, Pregnancy, and Pediatric Care

Along with Updated Statistical Information, Reports on Current Research Initiatives, a Glossary, and Directories of Internet, Hotline, and Other Resources

Edited by Dawn D. Matthews. 664 pages. 2003. 978-0-7808-0631-3.

"The 3rd edition of the *AIDS Sourcebook*, part of Omnigraphics' *Health Reference Series*, is a welcome update. . . . This resource is highly recommended for academic and public libraries."
— *American Reference Books Annual, 2004*

"Excellent sourcebook. This continues to be a highly recommended book. There is no other book that provides as much information as this book provides."
— *AIDS Book Review Journal, Dec-Jan '00*

"Recommended reference source."
— *Booklist, American Library Association, Dec '99*

Alcoholism Sourcebook, 2nd Edition

Basic Consumer Health Information about Alcohol Use, Abuse, and Dependence, Featuring Facts about the Physical, Mental, and Social Health Effects of Alcohol Addiction, Including Alcoholic Liver Disease, Pancreatic Disease, Cardiovascular Disease, Neurological Disorders, and the Effects of Drinking during Pregnancy

Along with Information about Alcohol Treatment, Medications, and Recovery Programs, in Addition to Tips for Reducing the Prevalence of Underage Drinking, Statistics about Alcohol Use, a Glossary of Related Terms, and Directories of Resources for More Help and Information

Edited by Amy L. Sutton. 653 pages. 2006. 978-0-7808-0942-0.

"This title is one of the few reference works on alcoholism for general readers. For some readers this will be a welcome complement to the many self-help books on the market. Recommended for collections serving general readers and consumer health collections."
— *E-Streams, Mar '01*

"This book is an excellent choice for public and academic libraries."
— *American Reference Books Annual, 2001*

"Recommended reference source."
— *Booklist, American Library Association, Dec '00*

"Presents a wealth of information on alcohol use and abuse and its effects on the body and mind, treatment, and prevention." — *SciTech Book News, Dec '00*

"Important new health guide which packs in the latest consumer information about the problems of alcoholism." — *Reviewer's Bookwatch, Nov '00*

SEE ALSO Drug Abuse Sourcebook

Allergies Sourcebook, 3rd Edition

Basic Consumer Health Information about Allergic Disorders, Such as Anaphylaxis, Hives, Eczema, Rhinitis, Sinusitis, and Conjunctivitis, and Their Triggers, Including Pollen, Mold, Dust Mites, Animal Dander, Insects, Chemicals, Food, Food Additives, and Medications;

Along with Advice about the Diagnosis and Treatment of Allergy Symptoms, a Glossary of Related Terms, a Directory of Resources for Help and Information, and Suggestions for Additional Reading

Edited by Amy L. Sutton. 598 pages. 2007. 978-0-7808-0950-5.

"This book brings a great deal of useful material together. . . . This is an excellent addition to public and consumer health library collections."
— *American Reference Books Annual, 2003*

"This second edition would be useful to laypersons with little or advanced knowledge of the subject matter. This book would also serve as a resource for nursing and other health care professions students. It would be useful in public, academic, and hospital libraries with consumer health collections." — *E-Streams, Jul '02*

■

Alternative Medicine Sourcebook

SEE Complementary & Alternative Medicine Sourcebook

■

Alzheimer's Disease Sourcebook, 3rd Edition

Basic Consumer Health Information about Alzheimer's Disease, Other Dementias, and Related Disorders, Including Multi-Infarct Dementia, AIDS Dementia Complex, Dementia with Lewy Bodies, Huntington's Disease, Wernicke-Korsakoff Syndrome (Alcohol-Related Dementia), Delirium, and Confusional States

Along with Information for People Newly Diagnosed with Alzheimer's Disease and Caregivers, Reports Detailing Current Research Efforts in Prevention, Diagnosis, and Treatment, Facts about Long-Term Care Issues, and Listings of Sources for Additional Information

Edited by Karen Bellenir. 645 pages. 2003. 978-0-7808-0666-5.

"This very informative and valuable tool will be a great addition to any library serving consumers, students and health care workers."
— *American Reference Books Annual, 2004*

"This is a valuable resource for people affected by dementias such as Alzheimer's. It is easy to navigate and includes important information and resources."
— *Doody's Review Service, Feb '04*

"Recommended reference source."
— *Booklist, American Library Association, Oct '99*

SEE ALSO *Brain Disorders Sourcebook*

Arthritis Sourcebook, 2nd Edition

Basic Consumer Health Information about Osteoarthritis, Rheumatoid Arthritis, Other Rheumatic Disorders, Infectious Forms of Arthritis, and Diseases with Symptoms Linked to Arthritis, Featuring Facts about Diagnosis, Pain Management, and Surgical Therapies

Along with Coping Strategies, Research Updates, a Glossary, and Resources for Additional Help and Information

Edited by Amy L. Sutton. 593 pages. 2004. 978-0-7808-0667-2.

"This easy-to-read volume is recommended for consumer health collections within public or academic libraries." — *E-Streams, May '05*

"As expected, this updated edition continues the excellent reputation of this series in providing sound, usable health information. . . . Highly recommended."
— *American Reference Books Annual, 2005*

"Excellent reference." — *The Bookwatch, Jan '05*

■

Asthma Sourcebook, 2nd Edition

Basic Consumer Health Information about the Causes, Symptoms, Diagnosis, and Treatment of Asthma in Infants, Children, Teenagers, and Adults, Including Facts about Different Types of Asthma, Common Co-Occurring Conditions, Asthma Management Plans, Triggers, Medications, and Medication Delivery Devices

Along with Asthma Statistics, Research Updates, a Glossary, a Directory of Asthma-Related Resources, and More

Edited by Karen Bellenir. 609 pages. 2006. 978-0-7808-0866-9.

"A worthwhile reference acquisition for public libraries and academic medical libraries whose readers desire a quick introduction to the wide range of asthma information." — *Choice, Association of College & Research Libraries, Jun '01*

"Recommended reference source."
— *Booklist, American Library Association, Feb '01*

"Highly recommended." — *The Bookwatch, Jan '01*

"There is much good information for patients and their families who deal with asthma daily."
— *American Medical Writers Association Journal, Winter '01*

"This informative text is recommended for consumer health collections in public, secondary school, and community college libraries and the libraries of universities with a large undergraduate population."
— *American Reference Books Annual, 2001*

■

Attention Deficit Disorder Sourcebook

Basic Consumer Health Information about Attention Deficit/Hyperactivity Disorder in Children and Adults,

Including Facts about Causes, Symptoms, Diagnostic Criteria, and Treatment Options Such as Medications, Behavior Therapy, Coaching, and Homeopathy

Along with Reports on Current Research Initiatives, Legal Issues, and Government Regulations, and Featuring a Glossary of Related Terms, Internet Resources, and a List of Additional Reading Material

Edited by Dawn D. Matthews. 470 pages. 2002. 978-0-7808-0624-5.

"Recommended reference source."
— Booklist, American Library Association, Jan '03

"This book is recommended for all school libraries and the reference or consumer health sections of public libraries." — American Reference Books Annual, 2003

■

Back & Neck Sourcebook, 2nd Edition

Basic Consumer Health Information about Spinal Pain, Spinal Cord Injuries, and Related Disorders, Such as Degenerative Disk Disease, Osteoarthritis, Scoliosis, Sciatica, Spina Bifida, and Spinal Stenosis, and Featuring Facts about Maintaining Spinal Health, Self-Care, Pain Management, Rehabilitative Care, Chiropractic Care, Spinal Surgeries, and Complementary Therapies

Along with Suggestions for Preventing Back and Neck Pain, a Glossary of Related Terms, and a Directory of Resources

Edited by Amy L. Sutton. 633 pages. 2004. 978-0-7808-0738-9.

"Recommended . . . an easy to use, comprehensive medical reference book." — E-Streams, Sep '05

"The strength of this work is its basic, easy-to-read format. Recommended." — Reference and User Services Quarterly, American Library Association, Winter '97

■

Blood & Circulatory Disorders Sourcebook, 2nd Edition

Basic Consumer Health Information about the Blood and Circulatory System and Related Disorders, Such as Anemia and Other Hemoglobin Diseases, Cancer of the Blood and Associated Bone Marrow Disorders, Clotting and Bleeding Problems, and Conditions That Affect the Veins, Blood Vessels, and Arteries, Including Facts about the Donation and Transplantation of Bone Marrow, Stem Cells, and Blood and Tips for Keeping the Blood and Circulatory System Healthy

Along with a Glossary of Related Terms and Resources for Additional Help and Information

Edited by Amy L. Sutton. 659 pages. 2005. 978-0-7808-0746-4.

"Highly recommended pick for basic consumer health reference holdings at all levels."
— The Bookwatch, Aug '05

"Recommended reference source."
— Booklist, American Library Association, Feb '99

"An important reference sourcebook written in simple language for everyday, non-technical users. "
— Reviewer's Bookwatch, Jan '99

■

Brain Disorders Sourcebook, 2nd Edition

Basic Consumer Health Information about Acquired and Traumatic Brain Injuries, Infections of the Brain, Epilepsy and Seizure Disorders, Cerebral Palsy, and Degenerative Neurological Disorders, Including Amyotrophic Lateral Sclerosis (ALS), Dementias, Multiple Sclerosis, and More

Along with Information on the Brain's Structure and Function, Treatment and Rehabilitation Options, Reports on Current Research Initiatives, a Glossary of Terms Related to Brain Disorders and Injuries, and a Directory of Sources for Further Help and Information

Edited by Sandra J. Judd. 625 pages. 2005. 978-0-7808-0744-0.

"Highly recommended pick for basic consumer health reference holdings at all levels."
— The Bookwatch, Aug '05

"Belongs on the shelves of any library with a consumer health collection." — E-Streams, Mar '00

"Recommended reference source."
— Booklist, American Library Association, Oct '99

SEE ALSO Alzheimer's Disease Sourcebook

■

Breast Cancer Sourcebook, 2nd Edition

Basic Consumer Health Information about Breast Cancer, Including Facts about Risk Factors, Prevention, Screening and Diagnostic Methods, Treatment Options, Complementary and Alternative Therapies, Post-Treatment Concerns, Clinical Trials, Special Risk Populations, and New Developments in Breast Cancer Research

Along with Breast Cancer Statistics, a Glossary of Related Terms, and a Directory of Resources for Additional Help and Information

Edited by Sandra J. Judd. 595 pages. 2004. 978-0-7808-0668-9.

"This book will be an excellent addition to public, community college, medical, and academic libraries."
— American Reference Books Annual, 2006

"It would be a useful reference book in a library or on loan to women in a support group."
— Cancer Forum, Mar '03

"Recommended reference source."
— Booklist, American Library Association, Jan '02

"This reference source is highly recommended. It is quite informative, comprehensive and detailed in nature, and yet it offers practical advice in easy-to-read language. It could be thought of as the 'bible' of breast cancer for the consumer." — *E-Streams, Jan '02*

"From the pros and cons of different screening methods and results to treatment options, *Breast Cancer Sourcebook* provides the latest information on the subject." — *Library Bookwatch, Dec '01*

"This thoroughgoing, very readable reference covers all aspects of breast health and cancer. . . . Readers will find much to consider here. Recommended for all public and patient health collections." — *Library Journal, Sep '01*

SEE ALSO *Cancer Sourcebook for Women, Women's Health Concerns Sourcebook*

■

Breastfeeding Sourcebook

Basic Consumer Health Information about the Benefits of Breastmilk, Preparing to Breastfeed, Breastfeeding as a Baby Grows, Nutrition, and More, Including Information on Special Situations and Concerns Such as Mastitis, Illness, Medications, Allergies, Multiple Births, Prematurity, Special Needs, and Adoption

Along with a Glossary and Resources for Additional Help and Information

Edited by Jenni Lynn Colson. 388 pages. 2002. 978-0-7808-0332-9.

"Particularly useful is the information about professional lactation services and chapters on breastfeeding when returning to work. . . . *Breastfeeding Sourcebook* will be useful for public libraries, consumer health libraries, and technical schools offering nurse assistant training, especially in areas where Internet access is problematic." — *American Reference Books Annual, 2003*

SEE ALSO *Pregnancy & Birth Sourcebook*

■

Burns Sourcebook

Basic Consumer Health Information about Various Types of Burns and Scalds, Including Flame, Heat, Cold, Electrical, Chemical, and Sun Burns

Along with Information on Short-Term and Long-Term Treatments, Tissue Reconstruction, Plastic Surgery, Prevention Suggestions, and First Aid

Edited by Allan R. Cook. 604 pages. 1999. 978-0-7808-0204-9.

"This is an exceptional addition to the series and is highly recommended for all consumer health collections, hospital libraries, and academic medical centers." — *E-Streams, Mar '00*

"This key reference guide is an invaluable addition to all health care and public libraries in confronting this ongoing health issue." — *American Reference Books Annual, 2000*

"Recommended reference source." — *Booklist, American Library Association, Dec '99*

SEE ALSO *Dermatological Disorders Sourcebook*

Cancer Sourcebook, 5th Edition

Basic Consumer Health Information about Major Forms and Stages of Cancer, Featuring Facts about Head and Neck Cancers, Lung Cancers, Gastrointestinal Cancers, Genitourinary Cancers, Lymphomas, Blood Cell Cancers, Endocrine Cancers, Skin Cancers, Bone Cancers, Metastatic Cancers, and More

Along with Facts about Cancer Treatments, Cancer Risks and Prevention, a Glossary of Related Terms, Statistical Data, and a Directory of Resources for Additional Information

Edited by Karen Bellenir. 1,133 pages. 2007. 978-0-7808-0947-5.

"With cancer being the second leading cause of death for Americans, a prodigious work such as this one, which locates centrally so much cancer-related information, is clearly an asset to this nation's citizens and others." — *Journal of the National Medical Association, 2004*

"This title is recommended for health sciences and public libraries with consumer health collections." — *E-Streams, Feb '01*

". . . can be effectively used by cancer patients and their families who are looking for answers in a language they can understand. Public and hospital libraries should have it on their shelves." — *American Reference Books Annual, 2001*

"Recommended reference source." — *Booklist, American Library Association, Dec '00*

SEE ALSO *Breast Cancer Sourcebook, Cancer Sourcebook for Women, Pediatric Cancer Sourcebook, Prostate Cancer Sourcebook*

■

Cancer Sourcebook for Women, 3rd Edition

Basic Consumer Health Information about Leading Causes of Cancer in Women, Featuring Facts about Gynecologic Cancers and Related Concerns, Such as Breast Cancer, Cervical Cancer, Endometrial Cancer, Uterine Sarcoma, Vaginal Cancer, Vulvar Cancer, and Common Non-Cancerous Gynecologic Conditions, in Addition to Facts about Lung Cancer, Colorectal Cancer, and Thyroid Cancer in Women

Along with Information about Cancer Risk Factors, Screening and Prevention, Treatment Options, and Tips on Coping with Life after Cancer Treatment, a Glossary of Cancer Terms, and a Directory of Resources for Additional Help and Information

Edited by Amy L. Sutton. 715 pages. 2006. 978-0-7808-0867-6.

"An excellent addition to collections in public, consumer health, and women's health libraries." — *American Reference Books Annual, 2003*

"Overall, the information is excellent, and complex topics are clearly explained. As a reference book for the consumer it is a valuable resource to assist them to make informed decisions about cancer and its treatments." — *Cancer Forum, Nov '02*

"Highly recommended for academic and medical reference collections." — *Library Bookwatch, Sep '02*

"This is a highly recommended book for any public or consumer library, being reader friendly and containing accurate and helpful information."
— *E-Streams, Aug '02*

"Recommended reference source."
— *Booklist, American Library Association, Jul '02*

SEE ALSO *Breast Cancer Sourcebook, Women's Health Concerns Sourcebook*

■

Cancer Survivorship Sourcebook

Basic Consumer Health Information about the Physical, Educational, Emotional, Social, and Financial Needs of Cancer Patients from Diagnosis, through Cancer Treatment, and Beyond, Including Facts about Researching Specific Types of Cancer and Learning about Clinical Trials and Treatment Options, and Featuring Tips for Coping with the Side Effects of Cancer Treatments and Adjusting to Life after Cancer Treatment Concludes

Along with Suggestions for Caregivers, Friends, and Family Members of Cancer Patients, a Glossary of Cancer Care Terms, and Directories of Related Resources

Edited by Karen Bellenir. 6561 pages. 2007. 978-0-7808-0985-7.

■

Cardiovascular Diseases & Disorders Sourcebook, 3rd Edition

Basic Consumer Health Information about Heart and Vascular Diseases and Disorders, Such as Angina, Heart Attacks, Arrhythmias, Cardiomyopathy, Valve Disease, Atherosclerosis, and Aneurysms, with Information about Managing Cardiovascular Risk Factors and Maintaining Heart Health, Medications and Procedures Used to Treat Cardiovascular Disorders, and Concerns of Special Significance to Women

Along with Reports on Current Research Initiatives, a Glossary of Related Medical Terms, and a Directory of Sources for Further Help and Information

Edited by Sandra J. Judd. 713 pages. 2005. 978-0-7808-0739-6.

"This updated sourcebook is still the best first stop for comprehensive introductory information on cardiovascular diseases."
— *American Reference Books Annual, 2006*

"Recommended for public libraries and libraries supporting health care professionals."
— *E-Streams, Sep '05*

"This should be a standard health library reference."
— *The Bookwatch, Jun '05*

"Recommended reference source."
— *Booklist, American Library Association, Dec '00*

"... comprehensive format provides an extensive overview on this subject."
— *Choice, Association of College & Research Libraries*

■

Caregiving Sourcebook

Basic Consumer Health Information for Caregivers, Including a Profile of Caregivers, Caregiving Responsibilities and Concerns, Tips for Specific Conditions, Care Environments, and the Effects of Caregiving

Along with Facts about Legal Issues, Financial Information, and Future Planning, a Glossary, and a Listing of Additional Resources

Edited by Joyce Brennfleck Shannon. 600 pages. 2001. 978-0-7808-0331-2.

"Essential for most collections."
— *Library Journal, Apr 1, 2002*

"An ideal addition to the reference collection of any public library. Health sciences information professionals may also want to acquire the *Caregiving Sourcebook* for their hospital or academic library for use as a ready reference tool by health care workers interested in aging and caregiving." — *E-Streams, Jan '02*

"Recommended reference source."
— *Booklist, American Library Association, Oct '01*

■

Child Abuse Sourcebook

Basic Consumer Health Information about the Physical, Sexual, and Emotional Abuse of Children, with Additional Facts about Neglect, Munchausen Syndrome by Proxy (MSBP), Shaken Baby Syndrome, and Controversial Issues Related to Child Abuse, Such as Withholding Medical Care, Corporal Punishment, and Child Maltreatment in Youth Sports, and Featuring Facts about Child Protective Services, Foster Care, Adoption, Parenting Challenges, and Other Abuse Prevention Efforts

Along with a Glossary of Related Terms and Resources for Additional Help and Information

Edited by Dawn D. Matthews. 620 pages. 2004. 978-0-7808-0705-1.

"A valuable and highly recommended resource for school, academic and public libraries whether used on its own or as a starting point for more in-depth research." — *E-Streams, Apr '05*

"Every week the news brings cases of child abuse or neglect, so it is useful to have a source that supplies so much helpful information. . . . Recommended. Public and academic libraries, and child welfare offices."
— *Choice, Association of College & Research Libraries, Mar '05*

"Packed with insights on all kinds of issues, from foster care and adoption to parenting and abuse prevention."
— *The Bookwatch, Nov '04*

SEE ALSO: *Domestic Violence Sourcebook*

Childhood Diseases & Disorders Sourcebook

Basic Consumer Health Information about Medical Problems Often Encountered in Pre-Adolescent Children, Including Respiratory Tract Ailments, Ear Infections, Sore Throats, Disorders of the Skin and Scalp, Digestive and Genitourinary Diseases, Infectious Diseases, Inflammatory Disorders, Chronic Physical and Developmental Disorders, Allergies, and More

Along with Information about Diagnostic Tests, Common Childhood Surgeries, and Frequently Used Medications, with a Glossary of Important Terms and Resource Directory

Edited by Chad T. Kimball. 662 pages. 2003. 978-0-7808-0458-6.

"This is an excellent book for new parents and should be included in all health care and public libraries."
— *American Reference Books Annual, 2004*

SEE ALSO: *Healthy Children Sourcebook*

Colds, Flu & Other Common Ailments Sourcebook

Basic Consumer Health Information about Common Ailments and Injuries, Including Colds, Coughs, the Flu, Sinus Problems, Headaches, Fever, Nausea and Vomiting, Menstrual Cramps, Diarrhea, Constipation, Hemorrhoids, Back Pain, Dandruff, Dry and Itchy Skin, Cuts, Scrapes, Sprains, Bruises, and More

Along with Information about Prevention, Self-Care, Choosing a Doctor, Over-the-Counter Medications, Folk Remedies, and Alternative Therapies, and Including a Glossary of Important Terms and a Directory of Resources for Further Help and Information

Edited by Chad T. Kimball. 638 pages. 2001. 978-0-7808-0435-7.

"A good starting point for research on common illnesses. It will be a useful addition to public and consumer health library collections."
— *American Reference Books Annual, 2002*

"Will prove valuable to any library seeking to maintain a current, comprehensive reference collection of health resources. . . . Excellent reference."
— *The Bookwatch, Aug '01*

"Recommended reference source."
— *Booklist, American Library Association, Jul '01*

Communication Disorders Sourcebook

Basic Information about Deafness and Hearing Loss, Speech and Language Disorders, Voice Disorders, Balance and Vestibular Disorders, and Disorders of Smell, Taste, and Touch

Edited by Linda M. Ross. 533 pages. 1996. 978-0-7808-0077-9.

"This is skillfully edited and is a welcome resource for the layperson. It should be found in every public and medical library." — *Booklist Health Sciences Supplement, American Library Association, Oct '97*

Complementary & Alternative Medicine Sourcebook, 3rd Edition

Basic Consumer Health Information about Complementary and Alternative Medical Therapies, Including Acupuncture, Ayurveda, Traditional Chinese Medicine, Herbal Medicine, Homeopathy, Naturopathy, Biofeedback, Hypnotherapy, Yoga, Art Therapy, Aromatherapy, Clinical Nutrition, Vitamin and Mineral Supplements, Chiropractic, Massage, Reflexology, Crystal Therapy, Therapeutic Touch, and More

Along with Facts about Alternative and Complementary Treatments for Specific Conditions Such as Cancer, Diabetes, Osteoarthritis, Chronic Pain, Menopause, Gastrointestinal Disorders, Headaches, and Mental Illness, a Glossary, and a Resource List for Additional Help and Information

Edited by Sandra J. Judd. 657 pages. 2006. 978-0-7808-0864-5.

"Recommended for public, high school, and academic libraries that have consumer health collections. Hospital libraries that also serve the public will find this to be a useful resource." — *E-Streams, Feb '03*

"Recommended reference source."
— *Booklist, American Library Association, Jan '03*

"An important alternate health reference."
— *MBR Bookwatch, Oct '02*

"A great addition to the reference collection of every type of library." — *American Reference Books Annual, 2000*

Congenital Disorders Sourcebook, 2nd Edition

Basic Consumer Health Information about Non-hereditary Birth Defects and Disorders Related to Prematurity, Gestational Injuries, Congenital Infections, and Birth Complications, Including Heart Defects, Hydrocephalus, Spina Bifida, Cleft Lip and Palate, Cerebral Palsy, and More

Along with Facts about the Prevention of Birth Defects, Fetal Surgery and Other Treatment Options, Research Initiatives, a Glossary of Related Terms, and Resources for Additional Information and Support

Edited by Sandra J. Judd. 647 pages. 2006. 978-0-7808-0945-1.

"Recommended reference source."
— *Booklist, American Library Association, Oct '97*

SEE ALSO *Pregnancy & Birth Sourcebook*

Contagious Diseases Sourcebook

Basic Consumer Health Information about Infectious Diseases Spread by Person-to-Person Contact through

Direct Touch, Airborne Transmission, Sexual Contact, or Contact with Blood or Other Body Fluids, Including Hepatitis, Herpes, Influenza, Lice, Measles, Mumps, Pinworm, Ringworm, Severe Acute Respiratory Syndrome (SARS), Streptococcal Infections, Tuberculosis, and Others

Along with Facts about Disease Transmission, Antimicrobial Resistance, and Vaccines, with a Glossary and Directories of Resources for More Information

Edited by Karen Bellenir. 643 pages. 2004. 978-0-7808-0736-5.

"This easy-to-read volume is recommended for consumer health collections within public or academic libraries." — E-Streams, May '05

"This informative book is highly recommended for public libraries, consumer health collections, and secondary schools and undergraduate libraries."
— American Reference Books Annual, 2005

"Excellent reference." — The Bookwatch, Jan '05

Death & Dying Sourcebook, 2nd Edition

Basic Consumer Health Information about End-of-Life Care and Related Perspectives and Ethical Issues, Including End-of-Life Symptoms and Treatments, Pain Management, Quality-of-Life Concerns, the Use of Life Support, Patients' Rights and Privacy Issues, Advance Directives, Physician-Assisted Suicide, Caregiving, Organ and Tissue Donation, Autopsies, Funeral Arrangements, and Grief

Along with Statistical Data, Information about the Leading Causes of Death, a Glossary, and Directories of Support Groups and Other Resources

Edited by Joyce Brennfleck Shannon. 653 pages. 2006. 978-0-7808-0871-3.

"Public libraries, medical libraries, and academic libraries will all find this sourcebook a useful addition to their collections."
— American Reference Books Annual, 2001

"An extremely useful resource for those concerned with death and dying in the United States."
— Respiratory Care, Nov '00

"Recommended reference source."
—Booklist, American Library Association, Aug '00

"This book is a definite must for all those involved in end-of-life care." — Doody's Review Service, 2000

Dental Care & Oral Health Sourcebook, 2nd Edition

Basic Consumer Health Information about Dental Care, Including Oral Hygiene, Dental Visits, Pain Management, Cavities, Crowns, Bridges, Dental Implants, and Fillings, and Other Oral Health Concerns, Such as Gum Disease, Bad Breath, Dry Mouth, Genetic and Developmental Abnormalities, Oral Cancers, Orthodontics, and Temporomandibular Disorders

Along with Updates on Current Research in Oral Health, a Glossary, a Directory of Dental and Oral Health Organizations, and Resources for People with Dental and Oral Health Disorders

Edited by Amy L. Sutton. 609 pages. 2003. 978-0-7808-0634-4.

"This book could serve as a turning point in the battle to educate consumers in issues concerning oral health."
— American Reference Books Annual, 2004

"Unique source which will fill a gap in dental sources for patients and the lay public. A valuable reference tool even in a library with thousands of books on dentistry. Comprehensive, clear, inexpensive, and easy to read and use. It fills an enormous gap in the health care literature." — Reference & User Services Quarterly, American Library Association, Summer '98

"Recommended reference source."
—Booklist, American Library Association, Dec '97

Depression Sourcebook

Basic Consumer Health Information about Unipolar Depression, Bipolar Disorder, Postpartum Depression, Seasonal Affective Disorder, and Other Types of Depression in Children, Adolescents, Women, Men, the Elderly, and Other Selected Populations

Along with Facts about Causes, Risk Factors, Diagnostic Criteria, Treatment Options, Coping Strategies, Suicide Prevention, a Glossary, and a Directory of Sources for Additional Help and Information

Edited by Karen Bellenir. 602 pages. 2002. 978-0-7808-0611-5.

"Depression Sourcebook is of a very high standard. Its purpose, which is to serve as a reference source to the lay reader, is very well served."
— Journal of the National Medical Association, 2004

"Invaluable reference for public and school library collections alike." — Library Bookwatch, Apr '03

"Recommended for purchase."
— American Reference Books Annual, 2003

Dermatological Disorders Sourcebook, 2nd Edition

Basic Consumer Health Information about Conditions and Disorders Affecting the Skin, Hair, and Nails, Such as Acne, Rosacea, Rashes, Dermatitis, Pigmentation Disorders, Birthmarks, Skin Cancer, Skin Injuries, Psoriasis, Scleroderma, and Hair Loss, Including Facts about Medications and Treatments for Dermatological Disorders and Tips for Maintaining Healthy Skin, Hair, and Nails

Along with Information about How Aging Affects the Skin, a Glossary of Related Terms, and a Directory of Resources for Additional Help and Information

Edited by Amy L. Sutton. 645 pages. 2005. 978-0-7808-0795-2.

"... comprehensive, easily read reference book."
—*Doody's Health Sciences Book Reviews, Oct '97*

SEE ALSO *Burns Sourcebook*

Diabetes Sourcebook, 3rd Edition

Basic Consumer Health Information about Type 1 Diabetes (Insulin-Dependent or Juvenile-Onset Diabetes), Type 2 Diabetes (Noninsulin-Dependent or Adult-Onset Diabetes), Gestational Diabetes, Impaired Glucose Tolerance (IGT), and Related Complications, Such as Amputation, Eye Disease, Gum Disease, Nerve Damage, and End-Stage Renal Disease, Including Facts about Insulin, Oral Diabetes Medications, Blood Sugar Testing, and the Role of Exercise and Nutrition in the Control of Diabetes

Along with a Glossary and Resources for Further Help and Information

Edited by Dawn D. Matthews. 622 pages. 2003. 978-0-7808-0629-0.

"This edition is even more helpful than earlier versions. . . . It is a truly valuable tool for anyone seeking readable and authoritative information on diabetes."
— *American Reference Books Annual, 2004*

"An invaluable reference." — *Library Journal, May '00*

Selected as one of the 250 "Best Health Sciences Books of 1999." — *Doody's Rating Service, Mar-Apr '00*

"Provides useful information for the general public."
— *Healthlines, University of Michigan Health Management Research Center, Sep/Oct '99*

". . . provides reliable mainstream medical information . . . belongs on the shelves of any library with a consumer health collection." — *E-Streams, Sep '99*

"Recommended reference source."
— *Booklist, American Library Association, Feb '99*

Diet & Nutrition Sourcebook, 3rd Edition

Basic Consumer Health Information about Dietary Guidelines and the Food Guidance System, Recommended Daily Nutrient Intakes, Serving Proportions, Weight Control, Vitamins and Supplements, Nutrition Issues for Different Life Stages and Lifestyles, and the Needs of People with Specific Medical Concerns, Including Cancer, Celiac Disease, Diabetes, Eating Disorders, Food Allergies, and Cardiovascular Disease

Along with Facts about Federal Nutrition Support Programs, a Glossary of Nutrition and Dietary Terms, and Directories of Additional Resources for More Information about Nutrition

Edited by Joyce Brennfleck Shannon. 633 pages. 2006. 978-0-7808-0800-3.

"This book is an excellent source of basic diet and nutrition information." — *Booklist Health Sciences Supplement, American Library Association, Dec '00*

"This reference document should be in any public library, but it would be a very good guide for beginning students in the health sciences. If the other books in this publisher's series are as good as this, they should all be in the health sciences collections."
— *American Reference Books Annual, 2000*

"This book is an excellent general nutrition reference for consumers who desire to take an active role in their health care for prevention. Consumers of all ages who select this book can feel confident they are receiving current and accurate information." — *Journal of Nutrition for the Elderly, Vol. 19, No. 4, 2000*

SEE ALSO *Digestive Diseases & Disorders Sourcebook, Eating Disorders Sourcebook, Gastrointestinal Diseases & Disorders Sourcebook, Vegetarian Sourcebook*

Digestive Diseases & Disorders Sourcebook

Basic Consumer Health Information about Diseases and Disorders that Impact the Upper and Lower Digestive System, Including Celiac Disease, Constipation, Crohn's Disease, Cyclic Vomiting Syndrome, Diarrhea, Diverticulosis and Diverticulitis, Gallstones, Heartburn, Hemorrhoids, Hernias, Indigestion (Dyspepsia), Irritable Bowel Syndrome, Lactose Intolerance, Ulcers, and More

Along with Information about Medications and Other Treatments, Tips for Maintaining a Healthy Digestive Tract, a Glossary, and Directory of Digestive Diseases Organizations

Edited by Karen Bellenir. 335 pages. 2000. 978-0-7808-0327-5.

"This title would be an excellent addition to all public or patient-research libraries."
— *American Reference Books Annual, 2001*

"This title is recommended for public, hospital, and health sciences libraries with consumer health collections." — *E-Streams, Jul-Aug '00*

"Recommended reference source."
— *Booklist, American Library Association, May '00*

SEE ALSO *Eating Disorders Sourcebook, Gastrointestinal Diseases & Disorders Sourcebook*

Disabilities Sourcebook

Basic Consumer Health Information about Physical and Psychiatric Disabilities, Including Descriptions of Major Causes of Disability, Assistive and Adaptive Aids, Workplace Issues, and Accessibility Concerns

Along with Information about the Americans with Disabilities Act, a Glossary, and Resources for Additional Help and Information

Edited by Dawn D. Matthews. 616 pages. 2000. 978-0-7808-0389-3.

"It is a must for libraries with a consumer health section." — *American Reference Books Annual, 2002*

"A much needed addition to the Omnigraphics *Health Reference Series*. A current reference work to provide people with disabilities, their families, caregivers or those who work with them, a broad range of information in one volume, has not been available until now. . . . It is recommended for all public and academic library reference collections." —*E-Streams, May '01*

"An excellent source book in easy-to-read format covering many current topics; highly recommended for all libraries." —*Choice, Association of College & Research Libraries, Jan '01*

"Recommended reference source."
—*Booklist, American Library Association, Jul '00*

■

Domestic Violence Sourcebook, 2nd Edition

Basic Consumer Health Information about the Causes and Consequences of Abusive Relationships, Including Physical Violence, Sexual Assault, Battery, Stalking, and Emotional Abuse, and Facts about the Effects of Violence on Women, Men, Young Adults, and the Elderly, with Reports about Domestic Violence in Selected Populations, and Featuring Facts about Medical Care, Victim Assistance and Protection, Prevention Strategies, Mental Health Services, and Legal Issues

Along with a Glossary of Related Terms and Resources for Additional Help and Information

Edited by Dawn D. Matthews. 628 pages. 2004. 978-0-7808-0669-6.

"Educators, clergy, medical professionals, police, and victims and their families will benefit from this realistic and easy-to-understand resource."
—*American Reference Books Annual, 2005*

"Recommended for all collections supporting consumer health information. It should also be considered for any collection needing general, readable information on domestic violence." —*E-Streams, Jan '05*

"This sourcebook complements other books in its field, providing a one-stop resource . . . Recommended."
—*Choice, Association of College & Research Libraries, Jan '05*

"Interested lay persons should find the book extremely beneficial. . . . A copy of *Domestic Violence and Child Abuse Sourcebook* should be in every public library in the United States."
—*Social Science & Medicine, No. 56, 2003*

"This is important information. The Web has many resources but this sourcebook fills an important societal need. I am not aware of any other resources of this type." —*Doody's Review Service, Sep '01*

"Recommended reference source."
—*Booklist, American Library Association, Apr '01*

"Important pick for college-level health reference libraries." —*The Bookwatch, Mar '01*

"Because this problem is so widespread and because this book includes a lot of issues within one volume, this work is recommended for all public libraries."
—*American Reference Books Annual, 2001*

SEE ALSO Child Abuse Sourcebook

■

Drug Abuse Sourcebook, 2nd Edition

Basic Consumer Health Information about Illicit Substances of Abuse and the Misuse of Prescription and Over-the-Counter Medications, Including Depressants, Hallucinogens, Inhalants, Marijuana, Stimulants, and Anabolic Steroids

Along with Facts about Related Health Risks, Treatment Programs, Prevention Programs, a Glossary of Abuse and Addiction Terms, a Glossary of Drug-Related Street Terms, and a Directory of Resources for More Information

Edited by Catherine Ginther. 607 pages. 2004. 978-0-7808-0740-2.

"Commendable for organizing useful, normally scattered government and association-produced data into a logical sequence."
—*American Reference Books Annual, 2006*

"This easy-to-read volume is recommended for consumer health collections within public or academic libraries." —*E-Streams, Sep '05*

"An excellent library reference."
—*The Bookwatch, May '05*

"Containing a wealth of information, this book will be useful to the college student just beginning to explore the topic of substance abuse. This resource belongs in libraries that serve a lower-division undergraduate or community college clientele as well as the general public." —*Choice, Association of College & Research Libraries, Jun '01*

"Recommended reference source."
—*Booklist, American Library Association, Feb '01*

SEE ALSO Alcoholism Sourcebook

■

Ear, Nose & Throat Disorders Sourcebook, 2nd Edition

Basic Consumer Health Information about Disorders of the Ears, Hearing Loss, Vestibular Disorders, Nasal and Sinus Problems, Throat and Vocal Cord Disorders, and Otolaryngologic Cancers, Including Facts about Ear Infections and Injuries, Genetic and Congenital Deafness, Sensorineural Hearing Disorders, Tinnitus, Vertigo, Ménière Disease, Rhinitis, Sinusitis, Snoring, Sore Throats, Hoarseness, and More

Along with Reports on Current Research Initiatives, a Glossary of Related Medical Terms, and a Directory of Sources for Further Help and Information

Edited by Sandra J. Judd. 659 pages. 2006. 978-0-7808-0872-0.

"Overall, this sourcebook is helpful for the consumer seeking information on ENT issues. It is recommended for public libraries."
— *American Reference Books Annual, 1999*

"Recommended reference source."
— *Booklist, American Library Association, Dec '98*

■

Eating Disorders Sourcebook, 2nd Edition

Basic Consumer Health Information about Anorexia Nervosa, Bulimia Nervosa, Binge Eating, Compulsive Exercise, Female Athlete Triad, and Other Eating Disorders, Including Facts about Body Image and Other Cultural and Age-Related Risk Factors, Prevention Efforts, Adverse Health Effects, Treatment Options, and the Recovery Process

Along with Guidelines for Healthy Weight Control, a Glossary, and Directories of Additional Resources

Edited by Joyce Brennfleck Shannon. 585 pages. 2007. 978-0-7808-0948-2.

"Recommended for health science libraries that are open to the public, as well as hospital libraries. This book is a good resource for the consumer who is concerned about eating disorders." — *E-Streams, Mar '02*

"This volume is another convenient collection of excerpted articles. Recommended for school and public library patrons; lower-division undergraduates; and two-year technical program students."
— *Choice, Association of College & Research Libraries, Jan '02*

"Recommended reference source."
— *Booklist, American Library Association, Oct '01*

SEE ALSO Diet & Nutrition Sourcebook, Digestive Diseases & Disorders Sourcebook, Gastrointestinal Diseases & Disorders Sourcebook

■

Emergency Medical Services Sourcebook

Basic Consumer Health Information about Preventing, Preparing for, and Managing Emergency Situations, When and Who to Call for Help, What to Expect in the Emergency Room, the Emergency Medical Team, Patient Issues, and Current Topics in Emergency Medicine

Along with Statistical Data, a Glossary, and Sources of Additional Help and Information

Edited by Jenni Lynn Colson. 494 pages. 2002. 978-0-7808-0420-3.

"Handy and convenient for home, public, school, and college libraries. Recommended."
— *Choice, Association of College & Research Libraries, Apr '03*

"This reference can provide the consumer with answers to most questions about emergency care in the United States, or it will direct them to a resource where the answer can be found."
— *American Reference Books Annual, 2003*

"Recommended reference source."
— *Booklist, American Library Association, Feb '03*

■

Endocrine & Metabolic Disorders Sourcebook

Basic Information for the Layperson about Pancreatic and Insulin-Related Disorders Such as Pancreatitis, Diabetes, and Hypoglycemia; Adrenal Gland Disorders Such as Cushing's Syndrome, Addison's Disease, and Congenital Adrenal Hyperplasia; Pituitary Gland Disorders Such as Growth Hormone Deficiency, Acromegaly, and Pituitary Tumors; Thyroid Disorders Such as Hypothyroidism, Graves' Disease, Hashimoto's Disease, and Goiter; Hyperparathyroidism; and Other Diseases and Syndromes of Hormone Imbalance or Metabolic Dysfunction

Along with Reports on Current Research Initiatives

Edited by Linda M. Shin. 574 pages. 1998. 978-0-7808-0207-0.

"Omnigraphics has produced another needed resource for health information consumers."
— *American Reference Books Annual, 2000*

"Recommended reference source."
— *Booklist, American Library Association, Dec '98*

■

Environmental Health Sourcebook, 2nd Edition

Basic Consumer Health Information about the Environment and Its Effect on Human Health, Including the Effects of Air Pollution, Water Pollution, Hazardous Chemicals, Food Hazards, Radiation Hazards, Biological Agents, Household Hazards, Such as Radon, Asbestos, Carbon Monoxide, and Mold, and Information about Associated Diseases and Disorders, Including Cancer, Allergies, Respiratory Problems, and Skin Disorders

Along with Information about Environmental Concerns for Specific Populations, a Glossary of Related Terms, and Resources for Further Help and Information

Edited by Dawn D. Matthews. 673 pages. 2003. 978-0-7808-0632-0.

"This recently updated edition continues the level of quality and the reputation of the numerous other volumes in Omnigraphics' *Health Reference Series*."
— *American Reference Books Annual, 2004*

"An excellent updated edition."
— *The Bookwatch, Oct '03*

"Recommended reference source."
— *Booklist, American Library Association, Sep '98*

"This book will be a useful addition to anyone's library." — *Choice Health Sciences Supplement, Association of College & Research Libraries, May '98*

". . . a good survey of numerous environmentally induced physical disorders . . . a useful addition to anyone's library."
— *Doody's Health Sciences Book Reviews, Jan '98*

Ethnic Diseases Sourcebook

Basic Consumer Health Information for Ethnic and Racial Minority Groups in the United States, Including General Health Indicators and Behaviors, Ethnic Diseases, Genetic Testing, the Impact of Chronic Diseases, Women's Health, Mental Health Issues, and Preventive Health Care Services

Along with a Glossary and a Listing of Additional Resources

Edited by Joyce Brennfleck Shannon. 664 pages. 2001. 978-0-7808-0336-7.

"Recommended for health sciences libraries where public health programs are a priority."
— *E-Streams, Jan '02*

"Not many books have been written on this topic to date, and the *Ethnic Diseases Sourcebook* is a strong addition to the list. It will be an important introductory resource for health consumers, students, health care personnel, and social scientists. It is recommended for public, academic, and large hospital libraries."
— *American Reference Books Annual, 2002*

"Recommended reference source."
— *Booklist, American Library Association, Oct '01*

"Will prove valuable to any library seeking to maintain a current, comprehensive reference collection of health resources. . . . An excellent source of health information about genetic disorders which affect particular ethnic and racial minorities in the U.S."
— *The Bookwatch, Aug '01*

Eye Care Sourcebook, 2nd Edition

Basic Consumer Health Information about Eye Care and Eye Disorders, Including Facts about the Diagnosis, Prevention, and Treatment of Common Refractive Problems Such as Myopia, Hyperopia, Astigmatism, and Presbyopia, and Eye Diseases, Including Glaucoma, Cataract, Age-Related Macular Degeneration, and Diabetic Retinopathy

Along with a Section on Vision Correction and Refractive Surgeries, Including LASIK and LASEK, a Glossary, and Directories of Resources for Additional Help and Information

Edited by Amy L. Sutton. 543 pages. 2003. 978-0-7808-0635-1.

". . . a solid reference tool for eye care and a valuable addition to a collection."
— *American Reference Books Annual, 2004*

Family Planning Sourcebook

Basic Consumer Health Information about Planning for Pregnancy and Contraception, Including Traditional Methods, Barrier Methods, Hormonal Methods, Permanent Methods, Future Methods, Emergency Contraception, and Birth Control Choices for Women at Each Stage of Life

Along with Statistics, a Glossary, and Sources of Additional Information

Edited by Amy Marcaccio Keyzer. 520 pages. 2001. 978-0-7808-0379-4.

"Recommended for public, health, and undergraduate libraries as part of the circulating collection."
— *E-Streams, Mar '02*

"Information is presented in an unbiased, readable manner, and the sourcebook will certainly be a necessary addition to those public and high school libraries where Internet access is restricted or otherwise problematic." — *American Reference Books Annual, 2002*

"Recommended reference source."
— *Booklist, American Library Association, Oct '01*

"Will prove valuable to any library seeking to maintain a current, comprehensive reference collection of health resources. . . . Excellent reference."
— *The Bookwatch, Aug '01*

SEE ALSO Pregnancy & Birth Sourcebook

Fitness & Exercise Sourcebook, 3rd Edition

Basic Consumer Health Information about the Physical and Mental Benefits of Fitness, Including Cardiorespiratory Endurance, Muscular Strength, Muscular Endurance, and Flexibility, with Facts about Sports Nutrition and Exercise-Related Injuries and Tips about Physical Activity and Exercises for People of All Ages and for People with Health Concerns

Along with Advice on Selecting and Using Exercise Equipment, Maintaining Exercise Motivation, a Glossary of Related Terms, and a Directory of Resources for More Help and Information

Edited by Amy L. Sutton. 663 pages. 2007. 978-0-7808-0946-8.

"This work is recommended for all general reference collections."
— *American Reference Books Annual, 2002*

"Highly recommended for public, consumer, and school grades fourth through college." — *E-Streams, Nov '01*

"Recommended reference source."
— *Booklist, American Library Association, Oct '01*

"The information appears quite comprehensive and is considered reliable. . . . This second edition is a welcomed addition to the series."
— *Doody's Review Service, Sep '01*

Food Safety Sourcebook

Basic Consumer Health Information about the Safe Handling of Meat, Poultry, Seafood, Eggs, Fruit Juices, and Other Food Items, and Facts about Pesticides, Drinking Water, Food Safety Overseas, and the Onset, Duration, and Symptoms of Foodborne Illnesses, Including Types of Pathogenic Bacteria, Parasitic Protozoa, Worms, Viruses, and Natural Toxins

Along with the Role of the Consumer, the Food Handler, and the Government in Food Safety; a Glossary, and Resources for Additional Help and Information

Edited by Dawn D. Matthews. 339 pages. 1999. 978-0-7808-0326-8.

"This book is recommended for public libraries and universities with home economic and food science programs." — E-Streams, Nov '00

"Recommended reference source."
— Booklist, American Library Association, May '00

"This book takes the complex issues of food safety and foodborne pathogens and presents them in an easily understood manner. [It does] an excellent job of covering a large and often confusing topic."
— American Reference Books Annual, 2000

■

Forensic Medicine Sourcebook

Basic Consumer Information for the Layperson about Forensic Medicine, Including Crime Scene Investigation, Evidence Collection and Analysis, Expert Testimony, Computer-Aided Criminal Identification, Digital Imaging in the Courtroom, DNA Profiling, Accident Reconstruction, Autopsies, Ballistics, Drugs and Explosives Detection, Latent Fingerprints, Product Tampering, and Questioned Document Examination

Along with Statistical Data, a Glossary of Forensics Terminology, and Listings of Sources for Further Help and Information

Edited by Annemarie S. Muth. 574 pages. 1999. 978-0-7808-0232-2.

"Given the expected widespread interest in its content and its easy to read style, this book is recommended for most public and all college and university libraries."
— E-Streams, Feb '01

"Recommended for public libraries."
— Reference & User Services Quarterly, American Library Association, Spring 2000

"Recommended reference source."
— Booklist, American Library Association, Feb '00

"A wealth of information, useful statistics, references are up-to-date and extremely complete. This wonderful collection of data will help students who are interested in a career in any type of forensic field. It is a great resource for attorneys who need information about types of expert witnesses needed in a particular case. It also offers useful information for fiction and nonfiction writers whose work involves a crime. A fascinating compilation. All levels."
— Choice, Association of College & Research Libraries, Jan '00

"There are several items that make this book attractive to consumers who are seeking certain forensic data. . . . This is a useful current source for those seeking general forensic medical answers."
— American Reference Books Annual, 2000

Gastrointestinal Diseases & Disorders Sourcebook, 2nd Edition

Basic Consumer Health Information about the Upper and Lower Gastrointestinal (GI) Tract, Including the Esophagus, Stomach, Intestines, Rectum, Liver, and Pancreas, with Facts about Gastroesophageal Reflux Disease, Gastritis, Hernias, Ulcers, Celiac Disease, Diverticulitis, Irritable Bowel Syndrome, Hemorrhoids, Gastrointestinal Cancers, and Other Diseases and Disorders Related to the Digestive Process

Along with Information about Commonly Used Diagnostic and Surgical Procedures, Statistics, Reports on Current Research Initiatives and Clinical Trials, a Glossary, and Resources for Additional Help and Information

Edited by Sandra J. Judd. 681 pages. 2006. 978-0-7808-0798-3.

". . . very readable form. The successful editorial work that brought this material together into a useful and understandable reference makes accessible to all readers information that can help them more effectively understand and obtain help for digestive tract problems."
— Choice, Association of College & Research Libraries, Feb '97

SEE ALSO Diet & Nutrition Sourcebook, Digestive Diseases & Disorders Sourcebook, Eating Disorders Sourcebook

■

Genetic Disorders Sourcebook, 3rd Edition

Basic Consumer Health Information about Hereditary Diseases and Disorders, Including Facts about the Human Genome, Genetic Inheritance Patterns, Disorders Associated with Specific Genes, Such as Sickle Cell Disease, Hemophilia, and Cystic Fibrosis, Chromosome Disorders, Such as Down Syndrome, Fragile X Syndrome, and Turner Syndrome, and Complex Diseases and Disorders Resulting from the Interaction of Environmental and Genetic Factors, Such as Allergies, Cancer, and Obesity

Along with Facts about Genetic Testing, Suggestions for Parents of Children with Special Needs, Reports on Current Research Initiatives, a Glossary of Genetic Terminology, and Resources for Additional Help and Information

Edited by Karen Bellenir. 777 pages. 2004. 978-0-7808-0742-6.

"This text is recommended for any library with an interest in providing consumer health resources."
— E-Streams, Aug '05

"This is a valuable resource for anyone wishing to have an understandable description of any of the topics or disorders included. The editor succeeds in making complex genetic issues understandable."
— Doody's Book Review Service, May '05

"A good acquisition for public libraries."
— American Reference Books Annual, 2005

■

Head Trauma Sourcebook

Basic Information for the Layperson about Open-Head and Closed-Head Injuries, Treatment Advances, Recovery, and Rehabilitation

Along with Reports on Current Research Initiatives

Edited by Karen Bellenir. 414 pages. 1997. 978-0-7808-0208-7.

Headache Sourcebook

Basic Consumer Health Information about Migraine, Tension, Cluster, Rebound and Other Types of Headaches, with Facts about the Cause and Prevention of Headaches, the Effects of Stress and the Environment, Headaches during Pregnancy and Menopause, and Childhood Headaches

Along with a Glossary and Other Resources for Additional Help and Information

Edited by Dawn D. Matthews. 362 pages. 2002. 978-0-7808-0337-4.

■

Healthy Aging Sourcebook

Basic Consumer Health Information about Maintaining Health through the Aging Process, Including Advice on Nutrition, Exercise, and Sleep, Help in Making Decisions about Midlife Issues and Retirement, and Guidance Concerning Practical and Informed Choices in Health Consumerism

Along with Data Concerning the Theories of Aging, Different Experiences in Aging by Minority Groups, and Facts about Aging Now and Aging in the Future; and Featuring a Glossary, a Guide to Consumer Help, Additional Suggested Reading, and Practical Resource Directory

Edited by Jenifer Swanson. 536 pages. 1999. 978-0-7808-0390-9.

SEE ALSO *Physical & Mental Issues in Aging Sourcebook*

■

Healthy Children Sourcebook

Basic Consumer Health Information about the Physical and Mental Development of Children between the Ages of 3 and 12, Including Routine Health Care, Preventative Health Services, Safety and First Aid,

Healthy Sleep, Dental Care, Nutrition, and Fitness, and Featuring Parenting Tips on Such Topics as Bedwetting, Choosing Day Care, Monitoring TV and Other Media, and Establishing a Foundation for Substance Abuse Prevention

Along with a Glossary of Commonly Used Pediatric Terms and Resources for Additional Help and Information.

Edited by Chad T. Kimball. 647 pages. 2003. 978-0-7808-0247-6.

SEE ALSO *Childhood Diseases & Disorders Sourcebook*

■

Healthy Heart Sourcebook for Women

Basic Consumer Health Information about Cardiac Issues Specific to Women, Including Facts about Major Risk Factors and Prevention, Treatment and Control Strategies, and Important Dietary Issues

Along with a Special Section Regarding the Pros and Cons of Hormone Replacement Therapy and Its Impact on Heart Health, and Additional Help, Including Recipes, a Glossary, and a Directory of Resources

Edited by Dawn D. Matthews. 336 pages. 2000. 978-0-7808-0329-9.

SEE ALSO *Cardiovascular Diseases & Disorders Sourcebook, Women's Health Concerns Sourcebook*

■

Hepatitis Sourcebook

Basic Consumer Health Information about Hepatitis A, Hepatitis B, Hepatitis C, and Other Forms of Hepatitis, Including Autoimmune Hepatitis, Alcoholic Hepatitis, Nonalcoholic Steatohepatitis, and Toxic Hepatitis, with

Facts about Risk Factors, Screening Methods, Diagnostic Tests, and Treatment Options

Along with Information on Liver Health, Tips for People Living with Chronic Hepatitis, Reports on Current Research Initiatives, a Glossary of Terms Related to Hepatitis, and a Directory of Sources for Further Help and Information

Edited by Sandra J. Judd. 597 pages. 2005. 978-0-7808-0749-5.

"Highly recommended."
— *American Reference Books Annual, 2006*

■

Household Safety Sourcebook

Basic Consumer Health Information about Household Safety, Including Information about Poisons, Chemicals, Fire, and Water Hazards in the Home

Along with Advice about the Safe Use of Home Maintenance Equipment, Choosing Toys and Nursery Furniture, Holiday and Recreation Safety, a Glossary, and Resources for Further Help and Information

Edited by Dawn D. Matthews. 606 pages. 2002. 978-0-7808-0338-1.

"This work will be useful in public libraries with large consumer health and wellness departments."
— *American Reference Books Annual, 2003*

"As a sourcebook on household safety this book meets its mark. It is encyclopedic in scope and covers a wide range of safety issues that are commonly seen in the home." — *E-Streams, Jul '02*

■

Hypertension Sourcebook

Basic Consumer Health Information about the Causes, Diagnosis, and Treatment of High Blood Pressure, with Facts about Consequences, Complications, and Co-Occurring Disorders, Such as Coronary Heart Disease, Diabetes, Stroke, Kidney Disease, and Hypertensive Retinopathy, and Issues in Blood Pressure Control, Including Dietary Choices, Stress Management, and Medications

Along with Reports on Current Research Initiatives and Clinical Trials, a Glossary, and Resources for Additional Help and Information

Edited by Dawn D. Matthews and Karen Bellenir. 613 pages. 2004. 978-0-7808-0674-0.

"Academic, public, and medical libraries will want to add the *Hypertension Sourcebook* to their collections."
— *E-Streams, Aug '05*

"The strength of this source is the wide range of information given about hypertension."
— *American Reference Books Annual, 2005*

■

Immune System Disorders Sourcebook, 2nd Edition

Basic Consumer Health Information about Disorders of the Immune System, Including Immune System Function and Response, Diagnosis of Immune Disorders, Information about Inherited Immune Disease, Acquired Immune Disease, and Autoimmune Diseases, Including Primary Immune Deficiency, Acquired Immunodeficiency Syndrome (AIDS), Lupus, Multiple Sclerosis, Type 1 Diabetes, Rheumatoid Arthritis, and Graves' Disease

Along with Treatments, Tips for Coping with Immune Disorders, a Glossary, and a Directory of Additional Resources.

Edited by Joyce Brennfleck Shannon. 671 pages. 2005. 978-0-7808-0748-8.

"Highly recommended for academic and public libraries." — *American Reference Books Annual, 2006*

"The updated second edition is a 'must' for any consumer health library seeking a solid resource covering the treatments, symptoms, and options for immune disorder sufferers. . . . An excellent guide."
— *MBR Bookwatch, Jan '06*

■

Infant & Toddler Health Sourcebook

Basic Consumer Health Information about the Physical and Mental Development of Newborns, Infants, and Toddlers, Including Neonatal Concerns, Nutrition Recommendations, Immunization Schedules, Common Pediatric Disorders, Assessments and Milestones, Safety Tips, and Advice for Parents and Other Caregivers

Along with a Glossary of Terms and Resource Listings for Additional Help

Edited by Jenifer Swanson. 585 pages. 2000. 978-0-7808-0246-9.

"As a reference for the general public, this would be useful in any library." — *E-Streams, May '01*

"Recommended reference source."
— *Booklist, American Library Association, Feb '01*

"This is a good source for general use."
— *American Reference Books Annual, 2001*

■

Infectious Diseases Sourcebook

Basic Consumer Health Information about Non-Contagious Bacterial, Viral, Prion, Fungal, and Parasitic Diseases Spread by Food and Water, Insects and Animals, or Environmental Contact, Including Botulism, E. Coli, Encephalitis, Legionnaires' Disease, Lyme Disease, Malaria, Plague, Rabies, Salmonella, Tetanus, and Others, and Facts about Newly Emerging Diseases, Such as Hantavirus, Mad Cow Disease, Monkeypox, and West Nile Virus

Along with Information about Preventing Disease Transmission, the Threat of Bioterrorism, and Current Research Initiatives, with a Glossary and Directory of Resources for More Information

Edited by Karen Bellenir. 634 pages. 2004. 978-0-7808-0675-7.

"This reference continues the excellent tradition of the *Health Reference Series* in consolidating a wealth of information on a selected topic into a format that is easy to use and accessible to the general public."
— *American Reference Books Annual, 2005*

"Recommended for public and academic libraries."
— *E-Streams, Jan '05*

Injury & Trauma Sourcebook

Basic Consumer Health Information about the Impact of Injury, the Diagnosis and Treatment of Common and Traumatic Injuries, Emergency Care, and Specific Injuries Related to Home, Community, Workplace, Transportation, and Recreation

Along with Guidelines for Injury Prevention, a Glossary, and a Directory of Additional Resources

Edited by Joyce Brennfleck Shannon. 696 pages. 2002. 978-0-7808-0421-0.

"This publication is the most comprehensive work of its kind about injury and trauma."
— *American Reference Books Annual, 2003*

"This sourcebook provides concise, easily readable, basic health information about injuries. . . . This book is well organized and an easy to use reference resource suitable for hospital, health sciences and public libraries with consumer health collections."
— *E-Streams, Nov '02*

"Practitioners should be aware of guides such as this in order to facilitate their use by patients and their families."
— *Doody's Health Sciences Book Review Journal, Sep-Oct '02*

"Recommended reference source."
— *Booklist, American Library Association, Sep '02*

"Highly recommended for academic and medical reference collections."
— *Library Bookwatch, Sep '02*

Kidney & Urinary Tract Diseases & Disorders Sourcebook

SEE Urinary Tract & Kidney Diseases & Disorders Sourcebook

Learning Disabilities Sourcebook, 2nd Edition

Basic Consumer Health Information about Learning Disabilities, Including Dyslexia, Developmental Speech and Language Disabilities, Non-Verbal Learning Disorders, Developmental Arithmetic Disorder, Developmental Writing Disorder, and Other Conditions That Impede Learning Such as Attention Deficit/Hyperactivity Disorder, Brain Injury, Hearing Impairment, Klinefelter Syndrome, Dyspraxia, and Tourette's Syndrome

Along with Facts about Educational Issues and Assistive Technology, Coping Strategies, a Glossary of Related Terms, and Resources for Further Help and Information

Edited by Dawn D. Matthews. 621 pages. 2003. 978-0-7808-0626-9.

"The second edition of Learning Disabilities Sourcebook far surpasses the earlier edition in that it is more focused on information that will be useful as a consumer health resource."
— *American Reference Books Annual, 2004*

"Teachers as well as consumers will find this an essential guide to understanding various syndromes and their latest treatments. [An] invaluable reference for public and school library collections alike."
— *Library Bookwatch, Apr '03*

Named "Outstanding Reference Book of 1999."
— *New York Public Library, Feb '00*

"An excellent candidate for inclusion in a public library reference section. It's a great source of information. Teachers will also find the book useful. Definitely worth reading."
— *Journal of Adolescent & Adult Literacy, Feb 2000*

"Readable . . . provides a solid base of information regarding successful techniques used with individuals who have learning disabilities, as well as practical suggestions for educators and family members. Clear language, concise descriptions, and pertinent information for contacting multiple resources add to the strength of this book as a useful tool."
— *Choice, Association of College & Research Libraries, Feb '99*

"Recommended reference source."
— *Booklist, American Library Association, Sep '98*

"A useful resource for libraries and for those who don't have the time to identify and locate the individual publications."
— *Disability Resources Monthly, Sep '98*

Leukemia Sourcebook

Basic Consumer Health Information about Adult and Childhood Leukemias, Including Acute Lymphocytic Leukemia (ALL), Chronic Lymphocytic Leukemia (CLL), Acute Myelogenous Leukemia (AML), Chronic Myelogenous Leukemia (CML), and Hairy Cell Leukemia, and Treatments Such as Chemotherapy, Radiation Therapy, Peripheral Blood Stem Cell and Marrow Transplantation, and Immunotherapy

Along with Tips for Life During and After Treatment, a Glossary, and Directories of Additional Resources

Edited by Joyce Brennfleck Shannon. 587 pages. 2003. 978-0-7808-0627-6.

"Unlike other medical books for the layperson, . . . the language does not talk down to the reader. . . . This volume is highly recommended for all libraries."
— *American Reference Books Annual, 2004*

". . . a fine title which ranges from diagnosis to alternative treatments, staging, and tips for life during and after diagnosis."
— *The Bookwatch, Dec '03*

Liver Disorders Sourcebook

Basic Consumer Health Information about the Liver and How It Works; Liver Diseases, Including Cancer, Cirrhosis, Hepatitis, and Toxic and Drug Related Diseases; Tips for Maintaining a Healthy Liver; Laboratory Tests, Radiology Tests, and Facts about Liver Transplantation

Along with a Section on Support Groups, a Glossary, and Resource Listings

Edited by Joyce Brennfleck Shannon. 591 pages. 2000. 978-0-7808-0383-1.

"A valuable resource."
— *American Reference Books Annual, 2001*

"This title is recommended for health sciences and public libraries with consumer health collections."
— *E-Streams, Oct '00*

"Recommended reference source."
— *Booklist, American Library Association, Jun '00*

■

Lung Disorders Sourcebook

Basic Consumer Health Information about Emphysema, Pneumonia, Tuberculosis, Asthma, Cystic Fibrosis, and Other Lung Disorders, Including Facts about Diagnostic Procedures, Treatment Strategies, Disease Prevention Efforts, and Such Risk Factors as Smoking, Air Pollution, and Exposure to Asbestos, Radon, and Other Agents

Along with a Glossary and Resources for Additional Help and Information

Edited by Dawn D. Matthews. 678 pages. 2002. 978-0-7808-0339-8.

"This title is a great addition for public and school libraries because it provides concise health information on the lungs."
— *American Reference Books Annual, 2003*

"Highly recommended for academic and medical reference collections." — *Library Bookwatch, Sep '02*

SEE ALSO Respiratory Diseases & Disorders Sourcebook

■

Medical Tests Sourcebook, 2nd Edition

Basic Consumer Health Information about Medical Tests, Including Age-Specific Health Tests, Important Health Screenings and Exams, Home-Use Tests, Blood and Specimen Tests, Electrical Tests, Scope Tests, Genetic Testing, and Imaging Tests, Such as X-Rays, Ultrasound, Computed Tomography, Magnetic Resonance Imaging, Angiography, and Nuclear Medicine

Along with a Glossary and Directory of Additional Resources

Edited by Joyce Brennfleck Shannon. 654 pages. 2004. 978-0-7808-0670-2.

"Recommended for hospital and health sciences libraries with consumer health collections."
— *E-Streams, Mar '00*

"This is an overall excellent reference with a wealth of general knowledge that may aid those who are reluctant to get vital tests performed."
— *Today's Librarian, Jan '00*

"A valuable reference guide."
— *American Reference Books Annual, 2000*

■

Men's Health Concerns Sourcebook, 2nd Edition

Basic Consumer Health Information about the Medical and Mental Concerns of Men, Including Theories about the Shorter Male Lifespan, the Leading Causes of Death and Disability, Physical Concerns of Special Significance to Men, Reproductive and Sexual Concerns, Sexually Transmitted Diseases, Men's Mental and Emotional Health, and Lifestyle Choices That Affect Wellness, Such as Nutrition, Fitness, and Substance Use

Along with a Glossary of Related Terms and a Directory of Organizational Resources in Men's Health

Edited by Robert Aquinas McNally. 644 pages. 2004. 978-0-7808-0671-9.

"A very accessible reference for non-specialist general readers and consumers." — *The Bookwatch, Jun '04*

"This comprehensive resource and the series are highly recommended."
— *American Reference Books Annual, 2000*

"Recommended reference source."
— *Booklist, American Library Association, Dec '98*

■

Mental Health Disorders Sourcebook, 3rd Edition

Basic Consumer Health Information about Mental and Emotional Health and Mental Illness, Including Facts about Depression, Bipolar Disorder, and Other Mood Disorders, Phobias, Post-Traumatic Stress Disorder (PTSD), Obsessive-Compulsive Disorder, and Other Anxiety Disorders, Impulse Control Disorders, Eating Disorders, Personality Disorders, and Psychotic Disorders, Including Schizophrenia and Dissociative Disorders

Along with Statistical Information, a Special Section Concerning Mental Health Issues in Children and Adolescents, a Glossary, and Directories of Resources for Additional Help and Information

Edited by Karen Bellenir. 661 pages. 2005. 978-0-7808-0747-1.

"Recommended for public libraries and academic libraries with an undergraduate program in psychology."
— *American Reference Books Annual, 2006*

"Recommended reference source."
— *Booklist, American Library Association, Jun '00*

Mental Retardation Sourcebook

Basic Consumer Health Information about Mental Retardation and Its Causes, Including Down Syndrome, Fetal Alcohol Syndrome, Fragile X Syndrome, Genetic Conditions, Injury, and Environmental Sources

Along with Preventive Strategies, Parenting Issues, Educational Implications, Health Care Needs, Employment and Economic Matters, Legal Issues, a Glossary, and a Resource Listing for Additional Help and Information

Edited by Joyce Brennfleck Shannon. 642 pages. 2000. 978-0-7808-0377-0.

"Public libraries will find the book useful for reference and as a beginning research point for students, parents, and caregivers."
— *American Reference Books Annual, 2001*

"The strength of this work is that it compiles many basic fact sheets and addresses for further information in one volume. It is intended and suitable for the general public. This sourcebook is relevant to any collection providing health information to the general public."
— *E-Streams, Nov '00*

"From preventing retardation to parenting and family challenges, this covers health, social and legal issues and will prove an invaluable overview."
— *Reviewer's Bookwatch, Jul '00*

■

Movement Disorders Sourcebook

Basic Consumer Health Information about Neurological Movement Disorders, Including Essential Tremor, Parkinson's Disease, Dystonia, Cerebral Palsy, Huntington's Disease, Myasthenia Gravis, Multiple Sclerosis, and Other Early-Onset and Adult-Onset Movement Disorders, Their Symptoms and Causes, Diagnostic Tests, and Treatments

Along with Mobility and Assistive Technology Information, a Glossary, and a Directory of Additional Resources

Edited by Joyce Brennfleck Shannon. 655 pages. 2003. 978-0-7808-0628-3.

". . . a good resource for consumers and recommended for public, community college and undergraduate libraries." — *American Reference Books Annual, 2004*

■

Muscular Dystrophy Sourcebook

Basic Consumer Health Information about Congenital, Childhood-Onset, and Adult-Onset Forms of Muscular Dystrophy, Such as Duchenne, Becker, Emery-Dreifuss, Distal, Limb-Girdle, Facioscapulohumeral (FSHD), Myotonic, and Ophthalmoplegic Muscular Dystrophies, Including Facts about Diagnostic Tests, Medical and Physical Therapies, Management of Co-Occurring Conditions, and Parenting Guidelines

Along with Practical Tips for Home Care, a Glossary, and Directories of Additional Resources

Edited by Joyce Brennfleck Shannon. 577 pages. 2004. 978-0-7808-0676-4.

"This book is highly recommended for public and academic libraries as well as health care offices that support the information needs of patients and their families."
— *E-Streams, Apr '05*

"Excellent reference." — *The Bookwatch, Jan '05*

■

Obesity Sourcebook

Basic Consumer Health Information about Diseases and Other Problems Associated with Obesity, and Including Facts about Risk Factors, Prevention Issues, and Management Approaches

Along with Statistical and Demographic Data, Information about Special Populations, Research Updates, a Glossary, and Source Listings for Further Help and Information

Edited by Wilma Caldwell and Chad T. Kimball. 376 pages. 2001. 978-0-7808-0333-6.

"The book synthesizes the reliable medical literature on obesity into one easy-to-read and useful resource for the general public."
— *American Reference Books Annual, 2002*

"This is a very useful resource book for the lay public."
— *Doody's Review Service, Nov '01*

"Well suited for the health reference collection of a public library or an academic health science library that serves the general population." — *E-Streams, Sep '01*

"Recommended reference source."
— *Booklist, American Library Association, Apr '01*

"Recommended pick both for specialty health library collections and any general consumer health reference collection." — *The Bookwatch, Apr '01*

■

Oral Health Sourcebook

SEE Dental Care & Oral Health Sourcebook

■

Osteoporosis Sourcebook

Basic Consumer Health Information about Primary and Secondary Osteoporosis and Juvenile Osteoporosis and Related Conditions, Including Fibrous Dysplasia, Gaucher Disease, Hyperthyroidism, Hypophosphatasia, Myeloma, Osteopetrosis, Osteogenesis Imperfecta, and Paget's Disease

Along with Information about Risk Factors, Treatments, Traditional and Non-Traditional Pain Management, a Glossary of Related Terms, and a Directory of Resources

Edited by Allan R. Cook. 584 pages. 2001. 978-0-7808-0239-1.

"This would be a book to be kept in a staff or patient library. The targeted audience is the layperson, but the therapist who needs a quick bit of information on a particular topic will also find the book useful."
— *Physical Therapy, Jan '02*

"This resource is recommended as a great reference source for public, health, and academic libraries, and is another triumph for the editors of Omnigraphics."
— *American Reference Books Annual, 2002*

"Recommended for all public libraries and general health collections, especially those supporting patient education or consumer health programs."
— *E-Streams, Nov '01*

"Will prove valuable to any library seeking to maintain a current, comprehensive reference collection of health resources. . . . From prevention to treatment and associated conditions, this provides an excellent survey."
— *The Bookwatch, Aug '01*

"Recommended reference source."
— *Booklist, American Library Association, Jul '01*

SEE ALSO *Healthy Aging Sourcebook, Physical & Mental Issues in Aging Sourcebook, Women's Health Concerns Sourcebook*

■

Pain Sourcebook, 2nd Edition

Basic Consumer Health Information about Specific Forms of Acute and Chronic Pain, Including Muscle and Skeletal Pain, Nerve Pain, Cancer Pain, and Disorders Characterized by Pain, Such as Fibromyalgia, Shingles, Angina, Arthritis, and Headaches

Along with Information about Pain Medications and Management Techniques, Complementary and Alternative Pain Relief Options, Tips for People Living with Chronic Pain, a Glossary, and a Directory of Sources for Further Information

Edited by Karen Bellenir. 670 pages. 2002. 978-0-7808-0612-2.

"A source of valuable information. . . . This book offers help to nonmedical people who need information about pain and pain management. It is also an excellent reference for those who participate in patient education."
— *Doody's Review Service, Sep '02*

"Highly recommended for academic and medical reference collections." — *Library Bookwatch, Sep '02*

"The text is readable, easily understood, and well indexed. This excellent volume belongs in all patient education libraries, consumer health sections of public libraries, and many personal collections."
— *American Reference Books Annual, 1999*

"The information is basic in terms of scholarship and is appropriate for general readers. Written in journalistic style . . . intended for non-professionals. Quite thorough in its coverage of different pain conditions and summarizes the latest clinical information regarding pain treatment." — *Choice, Association of College and Research Libraries, Jun '98*

"Recommended reference source."
— *Booklist, American Library Association, Mar '98*

■

Pediatric Cancer Sourcebook

Basic Consumer Health Information about Leukemias, Brain Tumors, Sarcomas, Lymphomas, and Other Cancers in Infants, Children, and Adolescents, Including Descriptions of Cancers, Treatments, and Coping Strategies

Along with Suggestions for Parents, Caregivers, and Concerned Relatives, a Glossary of Cancer Terms, and Resource Listings

Edited by Edward J. Prucha. 587 pages. 1999. 978-0-7808-0245-2.

"An excellent source of information. Recommended for public, hospital, and health science libraries with consumer health collections." — *E-Streams, Jun '00*

"Recommended reference source."
— *Booklist, American Library Association, Feb '00*

"A valuable addition to all libraries specializing in health services and many public libraries."
— *American Reference Books Annual, 2000*

SEE ALSO *Childhood Diseases & Disorders Sourcebook, Healthy Children Sourcebook*

■

Physical & Mental Issues in Aging Sourcebook

Basic Consumer Health Information on Physical and Mental Disorders Associated with the Aging Process, Including Concerns about Cardiovascular Disease, Pulmonary Disease, Oral Health, Digestive Disorders, Musculoskeletal and Skin Disorders, Metabolic Changes, Sexual and Reproductive Issues, and Changes in Vision, Hearing, and Other Senses

Along with Data about Longevity and Causes of Death, Information on Acute and Chronic Pain, Descriptions of Mental Concerns, a Glossary of Terms, and Resource Listings for Additional Help

Edited by Jenifer Swanson. 660 pages. 1999. 978-0-7808-0233-9.

"This is a treasure of health information for the layperson." — *Choice Health Sciences Supplement, Association of College & Research Libraries, May '00*

"Recommended for public libraries."
— *American Reference Books Annual, 2000*

"Recommended reference source."
— *Booklist, American Library Association, Oct '99*

SEE ALSO *Healthy Aging Sourcebook*

■

Podiatry Sourcebook, 2nd Edition

Basic Consumer Health Information about Disorders, Diseases, Deformities, and Injuries that Affect the Foot and Ankle, Including Sprains, Corns, Calluses, Bunions, Plantar Warts, Plantar Fasciitis, Neuromas, Clubfoot, Flat Feet, Achilles Tendonitis, and Much More

Along with Information about Selecting a Foot Care Specialist, Foot Fitness, Shoes and Socks, Diagnostic Tests and Corrective Procedures, Financial Assistance for Corrective Devices, a Glossary of Related Terms, and a Directory of Resources for Additional Help and Information

Edited by Ivy L. Alexander. 543 pages. 2007. 978-0-7808-0944-4.

"Recommended reference source."
— *Booklist, American Library Association, Feb '02*

"There is a lot of information presented here on a topic that is usually only covered sparingly in most larger comprehensive medical encyclopedias."
— *American Reference Books Annual, 2002*

∎

Pregnancy & Birth Sourcebook, 2nd Edition

Basic Consumer Health Information about Conception and Pregnancy, Including Facts about Fertility, Infertility, Pregnancy Symptoms and Complications, Fetal Growth and Development, Labor, Delivery, and the Postpartum Period, as Well as Information about Maintaining Health and Wellness during Pregnancy and Caring for a Newborn

Along with Information about Public Health Assistance for Low-Income Pregnant Women, a Glossary, and Directories of Agencies and Organizations Providing Help and Support

Edited by Amy L. Sutton. 626 pages. 2004. 978-0-7808-0672-6.

"Will appeal to public and school reference collections strong in medicine and women's health. . . . Deserves a spot on any medical reference shelf."
— *The Bookwatch, Jul '04*

"A well-organized handbook. Recommended."
— *Choice, Association of College & Research Libraries, Apr '98*

"Recommended reference source."
— *Booklist, American Library Association, Mar '98*

"Recommended for public libraries."
— *American Reference Books Annual, 1998*

SEE ALSO *Breastfeeding Sourcebook, Congenital Disorders Sourcebook, Family Planning Sourcebook*

∎

Prostate & Urological Disorders Sourcebook

Basic Consumer Health Information about Urogenital and Sexual Disorders in Men, Including Prostate and Other Andrological Cancers, Prostatitis, Benign Prostatic Hyperplasia, Testicular and Penile Trauma, Cryptorchidism, Peyronie Disease, Erectile Dysfunction, and Male Factor Infertility, and Facts about Commonly Used Tests and Procedures, Such as Prostatectomy, Vasectomy, Vasectomy Reversal, Penile Implants, and Semen Analysis

Along with a Glossary of Andrological Terms and a Directory of Resources for Additional Information

Edited by Karen Bellenir. 631 pages. 2005. 978-0-7808-0797-6.

Prostate Cancer Sourcebook

Basic Consumer Health Information about Prostate Cancer, Including Information about the Associated Risk Factors, Detection, Diagnosis, and Treatment of Prostate Cancer

Along with Information on Non-Malignant Prostate Conditions, and Featuring a Section Listing Support and Treatment Centers and a Glossary of Related Terms

Edited by Dawn D. Matthews. 358 pages. 2001. 978-0-7808-0324-4.

"Recommended reference source."
— *Booklist, American Library Association, Jan '02*

"A valuable resource for health care consumers seeking information on the subject. . . . All text is written in a clear, easy-to-understand language that avoids technical jargon. Any library that collects consumer health resources would strengthen their collection with the addition of the *Prostate Cancer Sourcebook*."
— *American Reference Books Annual, 2002*

SEE ALSO *Men's Health Concerns Sourcebook*

∎

Reconstructive & Cosmetic Surgery Sourcebook

Basic Consumer Health Information on Cosmetic and Reconstructive Plastic Surgery, Including Statistical Information about Different Surgical Procedures, Things to Consider Prior to Surgery, Plastic Surgery Techniques and Tools, Emotional and Psychological Considerations, and Procedure-Specific Information

Along with a Glossary of Terms and a Listing of Resources for Additional Help and Information

Edited by M. Lisa Weatherford. 374 pages. 2001. 978-0-7808-0214-8.

"An excellent reference that addresses cosmetic and medically necessary reconstructive surgeries. . . . The style of the prose is calm and reassuring, discussing the many positive outcomes now available due to advances in surgical techniques."
— *American Reference Books Annual, 2002*

"Recommended for health science libraries that are open to the public, as well as hospital libraries that are open to the patients. This book is a good resource for the consumer interested in plastic surgery."
— *E-Streams, Dec '01*

"Recommended reference source."
— *Booklist, American Library Association, Jul '01*

∎

Rehabilitation Sourcebook

Basic Consumer Health Information about Rehabilitation for People Recovering from Heart Surgery, Spinal Cord Injury, Stroke, Orthopedic Impairments, Amputation, Pulmonary Impairments, Traumatic Injury, and More, Including Physical Therapy, Occupational Therapy, Speech/Language Therapy, Massage Therapy, Dance Therapy, Art Therapy, and Recreational Therapy

Along with Information on Assistive and Adaptive Devices, a Glossary, and Resources for Additional Help and Information

Edited by Dawn D. Matthews. 531 pages. 1999. 978-0-7808-0236-0.

"This is an excellent resource for public library reference and health collections."
— American Reference Books Annual, 2001

"Recommended reference source."
— Booklist, American Library Association, May '00

Respiratory Diseases & Disorders Sourcebook

Basic Information about Respiratory Diseases and Disorders, Including Asthma, Cystic Fibrosis, Pneumonia, the Common Cold, Influenza, and Others, Featuring Facts about the Respiratory System, Statistical and Demographic Data, Treatments, Self-Help Management Suggestions, and Current Research Initiatives

Edited by Allan R. Cook and Peter D. Dresser. 771 pages. 1995. 978-0-7808-0037-3.

"Designed for the layperson and for patients and their families coping with respiratory illness. . . . an extensive array of information on diagnosis, treatment, management, and prevention of respiratory illnesses for the general reader." — Choice, Association of College & Research Libraries, Jun '96

"A highly recommended text for all collections. It is a comforting reminder of the power of knowledge that good books carry between their covers."
— Academic Library Book Review, Spring '96

"A comprehensive collection of authoritative information presented in a nontechnical, humanitarian style for patients, families, and caregivers."
— Association of Operating Room Nurses, Sep/Oct '95

SEE ALSO Lung Disorders Sourcebook

Sexually Transmitted Diseases Sourcebook, 3rd Edition

Basic Consumer Health Information about Chlamydial Infections, Gonorrhea, Hepatitis, Herpes, HIV/AIDS, Human Papillomavirus, Pubic Lice, Scabies, Syphilis, Trichomoniasis, Vaginal Infections, and Other Sexually Transmitted Diseases, Including Facts about Risk Factors, Symptoms, Diagnosis, Treatment, and the Prevention of Sexually Transmitted Infections

Along with Updates on Current Research Initiatives, a Glossary of Related Terms, and Resources for Additional Help and Information

Edited by Amy L. Sutton. 629 pages. 2006. 978-0-7808-0824-9.

"Recommended for consumer health collections in public libraries, and secondary school and community college libraries."
— American Reference Books Annual, 2002

"Every school and public library should have a copy of this comprehensive and user-friendly reference book."
— Choice, Association of College & Research Libraries, Sep '01

"This is a highly recommended book. This is an especially important book for all school and public libraries."
— AIDS Book Review Journal, Jul-Aug '01

"Recommended reference source."
— Booklist, American Library Association, Apr '01

Sleep Disorders Sourcebook, 2nd Edition

Basic Consumer Health Information about Sleep and Sleep Disorders, Including Insomnia, Sleep Apnea, Restless Legs Syndrome, Narcolepsy, Parasomnias, and Other Health Problems That Affect Sleep, Plus Facts about Diagnostic Procedures, Treatment Strategies, Sleep Medications, and Tips for Improving Sleep Quality

Along with a Glossary of Related Terms and Resources for Additional Help and Information

Edited by Amy L. Sutton. 567 pages. 2005. 978-0-7808-0743-3.

"This book will be useful for just about everybody, especially the 40 million Americans with sleep disorders."
— American Reference Books Annual, 2006

"Recommended for public libraries and libraries supporting health care professionals." — E-Streams, Sep '05

". . . key medical library acquisition."
— The Bookwatch, Jun '05

Smoking Concerns Sourcebook

Basic Consumer Health Information about Nicotine Addiction and Smoking Cessation, Featuring Facts about the Health Effects of Tobacco Use, Including Lung and Other Cancers, Heart Disease, Stroke, and Respiratory Disorders, Such as Emphysema and Chronic Bronchitis

Along with Information about Smoking Prevention Programs, Suggestions for Achieving and Maintaining a Smoke-Free Lifestyle, Statistics about Tobacco Use, Reports on Current Research Initiatives, a Glossary of Related Terms, and Directories of Resources for Additional Help and Information

Edited by Karen Bellenir. 621 pages. 2004. 978-0-7808-0323-7.

"Provides everything needed for the student or general reader seeking practical details on the effects of tobacco use." — The Bookwatch, Mar '05

"Public libraries and consumer health care libraries will find this work useful."
— American Reference Books Annual, 2005

Sports Injuries Sourcebook, 3rd Edition

Basic Consumer Health Information about Sprains and Strains, Fractures, Growth Plate Injuries, Overtraining Injuries, and Injuries to the Head, Face, Shoulders, Elbows, Hands, Spinal Column, Knees, Ankles, and Feet, and with Facts about Heat-Related Illness, Steroids and Sport Supplements, Protective Equipment, Diagnostic Procedures, Treatment Options, and Rehabilitation

Along with a Glossary of Related Terms and a Directory of Resources for Additional Help and Information

Edited by Sandra J. Judd. 651 pages. 2007. 978-0-7808-0949-9.

"This is an excellent reference for consumers and it is recommended for public, community college, and undergraduate libraries."
— *American Reference Books Annual, 2003*

"Recommended reference source."
— *Booklist, American Library Association, Feb '03*

■

Stress-Related Disorders Sourcebook

Basic Consumer Health Information about Stress and Stress-Related Disorders, Including Stress Origins and Signals, Environmental Stress at Work and Home, Mental and Emotional Stress Associated with Depression, Post-Traumatic Stress Disorder, Panic Disorder, Suicide, and the Physical Effects of Stress on the Cardiovascular, Immune, and Nervous Systems

Along with Stress Management Techniques, a Glossary, and a Listing of Additional Resources

Edited by Joyce Brennfleck Shannon. 610 pages. 2002. 978-0-7808-0560-6.

"Well written for a general readership, the *Stress-Related Disorders Sourcebook* is a useful addition to the health reference literature."
— *American Reference Books Annual, 2003*

"I am impressed by the amount of information. It offers a thorough overview of the causes and consequences of stress for the layperson. . . . A well-done and thorough reference guide for professionals and nonprofessionals alike." — *Doody's Review Service, Dec '02*

■

Stroke Sourcebook

Basic Consumer Health Information about Stroke, Including Ischemic, Hemorrhagic, Transient Ischemic Attack (TIA), and Pediatric Stroke, Stroke Triggers and Risks, Diagnostic Tests, Treatments, and Rehabilitation Information

Along with Stroke Prevention Guidelines, Legal and Financial Information, a Glossary, and a Directory of Additional Resources

Edited by Joyce Brennfleck Shannon. 606 pages. 2003. 978-0-7808-0630-6.

"This volume is highly recommended and should be in every medical, hospital, and public library."
— *American Reference Books Annual, 2004*

"Highly recommended for the amount and variety of topics and information covered." — *Choice, Nov '03*

■

Surgery Sourcebook

Basic Consumer Health Information about Inpatient and Outpatient Surgeries, Including Cardiac, Vascular, Orthopedic, Ocular, Reconstructive, Cosmetic, Gynecologic, and Ear, Nose, and Throat Procedures and More

Along with Information about Operating Room Policies and Instruments, Laser Surgery Techniques, Hospital Errors, Statistical Data, a Glossary, and Listings of Sources for Further Help and Information

Edited by Annemarie S. Muth and Karen Bellenir. 596 pages. 2002. 978-0-7808-0380-0.

"Large public libraries and medical libraries would benefit from this material in their reference collections."
— *American Reference Books Annual, 2004*

"Invaluable reference for public and school library collections alike." — *Library Bookwatch, Apr '03*

■

Thyroid Disorders Sourcebook

Basic Consumer Health Information about Disorders of the Thyroid and Parathyroid Glands, Including Hypothyroidism, Hyperthyroidism, Graves Disease, Hashimoto Thyroiditis, Thyroid Cancer, and Parathyroid Disorders, Featuring Facts about Symptoms, Risk Factors, Tests, and Treatments

Along with Information about the Effects of Thyroid Imbalance on Other Body Systems, Environmental Factors That Affect the Thyroid Gland, a Glossary, and a Directory of Additional Resources

Edited by Joyce Brennfleck Shannon. 599 pages. 2005. 978-0-7808-0745-7.

"Recommended for consumer health collections."
— *American Reference Books Annual, 2006*

"Highly recommended pick for basic consumer health reference holdings at all levels."
— *The Bookwatch, Aug '05*

■

Transplantation Sourcebook

Basic Consumer Health Information about Organ and Tissue Transplantation, Including Physical and Financial Preparations, Procedures and Issues Relating to Specific Solid Organ and Tissue Transplants, Rehabilitation, Pediatric Transplant Information, the Future of Transplantation, and Organ and Tissue Donation

Along with a Glossary and Listings of Additional Resources

Edited by Joyce Brennfleck Shannon. 628 pages. 2002. 978-0-7808-0322-0.

"Along with these advances [in transplantation technology] have come a number of daunting questions for potential transplant patients, their families, and their health care providers. This reference text is the best single tool to address many of these questions. . . . It will be a much-needed addition to the reference collections in health care, academic, and large public libraries."
— *American Reference Books Annual, 2003*

"Recommended for libraries with an interest in offering consumer health information." — *E-Streams, Jul '02*

"This is a unique and valuable resource for patients facing transplantation and their families."
— *Doody's Review Service, Jun '02*

Traveler's Health Sourcebook

Basic Consumer Health Information for Travelers, Including Physical and Medical Preparations, Transportation Health and Safety, Essential Information about Food and Water, Sun Exposure, Insect and Snake Bites, Camping and Wilderness Medicine, and Travel with Physical or Medical Disabilities

Along with International Travel Tips, Vaccination Recommendations, Geographical Health Issues, Disease Risks, a Glossary, and a Listing of Additional Resources

Edited by Joyce Brennfleck Shannon. 613 pages. 2000. 978-0-7808-0384-8.

"Recommended reference source."
— *Booklist, American Library Association, Feb '01*

"This book is recommended for any public library, any travel collection, and especially any collection for the physically disabled."
— *American Reference Books Annual, 2001*

SEE ALSO Worldwide Health Sourcebook

Urinary Tract & Kidney Diseases & Disorders Sourcebook, 2nd Edition

Basic Consumer Health Information about the Urinary System, Including the Bladder, Urethra, Ureters, and Kidneys, with Facts about Urinary Tract Infections, Incontinence, Congenital Disorders, Kidney Stones, Cancers of the Urinary Tract and Kidneys, Kidney Failure, Dialysis, and Kidney Transplantation

Along with Statistical and Demographic Information, Reports on Current Research in Kidney and Urologic Health, a Summary of Commonly Used Diagnostic Tests, a Glossary of Related Terms, and a Directory of Resources for Additional Help and Information

Edited by Ivy L. Alexander. 649 pages. 2005. 978-0-7808-0750-1.

"A good choice for a consumer health information library or for a medical library needing information to refer to their patients."
— *American Reference Books Annual, 2006*

Vegetarian Sourcebook

Basic Consumer Health Information about Vegetarian Diets, Lifestyle, and Philosophy, Including Definitions of Vegetarianism and Veganism, Tips about Adopting Vegetarianism, Creating a Vegetarian Pantry, and Meeting Nutritional Needs of Vegetarians, with Facts Regarding Vegetarianism's Effect on Pregnant and Lactating Women, Children, Athletes, and Senior Citizens

Along with a Glossary of Commonly Used Vegetarian Terms and Resources for Additional Help and Information

Edited by Chad T. Kimball. 360 pages. 2002. 978-0-7808-0439-5.

"Organizes into one concise volume the answers to the most common questions concerning vegetarian diets and lifestyles. This title is recommended for public and secondary school libraries." — *E-Streams, Apr '03*

"Invaluable reference for public and school library collections alike." — *Library Bookwatch, Apr '03*

"The articles in this volume are easy to read and come from authoritative sources. The book does not necessarily support the vegetarian diet but instead provides the pros and cons of this important decision. The Vegetarian Sourcebook is recommended for public libraries and consumer health libraries."
— *American Reference Books Annual, 2003*

SEE ALSO Diet & Nutrition Sourcebook

Women's Health Concerns Sourcebook, 2nd Edition

Basic Consumer Health Information about the Medical and Mental Concerns of Women, Including Maintaining Health and Wellness, Gynecological Concerns, Breast Health, Sexuality and Reproductive Issues, Menopause, Cancer in Women, Leading Causes of Death and Disability among Women, Physical Concerns of Special Significance to Women, and Women's Mental and Emotional Health

Along with a Glossary of Related Terms and Directories of Resources for Additional Help and Information

Edited by Amy L. Sutton. 746 pages. 2004. 978-0-7808-0673-3.

"This is a useful reference book, which makes the reader knowledgeable about several issues that concern women's health. It is recommended for public libraries and home library collections." — *E-Streams, May '05*

"A useful addition to public and consumer health library collections."
— *American Reference Books Annual, 2005*

"A highly recommended title."
— *The Bookwatch, May '04*

"Handy compilation. There is an impressive range of diseases, devices, disorders, procedures, and other physical and emotional issues covered . . . well organized, illustrated, and indexed." — *Choice, Association of College & Research Libraries, Jan '98*

SEE ALSO *Breast Cancer Sourcebook, Cancer Sourcebook for Women, Healthy Heart Sourcebook for Women, Osteoporosis Sourcebook*

▪

Workplace Health & Safety Sourcebook

Basic Consumer Health Information about Workplace Health and Safety, Including the Effect of Workplace Hazards on the Lungs, Skin, Heart, Ears, Eyes, Brain, Reproductive Organs, Musculoskeletal System, and Other Organs and Body Parts

Along with Information about Occupational Cancer, Personal Protective Equipment, Toxic and Hazardous Chemicals, Child Labor, Stress, and Workplace Violence

Edited by Chad T. Kimball. 626 pages. 2000. 978-0-7808-0231-5.

"As a reference for the general public, this would be useful in any library." —*E-Streams, Jun '01*

"Provides helpful information for primary care physicians and other caregivers interested in occupational medicine. . . . General readers; professionals."
—*Choice, Association of College & Research Libraries, May '01*

"Recommended reference source."
—*Booklist, American Library Association, Feb '01*

"Highly recommended." —*The Bookwatch, Jan '01*

▪

Worldwide Health Sourcebook

Basic Information about Global Health Issues, Including Malnutrition, Reproductive Health, Disease Dispersion and Prevention, Emerging Diseases, Risky Health Behaviors, and the Leading Causes of Death

Along with Global Health Concerns for Children, Women, and the Elderly, Mental Health Issues, Research and Technology Advancements, and Economic, Environmental, and Political Health Implications, a Glossary, and a Resource Listing for Additional Help and Information

Edited by Joyce Brennfleck Shannon. 614 pages. 2001. 978-0-7808-0330-5.

"Named an Outstanding Academic Title."
—*Choice, Association of College & Research Libraries, Jan '02*

"Yet another handy but also unique compilation in the extensive *Health Reference Series*, this is a useful work because many of the international publications reprinted or excerpted are not readily available. Highly recommended." —*Choice, Association of College & Research Libraries, Nov '01*

"Recommended reference source."
—*Booklist, American Library Association, Oct '01*

SEE ALSO *Traveler's Health Sourcebook*

629

Teen Health Series
Helping Young Adults Understand, Manage, and Avoid Serious Illness

List price $65 per volume. **School and library price $58 per volume.**

Alcohol Information for Teens
Health Tips about Alcohol and Alcoholism

Including Facts about Underage Drinking, Preventing Teen Alcohol Use, Alcohol's Effects on the Brain and the Body, Alcohol Abuse Treatment, Help for Children of Alcoholics, and More

Edited by Joyce Brennfleck Shannon. 370 pages. 2005. 978-0-7808-0741-9.

"Boxed facts and tips add visual interest to the well-researched and clearly written text."
— *Curriculum Connection, Apr '06*

Allergy Information for Teens
Health Tips about Allergic Reactions Such as Anaphylaxis, Respiratory Problems, and Rashes

Including Facts about Identifying and Managing Allergies to Food, Pollen, Mold, Animals, Chemicals, Drugs, and Other Substances

Edited by Karen Bellenir. 410 pages. 2006. 978-0-7808-0799-0.

Asthma Information for Teens
Health Tips about Managing Asthma and Related Concerns

Including Facts about Asthma Causes, Triggers, Symptoms, Diagnosis, and Treatment

Edited by Karen Bellenir. 386 pages. 2005. 978-0-7808-0770-9.

"Highly recommended for medical libraries, public school libraries, and public libraries."
— *American Reference Books Annual, 2006*

"It is so clearly written and well organized that even hesitant readers will be able to find the facts they need, whether for reports or personal information. . . . A succinct but complete resource."
— *School Library Journal, Sep '05*

Body Information for Teens
Health Tips about Maintaining Well-Being for a Lifetime

Including Facts about the Development and Functioning of the Body's Systems, Organs, and Structures and the Health Impact of Lifestyle Choices

Edited by Sandra Augustyn Lawton. 458 pages. 2007. 978-0-7808-0443-2.

Cancer Information for Teens
Health Tips about Cancer Awareness, Prevention, Diagnosis, and Treatment

Including Facts about Frequently Occurring Cancers, Cancer Risk Factors, and Coping Strategies for Teens Fighting Cancer or Dealing with Cancer in Friends or Family Members

Edited by Wilma R. Caldwell. 428 pages. 2004. 978-0-7808-0678-8.

"Recommended for school libraries, or consumer libraries that see a lot of use by teens."
— *E-Streams, May '05*

"A valuable educational tool."
— *American Reference Books Annual, 2005*

"Young adults and their parents alike will find this new addition to the *Teen Health Series* an important reference to cancer in teens."
— *Children's Bookwatch, Feb '05*

Complementary and Alternative Medicine Information for Teens
Health Tips about Non-Traditional and Non-Western Medical Practices

Including Information about Acupuncture, Chiropractic Medicine, Dietary and Herbal Supplements, Hypnosis, Massage Therapy, Prayer and Spirituality, Reflexology, Yoga, and More

Edited by Sandra Augustyn Lawton. 405 pages. 2006. 978-0-7808-0966-6.

Diabetes Information for Teens
Health Tips about Managing Diabetes and Preventing Related Complications

Including Information about Insulin, Glucose Control, Healthy Eating, Physical Activity, and Learning to Live with Diabetes

Edited by Sandra Augustyn Lawton. 410 pages. 2006. 978-0-7808-0811-9.

Diet Information for Teens, 2nd Edition

Health Tips about Diet and Nutrition

Including Facts about Dietary Guidelines, Food Groups, Nutrients, Healthy Meals, Snacks, Weight Control, Medical Concerns Related to Diet, and More

Edited by Karen Bellenir. 432 pages. 2006. 978-0-7808-0820-1.

"Full of helpful insights and facts throughout the book. . . . An excellent resource to be placed in public libraries or even in personal collections."
— American Reference Books Annual, 2002

"Recommended for middle and high school libraries and media centers as well as academic libraries that educate future teachers of teenagers. It is also a suitable addition to health science libraries that serve patrons who are interested in teen health promotion and education."
— E-Streams, Oct '01

"This comprehensive book would be beneficial to collections that need information about nutrition, dietary guidelines, meal planning, and weight control. . . . This reference is so easy to use that its purchase is recommended."
— The Book Report, Sep-Oct '01

"This book is written in an easy to understand format describing issues that many teens face every day, and then provides thoughtful explanations so that teens can make informed decisions. This is an interesting book that provides important facts and information for today's teens."
— Doody's Health Sciences Book Review Journal, Jul-Aug '01

"A comprehensive compendium of diet and nutrition. The information is presented in a straightforward, plain-spoken manner. This title will be useful to those working on reports on a variety of topics, as well as to general readers concerned about their dietary health."
— School Library Journal, Jun '01

Drug Information for Teens, 2nd Edition

Health Tips about the Physical and Mental Effects of Substance Abuse

Including Information about Marijuana, Inhalants, Club Drugs, Stimulants, Hallucinogens, Opiates, Prescription and Over-the-Counter Drugs, Herbal Products, Tobacco, Alcohol, and More

Edited by Sandra Augustyn Lawton. 468 pages. 2006. 978-0-7808-0862-1.

"A clearly written resource for general readers and researchers alike."
— School Library Journal

"This book is well-balanced. . . . a must for public and school libraries."
— VOYA: Voice of Youth Advocates, Dec '03

"The chapters are quick to make a connection to their teenage reading audience. The prose is straightforward and the book lends itself to spot reading. It should be useful both for practical information and for research, and it is suitable for public and school libraries."
— American Reference Books Annual, 2003

"Recommended reference source."
— Booklist, American Library Association, Feb '03

"This is an excellent resource for teens and their parents. Education about drugs and substances is key to discouraging teen drug abuse and this book provides this much needed information in a way that is interesting and factual."
— Doody's Review Service, Dec '02

Eating Disorders Information for Teens

Health Tips about Anorexia, Bulimia, Binge Eating, and Other Eating Disorders

Including Information on the Causes, Prevention, and Treatment of Eating Disorders, and Such Other Issues as Maintaining Healthy Eating and Exercise Habits

Edited by Sandra Augustyn Lawton. 337 pages. 2005. 978-0-7808-0783-9.

"An excellent resource for teens and those who work with them."
— VOYA: Voice of Youth Advocates, Apr '06

"A welcome addition to high school and undergraduate libraries." *— American Reference Books Annual, 2006*

"This book covers the topic in a lucid manner but delves deeper into every aspect of an eating disorder. A solid addition for any nonfiction or reference collection."
— School Library Journal, Dec '05

Fitness Information for Teens

Health Tips about Exercise, Physical Well-Being, and Health Maintenance

Including Facts about Aerobic and Anaerobic Conditioning, Stretching, Body Shape and Body Image, Sports Training, Nutrition, and Activities for Non-Athletes

Edited by Karen Bellenir. 425 pages. 2004. 978-0-7808-0679-5.

"Another excellent offering from Omnigraphics in their *Teen Health Series*. . . . This book will be a great addition to any public, junior high, senior high, or secondary school library."
— American Reference Books Annual, 2005

Learning Disabilities Information for Teens

Health Tips about Academic Skills Disorders and Other Disabilities That Affect Learning

Including Information about Common Signs of Learning Disabilities, School Issues, Learning to Live with a Learning Disability, and Other Related Issues

Edited by Sandra Augustyn Lawton. 337 pages. 2005. 978-0-7808-0796-9.

"This book provides a wealth of information for any reader interested in the signs, causes, and consequences of learning disabilities, as well as related legal rights and educational interventions. . . . Public and academic libraries should want this title for both students and general readers."

— American Reference Books Annual, 2006

■

Mental Health Information for Teens, 2nd Edition

Health Tips about Mental Wellness and Mental Illness

Including Facts about Mental and Emotional Health, Depression and Other Mood Disorders, Anxiety Disorders, Behavior Disorders, Self-Injury, Psychosis, Schizophrenia, and More

Edited by Karen Bellenir. 400 pages. 2006. 978-0-7808-0863-8.

"In both language and approach, this user-friendly entry in the *Teen Health Series* is on target for teens needing information on mental health concerns."

— Booklist, American Library Association, Jan '02

"Readers will find the material accessible and informative, with the shaded notes, facts, and embedded glossary insets adding appropriately to the already interesting and succinct presentation."

— School Library Journal, Jan '02

"This title is highly recommended for any library that serves adolescents and parents/caregivers of adolescents."

— E-Streams, Jan '02

"Recommended for high school libraries and young adult collections in public libraries. Both health professionals and teenagers will find this book useful."

— American Reference Books Annual, 2002

"This is a nice book written to enlighten the society, primarily teenagers, about common teen mental health issues. It is highly recommended to teachers and parents as well as adolescents."

— Doody's Review Service, Dec '01

■

Sexual Health Information for Teens

Health Tips about Sexual Development, Human Reproduction, and Sexually Transmitted Diseases

Including Facts about Puberty, Reproductive Health, Chlamydia, Human Papillomavirus, Pelvic Inflammatory Disease, Herpes, AIDS, Contraception, Pregnancy, and More

Edited by Deborah A. Stanley. 391 pages. 2003. 978-0-7808-0445-6.

"This work should be included in all high school libraries and many larger public libraries. . . . highly recommended."

— American Reference Books Annual, 2004

"*Sexual Health* approaches its subject with appropriate seriousness and offers easily accessible advice and information."

— School Library Journal, Feb '04

Skin Health Information for Teens

Health Tips about Dermatological Concerns and Skin Cancer Risks

Including Facts about Acne, Warts, Hives, and Other Conditions and Lifestyle Choices, Such as Tanning, Tattooing, and Piercing, That Affect the Skin, Nails, Scalp, and Hair

Edited by Robert Aquinas McNally. 429 pages. 2003. 978-0-7808-0446-3.

"This volume, as with others in the series, will be a useful addition to school and public library collections."

— American Reference Books Annual, 2004

"There is no doubt that this reference tool is valuable."

— VOYA: Voice of Youth Advocates, Feb '04

"This volume serves as a one-stop source and should be a necessity for any health collection."

— Library Media Connection

■

Sports Injuries Information for Teens

Health Tips about Sports Injuries and Injury Protection

Including Facts about Specific Injuries, Emergency Treatment, Rehabilitation, Sports Safety, Competition Stress, Fitness, Sports Nutrition, Steroid Risks, and More

Edited by Joyce Brennfleck Shannon. 405 pages. 2003. 978-0-7808-0447-0.

"This work will be useful in the young adult collections of public libraries as well as high school libraries."

— American Reference Books Annual, 2004

■

Suicide Information for Teens

Health Tips about Suicide Causes and Prevention

Including Facts about Depression, Risk Factors, Getting Help, Survivor Support, and More

Edited by Joyce Brennfleck Shannon. 368 pages. 2005. 978-0-7808-0737-2.

■

Tobacco Information for Teens

Health Tips about the Hazards of Using Cigarettes, Smokeless Tobacco, and Other Nicotine Products

Including Facts about Nicotine Addiction, Immediate and Long-Term Health Effects of Tobacco Use, Related Cancers, Smoking Cessation, Tobacco Use Prevention, and Tobacco Use Statistics

Edited by Karen Bellenir. 440 pages. 2007. 978-0-7808-0976-5.

Health Reference Series

Teen Health Series